DRUG

NATIONAL HEALTH SERVICE

ENGLAND AND WALES

SEPTEMBER 1990

0300M/1

Technical Specifications
are available singly from:

The Department of Health
Room 541
Portland Court
158–176 Gt. Portland St.
London W1N 5TB

To: General Medical Practitioners
   Pharmacy Contractors
   Appliance Contractors
   (Excluding Drug Stores)

PREFACE

AMENDMENTS TO THE DRUG TARIFF

SEPTEMBER 1990

1. Pursuant to Regulation 28(1) of the National Health Service (General Medical and Pharmaceutical Services) Regulations 1974, the Secretary of State for Health has amended the Drug Tariff with effect from 1 September 1990.

2. While every effort is made to ensure that each monthly publication of the Drug Tariff includes all amendments made by the Secretary of State to the price applicable to the relevant period, the need to observe printing deadlines sometimes defeats those efforts. Any omitted amendments will be effective from the date on which they come into force, even if publication of the details is unavoidably delayed.

3. **ADVANCE NOTICE**

Contractors should note the following changes to Part XVII effective from 1 October 1990.

   Additions

   Doxycyline Capsules 100 mg BP
   Paracetamol Tablets, Dispersible, DPF

   Deletions

   Ampicillin Tablets, Paediatric, BP
   Aspirin, Paracetamol and Codeine Tablets, DPF
   Aspirin Tablets, BP
   Benzocaine Lozenges, DPF
   Co-codamol Tablets, DPF
   Co-codamol Tablets, Dispersible, DPF
   Co-dydramol Tablets, DPF
   Co-trimoxazole Tablets, Double Strength, DPF
   Co-trimoxazole Tablets, Double Strength, Dispersible, DPF
   Mefenamic Acid Capsules, BP
   Pentazocine Tablets, BP.

4. Please note that you are now being supplied each month with Drug Tariff which incorporates all amendments to date. These are listed below:

NB All entries showing a change in price are indicated by ∇ for price reduction and Δ for price increases; changes to the text relating to code, product description, or the inclusion of a new product are indicated by a vertical line in the margin.

5. ADDITIONS

<u>Part VII – Drugs with Common Pack</u>
<u>Page 31</u>

Praxilene Capsules   100 pack

<u>Part IXB – Incontinence Appliances</u>
<u>Page 119 – Leg Bags</u>

Bard Ltd
    Uriplan Range
    750 ml, 4" inlet tube   DT75   10 @ 2120p

<u>Page 120</u>

Bradgate Unitech Ltd
    Careline Leg Bag

350 ml short tube	45-01SVC	10 @	1800p
350 ml long tube	45-02SVL	10 @	1800p
500 ml short tube	45-05SVC	10 @	1850p
500 ml long tube	45-06SVL	10 @	1850p
750 ml short tube	45-09SVC	10 @	1900p
750 ml long tube	45-10SVL	10 @	1900p

<u>Part IXC – Stoma Appliances</u>
<u>Page 187 – Colostomy Bags</u>

Palex (Cambridge Selfcare Diagnostics Ltd)
    Closed Stoma bag with
    CL Resin seal microporous
    adhesive and deodorising
    flatus filter

19mm starter hole	BCLF19	30 @	5100p
25mm precut	BCLF25	30 @	5100p
32mm precut	BCLF32	30 @	5100p
38mm precut	BCLF38	30 @	5100p
44mm precut	BCLF44	30 @	5100p
51mm precut	BCLF51	30 @	5100p
64mm precut	BCLF64	30 @	5100p

<u>Page 201 – Filters/Bridges</u>

Salt and Son Ltd
    Metal Bridges – ready-
    fixed to lightweight and
    LWU disposable bags   833052 20 @ 704p
    – for use with other
    disposable bags   833053 30 @ 1056p

<u>Part IXC – Stoma Appliances</u>
<u>Page 219 – Ileostomy Bags</u>

Salt and Son Ltd
    Cohflex Paediatric
    Drainable Bag   10mm starter   632310 30 @ 4460p

ADDITIONS contd

Page 243 – Stoma Caps/Dressings

Palex (Cambridge Selfcare Diagnostics Ltd)
    Mini Stoma Cap   MINI 1   30 @ 2450p

6.   DELETIONS

Part VIII – Basic Prices of Drugs
Page 41

Eugenol BP 1980

Page 43

Hydrotalcite Tablets BP, 500 mg   120 @ 174p   category C

Page 52

Starch Glycerin BPC 1963

Page 54

Vitamins B and C Injections BPC (1M weak/4ml)   10 @ 417p
                      (1M strong/7ml)   10 @ 450p
                      (1V strong/10ml) 10 @ 450p

Part IXA – Appliances
Page 89 – Hypodermic Equipment

(II)   Syringes for use with insulin of other strengths

Part IXB – Incontinence Appliances
Page 119 – Leg Bags

Aldington Laboratories Ltd
    Alden leg bag
        Dryaid leg bag 350ml   831035
        With 30 cm tube   831036
        Dryaid leg bag 500ml   831050
        With 30 cm tube   831051

Part IXC – Stoma Appliances
Page 183 – Colostomy Bags

Francol Surgical – Entire entry

Page 187 – Colostomy Bags

Salt and Son Ltd   Kombo Closed Bag with
                       Karaya Medium   delete 5 pack range
                       With Karaya and Filter delete 5 pack range
                       Kombo Drainable Bag with
                       Karaya Medium   delete 5 pack range

Page 188 – Colostomy Bags

Salt and Son Ltd	with Karaya and Filter	delete 5 pack range
	Solo Closed Bag	delete 10 pack range
	with Filter	delete entire 10 pack range

Page 188a	Solo Drainable Bag medium	delete 10 pack range
	with filter medium	delete 10 pack range
	Supasar Closed Bag Medium Starter 711644	
	Coloset Closed Bag	delete 10 pack range

Page 218 – Ileostomy Bags

Salt and Son Ltd	Light White Drainable Bags	
	Large	delete 10 pack range
	Small	delete 10 pack range
	Medium	delete 10 pack range
	Coloset Drainable Bag Medium Starter 711689	
	Light White Drainable Adhesive Bag	
	Large	delete 10 pack range
	Small	delete 10 pack range
	Medium	delete 10 pack range

Page 251 – Two Piece Ostomy Systems

Salt and Son Ltd	Clear Closed Bag Medium	delete 10 pack range
	Clear Drainable Bag Medium	delete 10 pack range
	Post—Operative Closed Bag	delete 10 pack range
	Pink Closed Bag	delete 10 pack range

Page 261 – Urostomy Bags

Salt and Son Ltd	Light White Urostomy Bag with realistic	
	Large	delete 10 pack range
	Light White Clear Urostomy Bag with realistic	
	Large	delete 10 pack range
	Small	delete 10 pack range
	Light White Urostomy Bag	
	Large	delete 10 pack range
Page 261a	Light White Clear Urostomy Bag	
	Large	delete 10 pack range
	Small	delete 10 pack range
	Light White Urostomy Adhesive Bag	
	Large	delete 10 pack range
Page 262	Light White Clear Urostomy Adhesive Bag	
	Small	delete 10 pack range

0300M/6

OTHER CHANGES

<u>Part II – "ZD" List</u>

<u>Page 5</u>

Controlled Drugs

<u>now reads</u>

Controlled Drugs in schedules 1, 2 and 3 of the Misuse of Drugs Regulations 1985.

<u>Page 7</u>

<u>Clause 9C</u>

Where insufficient information is available to price the prescription etc

<u>now reads</u>

Where insufficient information is available to enable the PPA or WPC to process the prescription, etc

<u>Part VIII – Basic Prices of Drugs</u>

<u>Page 35</u>
Aspirin BP (Powder) from category A to C

<u>Page 36</u>
Bismuth Subnitrate BPC from category B to C

<u>Page 37</u>
Calamine Lotion Oily BP 1980 500 ml @ 255p category B
<u>now reads</u>
Calamine Lotion Oily BP 1980 100 ml @ 35p category C

<u>Page 42</u>

Gentian, Alkaline Mixture BP 2 litre @ 349p category A

<u>now reads</u>

Gentian, Alkaline Mixture BP 200 ml @ 20p category E

Gentian, Infusion Compound Concentrated BP from category A to C

<u>Page 44</u>

Liquefied Phenol BP from category B to C

<u>Page 51</u>

Silver Nitrate BP from category B to C

Sodium Hydroxide BP (Pellets) from category B to C

<u>Part IXA – Appliance</u>

<u>Page 65 – Catheters</u>

Bard Uriplan <u>now reads</u> Bard Reliacath

CONTENTS

DRUG TARIFF

DEFINITIONS:

a.   Except where the context otherwise requires, the terms to which a meaning is assigned by the Regulations or the Terms of Service have the same meaning in this Tariff.

b.   The term contractor has the same meaning as chemist as defined in the Regulations.

c.   A pharmacy contractor is a person with whom the Family Practitioner Committee has made arrangements for the provision of pharmaceutical services in respect of the supply of drugs, appliances and chemical reagents.

d.   An appliance contractor is a person with whom the Family Practitioner Committee has made arrangements for the provision of pharmaceutical services so far as it relates to the supply of appliances included within Part IXA/B/C of this Tariff.

e.   A drug store contractor is a person with whom the Family Practitioner Committee has made arrangements for the provision of pharmaceutical services so far as it relates to the supply of medicinal products on a general sale list under or by virtue of the provisions of the Medicines Act.

f.   The term person includes a body of person corporate or unincorporate.

g.   The term Pricing Authority means, as the case may require, the Prescription Pricing Authority or the Welsh Pricing Committee.

h.   The term appliances as used in this Tariff includes dressings.

NB. In the preparation of this Tariff the Secretary of State for Health has consulted the Pharmaceutical Services Negotiating Committee.

PART I

REQUIREMENTS FOR THE SUPPLY OF DRUGS, APPLIANCES
AND CHEMICAL REAGENTS

CLAUSE 1. DRUGS

Any drug included in this Tariff or in the British National Formulary, Dental Practitioner's
Formulary, European Pharmaceopoeia, British Pharmacopoeia or the British Pharmaceutical Codex,
supplied as part of pharmaceutical services, must comply with the standard or formula specified
therein unless the prescriber has indicated to the contrary. Any drug supplied which is not so
included must be of a grade or quality not lower than that ordinarily used for medicinal purposes.

CLAUSE 2. APPLIANCES

The only appliances which may be supplied as part of the pharmaceutical services are those listed
in Part IXA/B/C of the Tariff and which comply with the specifications therein.

CLAUSE 3. CHEMICAL REAGENTS

The only chemical reagents which may be supplied as part of the pharmaceutical services are those
listed in Part IXR of the Tariff.

CLAUSE 4. DOMICILIARY OXYGEN THERAPY SERVICE

The requirements for the supply of domiciliary oxygen and its associated appliances together with
the arrangements for reimbursement of those contractors included on the Family Practitioner
Committee's lists of contractors authorised to provide this service, are set out in Part X of the
Tariff.

PART II

REQUIREMENTS ENABLING PAYMENTS TO BE
MADE FOR DRUGS, APPLIANCES AND
CHEMICAL REAGENTS

CLAUSE 5. CLAIMS FOR PAYMENT

Contractors shall endorse prescription forms as required in Clause 9 (Endorsement Requirements) of this Tariff. Contractors shall sort and despatch forms in such manner as the Family Practitioner Committee may direct. Contractors shall despatch the forms together with the appropriate claim form not later than the fifth day of the month following that in which the supply was made.

CLAUSE 6. CALCULATION OF PAYMENTS

A.   Pharmacy Contractors

Payment for services provided by pharmacy contractors in respect of the supply of drugs, appliances and chemical reagents supplied against prescriptions at each separate place of business shall comprise:-

(i)   (a)   The total of the prices of the drugs, appliances and chemical reagents so supplied calculated in accordance with the requirements of this Tariff

LESS

*(b)   An amount, based on the total of the prices at (i)(a) above, calculated from the table at Part V ("Deduction Scale")

PLUS

(c)   An on cost allowance of 5% of the total of prices at (i)(a) above, that is before the subtraction of the amount calculated as at (i)(b)

AND

(ii)   The appropriate professional fee as set out in Part IIIA

AND

(iii)   The allowance for containers and specified measuring devices as set out in Part IV.

*NOTE

No deduction will be made in respect of prescriptions for items listed on page 5 for which the contractor has not been able to obtain a discount:

"ZD" LIST

Alternative Medicines
Borderline Substance Foods
CAPD Fluids
Cesamet Capsules 1mg (Lilly)
Clomid Tablets (Merrell Dow)
Controlled Drugs in schedules 1, 2 and 3 of
   the Misuse of Drugs Regulations 1985 |
Covermark Products listed in
   Drug Tariff (Charles Fox)
Cytosar Injection (Upjohn)
Dermacolor Products listed in
   Drug Tariff (Stiefel)
Drug available only on a named
   patient basis: eg
      Cystrin Tablets (Tillots Labs)
      Ditropan Tablets (Smith & Nephew)
      Ospolot Tablets 50 mg & 200 mg (Bayer)
Eraldin Injection (ICI)
Eye Drops (Special Formulae)
Fertiral (Hoechst)
Flolan
Fungizone tissue culture (Squibb)
Furamide Tablets (Boots)
Gammabulin (Immuno)
Gammimune-N (Cutler)
Gonadotrophon LH Injection (Paines and Byrne)
Healonid Injection (Pharmacia (GB) Ltd)
Homoeopathic Products
HRF Injection (Wyeth)
HSL Catarrh vaccine
   (Harley St Labs)

Intraglobulin (Biotest Folex)
Intron-A Injection (Kirby Warrick)
Iscador Injection (Weleda)
Kabiglobulin (KabiVitrum)
* Keromask Products listed in
   Drug Tariff (Innoxa)
Lithium Citrate Syrup (RP Drugs)
Made to measure elastic hosiery & trusse:
Natures Own products
Ospolot suspension (Bayer)
Products manufactured by
   Geistlich Sons Ltd
Rabies vaccines, Merieux inactivated
       (Servier)
Relefact LH-RH (Hoechst)
Relefact LH-RH/TRH (Hoechst)
Roferon - A Injection (Roche)
Sandimmun Infusion   (Sandoz)
Sandimmun Oral Solution (")
Sandoglobulin   (")
SDV
Somatonorm Injection (KabiVitrum)
Special formulations
Tenormin Injection (Stuart)
Tiscar Injection/Infusion (Beecham)
TPN's
Veil Cover Cream
Wellferon Injection (Wellcome)

Contractors who have not received discount in respect of the above products shoul' endorse the prescription "ZD". The prescription price reimbursement will then have no discoun' deduction applied.

* Part XV

CLAUSE 6 - cont

B.   Appliance Contractors

Payment for services provided by appliance contractors in respect of the supply of appliances so supplied against prescriptions at each separate place of business, shall comprise:-

(i)   The total of the prices of the appliances, calculated in accordance with Part IXA/B/C

PLUS

(ii)   An amount based on the number of prescriptions against which supply is made each month, calculated from the Table at Part VIB ("Oncost Allowance" scale) and applied to the toal of the prices at (i) above.

PROVIDED THAT

(a) Where prescription forms are received by the Pricing Authority from two or more contractors whose names are separately entered on the pharmaceutical list for the supply of appliances only in respect of the provision of services at the same place of business, all such prescription forms shall be aggregated for the purpose of the calculation as at (ii) above and the rate so calculated shall be applied to the total of the prices calculated in accordance with (i) above in respect of the prescriptions received from each of those persons.

(b) A contractor's name shall not be entered on the Pharmaceutical List separately for the same place of business in respect of (1) the supply of appliances, (2) the supply of drugs and appliances, or (3) the supply of drugs, except in the case of a contractor for whom separate entries on the Pharmaceutical List relating to the same place of business were allowed prior to the first day of November 1961.

(c) Where a contractor's name is entered on the Pharmaceuticai List in respect of the provision of services at more than one place of business, the calculation as at (ii) above shall be made separately in relation to the total of the prices calculated in accordance with (i) above in respect of prescriptions received in respect of the services provided at each place of business.

AND

(iii) The appropriate fees as set out in Part IIIB.

C.   Drug Store Contractors

Payments to drug store contractors for pharmaceutical services relating to drugs supplied against prescriptions at each separate place of business are made on the same basis as payments to pharmacy contractors set out in Clause 6A(i)(a). plus an on-cost of 10.5% and attract the fee set out in Part IIIA(1) and the container allowances set out in Part IV.

CLAUSE 7. PAYMENTS FOR DRUGS, APPLIANCES AND CHEMICAL REAGENTS

A.   The price on which payment is based for a quantity of a drug, appliance or chemical reagent supplied is calculated proportionately from the basic price (see Clause 8 — Basic Price).

B.   Subject to the provisions of Clause 10 (Quantity to be supplied) payment will be calculated on the basis that the exact quantity ordered by the prescriber has been supplied.

C.   Where a prescription form has been returned to the contractor for endorsement or elucidation and it is returned to the Pricing Authority unendorsed, or incompletely endorsed, or without further explanation, then the price for the drug, appliance or chemical reagent which it orders shall be determined by the Secretary of State.

D.   If a contractor's overall supply of a product appears to justify payment being based on the cost of a larger size than that normally required pursuant to orders on prescription forms and notice has been given to that effect to the contractor, the basic price will be the price of that larger size, the prescription form being deemed to have been so endorsed.

CLAUSE 8. BASIC PRICE

A.   The basic price for those drugs, appliances and chemical reagents ordered by a name included in Parts VIII and IX or by a synonymn of that name shall be the price listed in the Drug Tariff.

B.   (i)   The basic price for any other drug shall be the List Price charged by the manufacturer, wholesaler or supplier for the pack from which it was supplied. In default of any such List Price, the price shall be determined by the Secretary of State.

      (ii)   For the purposes of this Tariff the term List Price means the price published by the manufacturer or manufacturer's authorised agent for the drug appliance or chemical reagent in question when supplied to contractors.

CLAUSE 9. ENDORSEMENT REQUIREMENTS

A.   Contractors shall endorse prescription forms for drugs, appliances and chemical reagents listed in this Tariff as required by this Clause and when so required by the provisions of Part II Clauses 10 (Quantity to be Supplied) and 11 (Broken Bulk), Part III (Fees), and Note 2 to Part IXA/B/C (Appliances).

B.   Every other prescription form shall be endorsed by the contractor with the pack size from which its order was supplied and, if the order is in pharmacopoeial or 'generic' form, with the brand name or the name of the manufacturer or wholesaler from whom the supply was purchased. Where additional specific endorsement is necessary contractors shall endorse prescription forms when so required by the provisions of Part II Clauses 10 (Quantity to be Supplied) and 11 (Broken Bulk), Part III (Fees).

C.   Where insufficient information is available to enable the PPA or WPC to process the prescription, the form shall be returned to the contractor who shall endorse the prescription form with the information requested.

D.   Where a contractor supplies a quantity at variance with that ordered, ie. under the provisions set out in Clause 10 (Quantity to be Supplied), the prescription shall be endorsed with the quantity supplied. An exception to this requirement is where a drug is supplied in a Calendar Pack and the quantity ordered differs from that pack. In such cases and in the absence of an endorsement to the contrary, the contractor will be deemed to have supplied the quantity available in the nearest number of packs or sub-packs to that ordered.

CLAUSE 10. QUANTITY TO BE SUPPLIED

A.   Subject to the requirements of the Weights and Measures (Equivalents for Dealing with Drugs) Regulations, 1970, with regard to the supply in metric quantities of orders expressed in imperial quantities, payment will normally be calculated on the basis that the exact quantity ordered by the prescriber has been supplied, except only of those preparations referred to in B and C below:

B.   Drugs and Chemical Reagents in Special Containers

Where the quantity ordered by the prescriber does not coincide with that of an original pack and the drug or chemical reagent is:

    (i)   Sterile

    (ii)   Effervescent or hygroscopic, or

* (iii) (a) Liquid preparations for addition to bath water

          (b) Coal Tar preparations

          (c) Viscous external preparations

    (iv) Packed in a collapsible tube, pressurised aerosol, spray, puffer pack, squeeze pack, castor, shaker, roll-on bottle, drop-bottle, container with an integral means of application, or any other container from which it is not practicable to dispense the exact quantity;

the contractor shall supply in the special container or containers the quantity nearest to that ordered and endorse the prescription form with the number and size of those containers. Although payment will normally be based on the quantity nearest to that ordered, some items are available in a larger size pack or container than that normally required pursuant to orders on prescription forms. Where the amount ordered on a prescription form, or the frequency of supply, justifies supply from such larger size pack or container, payment will be based on the cost of that larger size in the absence of endorsement.

C.   Calendar Packs (including Oral Contraceptives)

    (i)   A calendar pack is a blister or strip pack showing the days of the week or month against each of the several units in the pack. Although payment is normally based on the number of packs or sub-packs nearest to the quantity ordered (see Clause 9D (Endorsement Requirements)) there may be occasions when, in the pharmacist's professional opinion, the prescriber's intention is that an exact quantity should be supplied, or that sufficient packs or sub-packs should be supplied to cover the quantity ordered. In such cases the contractor should supp,y accordingly and endorse the prescription form with the quantity supplied. Payment will then be based on the quantity shown by the endorsement.

    (ii)   Payment for a Calendar Pack or Original Pack will be based on the smallest pack size available when one or a number of such packs are ordered. Some original packs contain more than one monthly cycle and prescriptions ordering three or more such packs will be returned to the contractor for clarification.

* Products included in Clause 10B(iii) are listed on page 8a

PART II

Products included in Clause 10B(iii) are listed below.

Liquid preparations for external use:

Sub Para	Name	Pack(s)
(a)	Alpha Keri Bath Oil	(240 ml and 480ml)
(b)	Alphosyl Lotion	(250 ml)
(b)	Alphosyl Shampoo	(125 ml)
(a)	Aveeno Emulave Fluid	(150 ml)
(a)	Aveeno Oilated Sachet	(30 g)
(a)	Aveeno Regular Sachet	(50 g)
(a)	Balneum Bath Additive	(225 ml and 500 ml)
(b)	Balneum with Tar	(225 ml)
(c)	Ceanel concentrate	(50 ml, 150 ml and 500 ml)
(b)	Gelcotar Gel	(50 g and 500 g)
(b)	Gelcotar Liquid Tar Shampoo	(150 ml and 350 ml)
(b)	Genisol Shampoo	(58 ml and 250 ml)
(a)	Hydromol Emollient Bath Additive	(150 ml and 350 ml)
(c)	Keri Tharapeutic Lotion	(190 ml and 380 ml)
(c)	Lacticare Lotion	(150 ml)
(c)	Oilatum Emollient	(150 ml and 350 ml)
(c)	Phisohex Medicated Face Wash	(150 ml)
(b)	Polytar Emollient	(350 ml)
(b)	Polytar Liquid	(65 ml, 150 ml and 350 ml)
(b)	Polytar Plus	(350 ml)
(b)	Psoriderm Bath Emulsion	(200 ml)
(b)	Psoriderm Cream	(225 ml)
(b)	Psoriderm Scalp Lotion Shampoo	(250 ml)
(c)	Quinoderm Lotio-Gel(5%)	(30 ml)
(c)	Quinoderm Lotio-Gel(10%)	(30 ml)
(c)	Seba Med Liquid Cleanser	(150 ml and 500 ml)
(a)	Ster-Zac Bath Concentrate	(28.5 ml)
(b)	T/Gel Shampoo	(125 ml and 200 ml)
(c)	Unguentum Merck	(200 ml dispenser)

CLAUSE 11. BROKEN BULK

A.   This Clause applies to drugs, appliances and chemical reagents other than those listed in Category A of Part VIII, and items supplied in special containers covered by Clause 10B (Quantity to be supplied) or Part IX of this Tariff except for Stoma and Incontinence appliances, ie Part IXB and IXC.

B.   When the quantity ordered on a prescription form is other than the minimum quantity the manufacturer, wholesaler or supplier is prepared to supply and the contractor, having purchased such minimum quantity as may be necessary to supply the quantity ordered cannot readily dispose of the remainder, payment will be made for the whole of the quantity purchased. Subsequent prescriptions, received during the next six months, will be deemed to have been supplied from the remainder and no further payment will be made to drug costs other than fees and container allowances until that remainder has been used up. Thereafter contractors must endorse prescription forms to indicate when a claim for payment is being made.

C.   Broken bulk can be claimed on calendar packs only when part of the contents are prescribed for post-coital contraception.

CLAUSE 12. OUT OF POCKET EXPENSES

Where, in exceptional circumstances, out-of-pocket expenses have been incurred in obtaining a drug, appliance or chemical reagent other than those priced in Part VIII Category A and Part IX of the Tariff and not required to be frequently supplied by the contractor, or where out-of-pocket expenses have been incurred in obtaining oxygen from a manufacturer, wholesaler or supplier specially for supply against a prescription, payment of the amount by which such expenses on any occasion exceed 10p may be made where the contractor sends a claim giving full particulars to the Pricing Authority with the appropriate prescription form.

CLAUSE 13. DRUG PREPARATIONS REQUIRING RECONSTITUTION FROM GRANULES OR POWDER

A.   This clause applies to a drug preparation requiring reconstitution from granules or powder by the contractor and resulting in a liquid of limited stability.

B.   When the quantity reconstituted from an original pack or packs is unavoidably greater than the quantity ordered, and it has not been possible for the contractor to use the remainder for or towards supplying against another prescription (see Clause 11 – Broken Bulk) payment, which attracts the standard professional fee (but see also Part IIIA, E), will be calculated from the Basic Price of the preparation and will be based on the nearest pack or number of packs necessary to cover the quantity ordered.

PART IIIA

PROFESSIONAL FEES (Pharmacy Contractors)
See Part II, Clause 6A(ii) (Page 4)

	Fee per prescription p	*Endorsements required by contractors
1. ALL PRESCRIPTIONS (except the Special Fee at 3) attract a Professional Fee which will have 3 values as follows:		
For the first 1400 prescriptions dispensed per month	144.5	NIL
For the next 5250 prescriptions dispensed	66.3	NIL
For prescriptions dispensed thereafter	73.3	NIL

2. ADDITIONAL FEES:

A. PREPARATIONS WHEN EXTEMPORANEOUSLY DISPENSED <u>AND ENDORSED.</u>

  (a) "Extemporaneously dispensed"

(i) Unit dosage forms, eg sachets capsules, pills, lozenges, pastiles, pessaries, powders	225 per 10 or part thereof	"Extemporaneously dispensed"
(ii) Liquids being 'special formula preparations', eg mixtures, lotions, nasal drops (not including dilutions)......	110	"Extemporaneously dispensed"
(iii) Liquid preparations prepared by straight forward dilution (not including reconstitution)	60	"Extemporaneously dispensed"
(iv) Special formula powders	110	"Extemporaneously dispensed"
(v) Ointments, creams pastes being 'special formula preparations' (not including dilutions)	225	"Extemporaneously dispensed"
(vi) Ointments, creams, pastes prepared by dilution or admixture of standard or proprietary ointments, creams and pastes	110	"Extemporaneously dispensed"

  (b) "Aseptically dispensed"
Preparations when aseptically dispensed (excluding proprietary preparations)

(i) Unit dosage forms, eg Injections	1115 per 10 or part thereof	"Aseptically dispensed"
(ii) Non-unit dosage forms, eg Eye Drops	670	"Aseptically dispensed"

  (c) "Extemporaneously sterilised"
Liquids, semi-solids, solids prepared with a BP sterilization process ....

	670	"Extemporaneously sterilised"

* see page 12

PART IIIA

PROFESSIONAL FEES (Pharmacy Contractors) – cont
See Part II, Clause 6A(ii) (page 4)

	Fee per prescription p	*Endorsements required by contractors
B. APPLIANCES AND DRESSINGS		
(a) (i) Elastic Hosiery (Compression Hosiery) requiring measurement and endorsed "measured and fitted"	110	"Measured and fitted"
(ii) Repairs to Elastic Hosiery	60	NIL
(b) (i) Trusses requiring measurement and endorsed "measured and fitted"	170	"Measured and fitted"
(ii) Repairs to Trusses	60	NIL
(c) Stoma Appliances, Suprapubic Belts, Incontinence Appliances		
(i) Replacement of complete appliance and/or)) ii) One or more types of spare parts and) accessories ....)	110	NIL
C. BULK PRESCRIPTIONS for schools or institutions supplied in accordance with the regulations	560	NIL
D. Where liquid preparations extemporaneously dispensed other than at 2A(b) and A(c) above are ordered by the prescriber to be supplied in more than one container, each extra quantity ordered	110	NIL
E. Where a preparation which requires the addition of a vehicle/diluent by the pharmacy contractor results in a liquid of stability of less than 14 days, and for pharmaceutical reasons necessitates supply in more than one container and the prescription form is endorsed with the number of extra quantities supplied, for each extra supply	110	Number of extra containers supplied
F. Where the prescription is for a Controlled Drug in Schedule 1.2 or 3 of the Misuse of Drugs Regulations 1985 and is endorsed "CD" by the contractor	110	"CD"

* see page 12

PROFESSIONAL FEES (Pharmacy Contractors) – cont
See Part II, Clause 6A(ii) (page 4)

G. When the prescription has been dispensed at a time when the premises are not open for dispensing on the day or (in the case of a prescription dispensed after midnight) the day following that on which it was written and

		FEE PER CALL-OUT		* Endorsements required by contractors
		Resident	Non-Resident†	
(i)	Is endorsed "urgent" by the prescriber and dispensed between the time the premises close for dispensing and 11 pm on days other than Sundays and public holidays	P	P	Time and date. Where appropriate "non-resident"
		600	1475	
	OR			
(ii)	Is endorsed "urgent" by the prescriber or "dispensed urgently" by the contractor and is signed by the patient (or his representative) and dispensed between 11 pm and the time the premises open for dispensing or on Sundays and public holidays			Time and date. Where appropriate "non-resident" Where appropriate "dispensed urgently" (signature of patient or representative required)
		775	1775	

Urgent fees are not payable for prescriptions despensed after the hours of opening required under a scheme proposed by a Family Practitioner Committee but before the actual closing of the pharmacy and the contractor still being present.

ALL "URGENT" PRESCRIPTIONS MUST BE ENDORSED WITH THE TIME AND DATE OF DISPENSING

† In order to qualify for the non-resident rates, a contractor who normally lives elsewhere than on his business premises will need to have left those premises and to return to open them to dispense an "urgent" prescription. In the absence of an endorsement 'non-resident' on 'urgent' prescription forms, payments will automatically be made at the 'resident' rate.

*Abbreviated endorsements, eg "Extemp prep" are acceptable. Endorsements under this heading apply only to claims for the appropriate professional fee. Further endorsement may be necessary for other purposes eg Part II Clause 8 (Basic Price), Clause 9 (Endorsement Requirements) and Notes to Part VIII (page 33).

H. FEE RELATED TO THRESHOLD QUANTITY

An additional fee of 30p will be paid in respect of each prescription with the exception of bulk prescriptions, for an oral solid dose preparation (as listed below, pages 13 to 22) where the quantity ordered exceeds the threshold listed against the preparation.

3. Special Fee – see page 22

Drug	Threshold quantity	Drug	Threshold quantity
Abicol tab	91	Antepsin tab 1g	138
Acepril tab 25mg	119	Anturan tab 100mg	135
Acepril tab 50mg	132	Anturan tab 200mg	160
Achromycin cap 250mg	49	Apisate tab	55
Achromycin tab 250mg	48	Apresoline tab 25mg	133
Actidil tab 2.5mg	75	Apresoline tab 50mg	135
Acupan tab 30mg	104	Aprinox tab 2.5mg	55
Adalat cap 10mg	147	Aprinox tab 5mg	59
Adalat cap 5mg	132	Apsifen tab 600mg	95
Adalat Retard tab 20mg	104	Arelix cap 6mg	54
Aldactide 25 tab	81	Artane Sustets 5mg	75
Aldactide 50 tab	67	Artane tab 2mg	125
Aladctone tab 100mg	57	Artane tab 5mg	116
Aldactone tab 25mg	98	Ascorbic acid tab 25mg	83
Aldactone tab 50mg	65	Ascorbic acid tab 50mg	99
Aldomet tab 125mg	125	Ascorbic acid tab 100mg	95
Aldomet tab 250mg	138	Ascorbic acid tab 200mg	88
Aldomet tab 500mg	140	Ascorbic acid tab 500mg	94
Allegron tab 25mg	115	Aspirin Nuseal 300mg	102
Allopurinol tab 100mg	106	Aspirin Nuseal 600mg	120
Allopurinol tab 300mg	57	Aspirin tab 75mg	63
Aloxiprin tab 600mg	165	Aspirin tab 300mg	87
Alrheumat cap 50mg	120	Aspirin tab disp 75mg	65
Alu-Cap cap 475mg	283	Aspirin tab disp 300mg	101
Aluminium hydroxide tab 500mg	145	Atarax tab 10mg	88
Alunex tab 4mg	62	Atarax tab 25mg	96
Alupent tab 20mg	129	Atenolol tab 50mg	60
Aluzine tab 20mg	60	Atenolol tab 100mg	59
Ambaxin tab 400mg	24	Atromid-S cap 500mg	154
Amfipen cap 250mg	33	Augmentin tab disp	30
Amilco tab	64	Augmentin tab 375mg	31
Amiloride HCl tab 5mg	72	Aventyl Pulvules 25mg	114
Aminophylline tab 100mg	109	Avloclor tab 250mg	48
Amitriptyline tab 10mg	102	Avomine tab 25mg	68
Amitriptyline tab 25mg	99	Azathioprine tab 50mg	114
Amitriptyline tab 50mg	72	Bactrim tab disp	40
Amoxil cap 250mg	29	Bactrim drapsule	35
Amoxil cap 500mg	29	Bactrim tab double strength	22
Amoxil tab disp 500mg	26	Baratol tab 25mg	116
Amoxycillin cap 250mg	29	Baxan cap 500mg	19
Amoxycillin cap 500mg	30	Baycaron tab 25mg	68
Ampicillin cap 250mg	34	Benadryl cap 25mg	94
Ampicillin cap 500mg	35	Bendogen tab 10mg	155
Amytal tab 15mg	90	Bendrofluazide tab 2.5mg	63
Amytal tab 30mg	119	Bendrofluazide tab 5mg	63
Amytal tab 50mg	120	Benemid tab 500mg	109
Amytal tab 100mg	91	Benoral tab 750mg	166
Anafranil cap 10mg	105	Benorylate tab 750mg	150
Anafranil cap 25mg	107	Bentex tab 2mg	125
Anafranil cap 50mg	92	Bentex tab 5mg	116
Anafranil SR tab 75mg	53	Benzhexol tab 2mg	125
Androcur tab 50mg	127	Benzhexol tab 5mg	116
Antabuse 200 tab	65	Beta-Cardone tab 40mg	118
Antepar tab 500mg	41	Beta-Cardone tab 80mg	87
		Betaloc tab 100mg	105

Drug	Threshold quantity	Drug	Threshold quantity
Betaloc tab 50mg	103	Charcoal tab BPC34	182
Betaloc-SA tab	66	Chloractil tab 25mg	109
Bethanidine sulph tab 10mg	155	Chloractil tab 50mg	107
Betim tab 10mg	92	Chloractil tab 100mg	103
Betnelan tab 0.5mg	71	Chlordiazepoxide cap 5mg	95
Betnesol tab 0.5mg	67	Chlordiazepoxide cap 10mg	105
Bezalip tab 200mg	133	Chlordiazepoxide tab 5mg	94
Blocadren tab 10mg	92	Chlordiazepoxide tab 10mg	103
Bolvidon tab 10mg	87	Chlordiazepoxide tab 25mg	97
Bolvidon tab 20mg	67	Chlorpheniramine tab 4mg	62
Bolvidon tab 30mg	62	Chlorpromazine tab 25mg	109
Bradilan tab 250mg	164	Chlorpromazine tab 50mg	107
Bradosol 1oz	45	Chlorpromazine tab 100mg	103
Brevinor tab	131	Chlorpropamide tab 100mg	85
Bricanyl SA tab	81	Chlorpropamide tab 250mg	79
Bricanyl tab 5mg	116	Choledyl tab 100mg	126
Brinaldix K tab	86	Choledyl tab 200mg	132
Broxil cap 250mg	33	Chymocyclar cap	48
Brufen tab 200mg	126	Chymoral forte tab	51
Brufen tab 400mg	116	Chymoral tab	55
Brufen tab 600mg	95	Cinobac cap 500mg	24
Burinex K tab	77	Clinoril tab 100mg	124
Burinex tab 1mg	80	Clinoril tab 200mg	93
Burinex tab 5mg	60	Clobazam cap 10mg	97
Buscopan tab	77	Clomid tab 50mg	30
Cafergot tab	51	Co-Betaloc tab	77
Calciferol tab high strength	92	Co-codamol tab	114
Calciferol tab strong 50000u	69	Co-codamol tab disp	114
Calcium gluconate tab 600mg	128	Co-codaprin tab	122
Calcium lactate tab 300mg	126	Co-codaprin tab disp	113
Calcium with vitamin D tab	98	Co-danthrusate cap	78
Calthor tab 250mg	34	Codeine phosphate tab 15mg	100
Calthor tab 500mg	33	Codeine phosphate tab 30mg	108
Camcolit tab 250mg	144	Codeine phosphate tab 60mg	134
Camcolit tab 400mg	91	Co-dydramol tab	111
Capoten tab 25mg	119	Cogentin tab 2mg	73
Capoten tab 50mg	132	Colchicine tab 0.5mg	90
Catapres Perlonget 0.25mg	77	Colofac tab 135mg	107
Catapres tab 0.3mg	144	Colpermin cap 0.2ml	119
Catapres tab 0.1mg	139	Comox tab disp	40
Caved S tab	157	Comox tab forte	22
Cedilanid tab	75	Concordin tab 10mg	124
Cedocard Retard tab 20mg	108	Concordin tab 5mg	106
Cedocard Retard tab 40mg	100	Conova 30 tab	136
Cedocard tab 5mg	127	Co-proxamol tab	125
Cedocard-10 tab 10mg	153	Cordarone X tab 200mg	65
Cedocard-20 tab 20mg	141	Cordilox tab 120mg	138
Celevac tab	212	Cordilox tab 160mg	98
Cellucon tab	212	Cordilox tab 40mg	146
Centyl K tab	71	Cordilox tab 80mg	139
Ceporex cap 250mg	35	Corgard tab 40mg	76
Ceporex cap 500mg	29	Corgard tab 80mg	74
Ceporex tab 250mg	34	Corgaretic tab 40mg	70
Ceporex tab 500mg	29	Corgaretic tab 80mg	64
Cetiprin tab 100mg	151	Corlan pellets	37

0303M/3

Drug	Threshold quantity	Drug	Threshold quantity
Cortelan tab 25mg	93	Dindevan tab 50mg	146
Cortisone acetate MSD tab 25mg	93	Dioctyl tab 100mg	109
Cortistab tab 5mg	198	Disipal tab 50mg	133
Cortistab tab 25mg	93	Distaclor cap 250mg	30
Cortisyl tab 25mg	93	Distamine tab 125mg	114
Co-trimoxazole tab	39	Distamine tab 250mg	98
Co-trimoxazole tab disp	40	Distaquaine VK tab 250mg	37
Co-trimoxazole tab forte	22	Diumide-K tab	64
Cyclophosphamide tab 50mg	84	Diurexan tab 20mg	63
Cyclospasmol cap 400mg	133	Dixarit tab 0.025mg	139
Cyclospasmol tab 400mg	134	Dolmatil tab 200mg	118
Dalacin cap 150mg	38	Dolobid tab 250mg	103
Daneral SA tab	57	Dolobid tab 500mg	76
Danol cap 100mg	86	Domical tab 50mg	72
Danol cap 200mg	81	Doxatet tab 100mg	13
Dantrium cap 25mg	180	Doxylar cap 100mg	14
Daonil tab 5mg	108	Dramamine tab 50mg	94
Dapsone tab 50mg	102	Duphaston tab 10mg	85
Dapsone tab 100mg	81	Duromine cap 15mg	47
Daraprim tab	30	Duromine cap 30mg	45
De-Noltab 120mg	150	Duvadilan 20mg tab	138
Decadron tab 0.5mg	133	Duvadilan Retard cap	87
Decaserpyl plus tab	111	Dyazide tab 50mg	61
Declinax tab 10mg	127	Dytac cap 50mg	80
Declinax tab 20mg	125	Dytide cap	70
Defencin cap 40mg	88	Economycin cap 250mg	49
Deltacortril tab ec 2.5mg	108	Effercitrate tab	56
Deltacortril tab ec 5mg	90	Elantan tab 20mg	111
Dequadin loz	48	Elantan tab 40mg	113
Deseril tab 1mg	128	Eldepryl tab 5mg	68
Deteclo tab	25	Eltroxin tab 0.05mg	113
Dexedrine tab 5mg	98	Eltroxin tab 0.1mg	101
Dextropropoxyphene cap 65mg	106	Emeside cap 250mg	147
Diabinese tab 100mg	91	Endoxana tab 50mg	84
Diabinese tab 250mg	89	Epanutin cap 25mg	90
Diamicron tab 80mg	90	Epanutin cap 50mg	116
Diamorphine HCl tab 10mg	170	Epanutin cap 100mg	135
Diamox Sustets 500mg	74	Ephedrine HCl tab 30mg	114
Diamox tab 250mg	91	Ephynal tab 200mg	130
Diane tab	107	Ephynal tab 50mg	137
Diatensic tab 50mg	73	Epilim tab crushable 100mg	205
Diazepam tab 2mg	87	Epilim tab ec 200mg	173
Diazepam tab 5mg	85	Epilim tab ec 500mg	149
Diazepam tab 10mg	72	Equanil tab 200mg	102
Dibenyline cap 10mg	90	Equanil tab 400mg	104
Diconal tab	63	Ergometrine tab 0.5mg	22
Dicynene tab 250mg	61	Erymax cap 250mg	34
Dicynene tab 500mg	53	Erythrocin tab 250mg	38
Digoxin tab 0.0625mg	65	Erythrocin tab 500mg	26
Digoxin tab 0.125mg	61	Erythromid tab 250mg	39
Digoxin tab 0.25mg	62	Erythromycin tab 250mg	41
Dihydrocodeine tab 30mg	102	Erythromycin tab 500mg	32
Dimotane LA tab 12mg	66	Erythroped A tab 500mg	31
Dimotane tab 4mg	68	Esbatal tab 10mg	155
Dindevan tab 10mg	153	Esidrex tab 25mg	69

Drug	Threshold quantity	Drug	Threshold quantity
Esidrex tab 50mg	61	Franol plus tab	135
Esidrex K tab	71	Franol tab	127
Estrovis tab 4mg	2	Froben tab 100mg	108
Ethinyloestradiol tab 0.01mg	91	Froben tab 50mg	117
Euglucon tab 2.5mg	90	Frumil tab	61
Euglucon tab 5mg	109	Frusemide tab 20mg	60
Eugynon 30 tab	133	Frusemide tab 40mg	77
Eugynon 50 tab	65	Frusemide tab 500mg	43
Exirel cap 15mg	125	Frusene tab 40mg	62
Exirel tab 10mg	121	Fucidin tab ec 250mg	95
Fabahistin tab 50mg	76	Fulcin tab 125mg	155
Fansidar tab	18	Fulcin tab 500mg	75
Farlutal tab 100mg	134	Fungilin loz 10mg	43
Fectrim tab disp	40	Furadantin tab 100mg	45
Fectrim tab forte	22	Furadantin tab 50mg	66
Fefol span	60	Gamanil tab 70mg	78
Feldene cap 10mg	85	Gastrocote tab	146
Feldene cap 20mg	49	Gastrozepin tab 50mg	93
Feldene tab disp 10mg	61	Gaviscon tab	140
Feldene tab disp 20mg	46	Glibenclamide tab 2.5mg	71
Femulen tab	154	Glibenclamide tab 5mg	101
Fenbid cap 300mg	117	Glibenese tab 5mg	118
Fenopron tab 300mg	128	Glucophage tab 850mg	104
Fenopron tab 600mg	105	Glucophage tab 500mg	126
Fentazin tab 2mg	107	Glurenorm tab 30mg	133
Fentazin tab 4mg	122	Glyceryl trinitrate tab 0.5mg	134
Feospan span	60	Glyceryl trinitrate tab 0.6mg	134
Fergon tab	115	Grisovin tab 500mg	75
Ferrocontin Continus tab	57	Grisovin tab 125mg	155
Ferrocontin Folic Continus tab	59	Gynovlar 21 tab	133
Ferrograd-Folic tab	61	Haldol tab 5mg	101
Ferrogradumet tab 325mg	56	Haldol tab 10mg	124
Ferromyn S tab	118	Half-Inderal LA cap 80mg	56
Ferromyn tab	119	Halibut liver oil cap BP	109
Ferrous gluconate tab 300mg	113	Haloperidol tab 1.5mg	115
Ferrous sulphate co tab	119	Haloperidol tab 5mg	101
Ferrous sulphate tab 200mg	111	Haloperidol tab 10mg	124
Ferrous sulphate tab 300mg	83	Harmogen tab	77
Fersaday tab	53	Heminevrin cap	79
Fersamal tab 200mg	114	Hexopal forte tab 750mg	137
Flagyl tab 200mg	33	Hexopal tab 500mg	147
Flagyl tab 400mg	30	Hibitane loz	37
Florinef tab 0.1mg	68	Hiprex tab 1g	79
Floxapen cap 250mg	37	Hismanal tab 10mg	47
Floxapen cap 500mg	34	Histryl span 5mg	73
Fluanxol tab 0.5mg	82	Honvan tab	102
Fluanxol tab 1mg	57	Hydergine tab 1.5mg	130
Flucloxacillin cap 250mg	39	Hydergine tab 4.5mg	63
Flucloxacillin cap 500mg	46	Hydralazine HCl tab 25mg	138
Folex 350 tab	58	Hydralazine HCl tab 50mg	132
Folic acid tab 5mg	83	Hydrenox tab 50mg	92
Folicin tab	87	Hydromet tab	117
Fortunan tab 1.5mg	115	Hydrocortistab tab 20mg	93
Fortunan tab 5mg	101	Hydrocortone tab 10mg	133
Fortunan tab 10mg	124	Hydrocortone tab 20mg	93

0303M/7

Drug	Threshold quantity	Drug	Threshold quantity
HydroSaluric tab 25mg	69	Kelfizine W tab 2g	7
HydroSaluric tab 50mg	61	Kemadrin tab 5mg	118
Hygroton K tab	77	Kerlone tab 20mg	47
Hygroton tab 100mg	54	Ketovite tab	133
Hygroton tab 50mg	62	Kinidin durules	136
Hypovase tab 0.5mg	128	Kloref tab	142
Hypovase tab 1mg	142	Labetolol tab 100mg	125
Hypovase tab 2mg	143	Labetolol tab 200mg	135
Hypovase tab 5mg	140	Labetolol tab 400mg	132
Ibumetin tab 600mg	95	Labrocol tab 100mg	125
Ibuprofen tab 200mg	112	Labrocol tab 200mg	135
Ibuprofen tab 400mg	104	Labrocol tab 400mg	132
Ibuprofen tab 600mg	95	Lanitop tab	70
Ilosone cap 250mg	36	Lanoxin 0.125mg tab	65
Imipramine tab 10mg	104	Lanoxin PG tab	75
Imipramine tab 25mg	123	Lanoxin tab 0.25mg	62
Imodium cap 2mg	47	Larapam cap 10mg	85
Imperacin tab 250mg	53	Larapam cap 20mg	49
Imuran tab 50mg	114	Laratrim fte tab	22
Inderal LA cap 160mg	65	Largactil tab 100mg	103
Inderal tab 10mg	157	Largactil tab 10mg	108
Inderal tab 160mg	129	Largactil tab 25mg	109
Inderal tab 40mg	129	Largactil tab 50mg	107
Inderal tab 80mg	137	Lasikal tab	78
Inderetic cap	86	Lasilactone cap	73
Inderex cap	66	Lasix tab 20mg	60
Indocid cap 25mg	117	Lasix tab 40mg	75
Indocid cap 50mg	109	Lasma tab 300mg	80
Indocid-R cap 75mg	63	Ledercort tab 2mg	88
Indolar SR cap	63	Ledercort tab 4mg	68
Indomethacin cap BP 25mg	113	Lederfen cap 300mg	113
Indomethacin cap BP 50mg	100	Lederfen tab 300mg	111
Indomod cap 75mg	63	Lentizol cap 25mg	65
Innovace tab 10mg	59	Lentizol cap 50mg	57
Innovace tab 20mg	62	Lioresal tab 10mg	159
Innovace tab 5mg	68	Liskonium tab 450mg	95
Ionamin 15mg cap	48	Loestrin 20 tab	126
Ionamin 30mg cap	47	Loestrin 30 tab	121
Ipral tab 100mg	41	Lomotil tab	67
Ipral tab 200mg	22	Loniten tab 10mg	134
Ismelin tab 10mg	116	Lopresor SR tab 200mg	66
Ismelin tab 25mg	91	Lopresor tab 100mg	105
Ismo 20 tab	111	Lopresor tab 50mg	103
Isoket Retard tab 20mg	108	Lopresoretic tab	79
Isoket Retard tab 40mg	100	Lorazepam 1mg	84
Isoniazid tab 100mg	122	Lorazepam 2.5mg	91
Isordil tab sublingual 5mg	127	Lormetazepam 1mg	49
Isordil tab 10mg	153	Ludiomil tab 25mg	80
Isordil tab 30mg	152	Ludiomil tab 50mg	63
Isordil Tembids 40mg	116	Ludiomil tab 75mg	51
Kalspare tab	56	Macrodantin cap 100mg	45
Keflex cap 250mg	35	Macrodantin cap 50mg	49
Keflex cap 500mg	29	Madopar cap 125	160
Keflex tab 250mg	34	Madopar cap 62.5mg	158
Keflex tab 500mg	29	Madopar caps 250mg	148

Drug	Threshold quantity	Drug	Threshold quantity
Magnapen cap 500mg	38	Molipaxin cap 50mg	101
Magnesium trisilicate co tab	143	Monit tab 20mg	111
Maloprim tab	24	Mono-Cedocard 20 tab	111
Marevan tab 1mg	114	Mono-Cedocard 40 tab	113
Marevan tab 3mg	87	Monotrim tab 100mg	38
Marevan tab 5mg	74	Monotrim tab 200mg	23
Marplan tab 10mg	113	Monovent tab 5mg	116
Marvelon tab	126	Motilium tab 10mg	73
Maxolon tab 10mg	70	Motipress tab	51
Medrone tab 4mg	69	Motival tab	99
Megaclor tab 170mg	82	Motrin tab 400mg	110
Melleril tab 100mg	100	Motrin tab 600mg	95
Melleril tab 10mg	108	MST continus tab 10mg	89
Melleril tab 25mg	101	MST continus tab 30mg	90
Melleril tab 50mg	95	MST continus tab 60mg	92
Meprobamate tab 200mg	91	Myambutol 100mg tab	111
Meprobamate tab 400mg	95	Myambutol 400mg tab	101
Meptid tab 200mg	90	Mycardol tab	141
Merbentyl tab 10mg	78	Mysoline tab	133
Merocaine loz	43	Mysteclin cap	43
Merocet loz	45	Mysteclin tab	44
Mestinon tab	251	Nacton forte tab 4mg	129
Metenix 5 tab	61	Nacton tab 2mg	141
Metformin tab 500mg	118	Nalcrom cap 100mg	186
Metformin tab 850mg	99	Naprosyn tab 250mg	105
Methyldopa tab 125mg	125	Naprosyn tab 500mg	83
Methyldopa tab 250mg	135	Naproxen tab 250mg	97
Methyldopa tab 500mg	138	Naproxen tab 500mg	76
Metoclopramide tab 10mg	74	Nardil tab	114
Metrolyl tab 400mg	30	Narphen tab 5mg	106
Metronidazole tab 200mg	28	Natrilix tab 2.5mg	58
Metronidazole tab 400mg	30	Navidrex-K tab	78
Mexitil cap 200mg	144	Navidrex tab 0.5mg	74
Microgynon 30 tab	133	Negram tab 500mg	74
Micronor tab	152	Neo-Mercazole tab 5mg	152
Microval tab	178	Neo-Naclex-K tab	78
Midamor tab 5mg	80	Neo-Naclex tab 5mg	65
Midrid cap	68	Neocon tab	123
Migraleve tab pink	44	Neogest tab	180
Migraleve tab yellow	42	Nephril tab 1mg	70
Migravess forte tab	57	Nethaprin Dospan tab	84
Migravess tab	59	Neulactil tab 2.5mg	131
Migril tab	52	Nicotinamide tab 50mg	121
Minilyn tab	143	Nicotinic acid tab 50mg	152
Minocin tab 100mg	73	Nitoman tab 25mg	130
Minocin tab 50mg	90	Nitrazepam tab 5mg	65
Minodiab tab 5mg	118	Nitrazepam tab 10mg	58
Minovlar tab	136	Nitrocontin tab 2.6mg	95
Miraxid tab	32	Nitrofurantoin tab 50mg	66
Mixogen tab	79	Nitrofurantoin tab 100mg	45
Moditen tab 1mg	68	Nivaquine tab 200mg	41
Moducren tab	66	Nizoral tab 200mg	33
Moduret 25 tab	56	Noctec cap 500mg	63
Moduretic tab	64	Noludar tab 200mg	76
Molipaxin cap 100mg	89	Nolvadex-D tab 20mg	81

Drug	Threshold quantity	Drug	Threshold quantity
Nolvadex tab 10mg	118	Paracetamol tab sol 500mg	115
Nordox cap 100mg	14	Paramax tab	67
Norflex tab 100mg	67	Parlodel cap 10mg	135
Norgeston tab	208	Parlodel tab 2.5mg	126
Noriday tab	156	Parnate tab	109
Norimin tab	129	Paroven cap 250mg	122
Norinyl-1 tab	127	Parstelin tab	101
Norval tab 10mg	87	Paxofen tab 600mg	95
Norval tab 20mg	67	Penbritin cap 250mg	37
Norval tab 30mg	62	Penbritin cap 500mg	36
Nuelin SA tab 175mg	96	Pendramine tab 125mg	114
Nuelin SA-250 tab	93	Pendramine tab 250mg	98
Nuelin tab 125mg	126	Penicillin VK cap 250mg	38
Nutrizym tab	319	Penicillin VK tab 125mg	34
Nystan tab oral	55	Penicillin VK tab 250mg	36
Nystan pastilles	47	Pentazocine cap 50mg	101
One-alpha cap 1mcg	67	Pentazocine tab 25mg	118
One-alpha cap 0.25mcg	69	Periactin tab 4mg	95
Opilon tab 40mg	143	Persantin tab 100mg	141
Optimax tab	152	Persantin tab 25mg	195
Optimax WV tab 500mg	143	Pertofran tab 25mg	143
Optimine tab 1mg	62	Pethidine tab 50mg	57
Oradexon tab 0.5mg	133	Phazyme tab	123
Oradexon tab 2mg	133	Phenergan tab 10mg	67
Orap tab 2mg	99	Phenergan tab 25mg	63
Orap tab 4mg	76	Phenobarbitone tab 15mg	115
Orimeten tab 250mg	120	Phenobarbitone tab 30mg	124
Ortho-Novin tab 1/50	123	Phenobarbitone tab 60mg	110
Orudis cap 100mg	98	Phenobarbitone tab 100mg	85
Orudis cap 50mg	120	Phenytoin tab 50mg	115
Oruvail 200 cap	47	Phenytoin tab 100mg	142
Oruvail cap 100mg	79	Phyllocontin tab forte 350mg	95
Ossopan 800 tab	148	Phyllocontin tab paed	104
Ovran tab	108	Phyllocontin tab 225mg	107
Ovran-30 tab	130	Physeptone tab 5mg	48
Ovranette tab	137	Piriton spandets	63
Ovysmen tab	129	Piriton tab 4mg	62
Oxazepam cap 30mg	83	Plaquenil tab 200mg	79
Oxazepam tab 10mg	86	Ponderax PA cap 60mg	57
Oxazepam tab 15mg	100	Pondocillin tab 500mg	18
Oxazepam tab 30mg	83	Ponstan cap 250mg	89
Oxprenolol tab 20mg	129	Ponstan tab disp 250mg	98
Oxprenolol tab 40mg	122	Ponstan tab forte 500mg	79
Oxprenolol tab 80mg	127	Potassium chloride tab slow 600mg	111
Oxprenolol tab 160mg	93	Potassium tab effervescent	166
Oxytetracycline tab 250mg	58	Praxilene cap 100mg	156
Pacitron tab 500mg	143	Prednesol tab 5mg	87
Palaprin forte tab	233	Prednisolone tab 1mg	145
Palfium tab 10mg	90	Prednisolone tab 5mg	82
Palfium tab 5mg	75	Prednisone tab 1mg	155
Paludrine tab 100mg	180	Prednisone tab 5mg	83
Pancrex V cap	356	Pregaday tab	59
Pancrex V tab forte	514	Premarin tab 1.25mg	75
Pancrex V tab	417	Premarin tab 2.5mg	108
Paracetamol tab 500mg	127	Premarin tab 625mcg	76

Drug	Threshold quantity	Drug	Threshold quantity
Prestim tab	77	Sandocal tab	110
Priadel tab	102	Sanomigran tab 0.5mg	105
Primalan tab 5mg	64	Sanomigran tab 1.5mg	55
Primolut N tab 5mg	84	Saventrine tab 30mg	148
Primperan tab 10mg	70	Secadrex tab	66
Pro-Actidil tab 10mg	56	Seconal sodium Pulvules 100mg	92
Pro-Banthine tab 15mg	102	Sectral cap 100mg	113
Progesic tab 200mg	103	Sectral cap 200mg	103
Progynova tab 1mg	68	Sectral tab 400mg	67
Progynova tab 2mg	77	Securon tab 120mg	96
Propranolol tab 10mg	150	Selexid tab 200mg	28
Propranolol tab 40mg	128	Semi-Daonil tab 2.5mg	72
Propranolol tab 80mg	135	Senna tab 7.5mg	109
Propranolol tab 160mg	127	Septrin tab disp	40
Prothiaden cap 25mg	98	Septrin tab forte	22
Prothiaden tab 75mg	52	Septrin tab paed	74
Pro-Vent cap 300mg	73	Septrin tab	40
Provera tab 5mg	69	Serc tab 8mg	128
Provera tab 100mg	134	Serenace cap 0.5mg	102
Pro-Viron tab 25mg	118	Serenace tab 1.5mg	115
Pyridium tab 100mg	95	Serenace tab 5mg	101
Pyridoxine tab 10mg	71	Serenace tab 10mg	124
Pyridoxine tab 20mg	102	Serophene tab 50mg	30
Pyridoxine tab 50mg	111	Serpasil-Esidrex tab	117
Pyrogastrone tab	148	Serpasil tab 0.25mg	113
Quinidine sulph tab 200mg	103	Sinemet-Plus tab	153
Quinine bisulph tab 300mg	63	Sinemet-110 tab	145
Quinine sulph tab 200mg	61	Sinemet-275 tab	140
Quinine sulph tab 300mg	57	Sinequan cap 10mg	98
Rastinon tab 500mg	128	Sinequan cap 25mg	101
Rautrax tab	93	Sinequan cap 50mg	73
Rauwiloid tab	113	Sinequan cap 75mg	52
Rheumacin SR cap	63	Sinthrome tab 1mg	124
Rheumox caps 300mg	110	Sloprolol cap	65
Rheumox tab 600mg	82	Slo-Phyllin 125mg	87
Rifadin cap 300mg	68	Slo-Phyllin 250mg	87
Rifinah 300 tab	93	Slo-Phyllin 60mg	96
Rimactane cap 300mg	68	Slow-Fe Folic	57
Rimactazid 300 tab	93	Slow-K tab 600mg	118
Rivotril tab 0.5mg	144	Slow-Fe tab	62
Rivotril tab 2mg	104	Slow Trasicor tab 160mg	69
Ro-A-Vit tab	96	Sodium Amytal Pulvules 60mg	108
Robaxin tab 750mg	92	Sodium Amytal Pulvules 200mg	78
Ronicol tab 25mg	134	Sodium amytal tab 200mg	81
Ronicol Timespan tab	89	Soneryl tab 100mg	82
Rynacrom cap	149	Soni-Slo cap 40mg	116
Rythmodan cap 100mg	142	Sorbichew tab 5mg	108
Rythmodan Retard tab	92	Sorbid SA tab 40mg	100
Sabidal SR tab 270mg	103	Sorbitrate tab 10mg	153
Salazopyrin EN tab	198	Sorbitrate tab 20mg	141
Salazopyrin tab	199	Sotacor tab 160mg	65
Salbutamol tab 2mg	111	Sotacor tab 80mg	87
Salbutamol tab 4mg	116	Sotazide tab	66
Saluric tab 0.5mg	75	Spasmonal tab	85
Sando-K tab	120	Spiroctan cap 100mg	52

0303M/15

Drug	Threshold quantity	Drug	Threshold quantity
Spiroctan tab 25mg	77	Tenoretic tab	59
Spiroctan tab 50mg	69	Tenormin LS tab 50mg	58
Spironolactone tab 25mg	95	Tenormin tab 100mg	58
Spironolactone tab 50mg	65	Tenuate dospan tab 75mg	49
Spironolactone tab 100mg	56	Teronac tab 2mg	46
Spiroprop tab	80	Terramycin tab 250mg	43
Stelabid tab	85	Terramycin cap 250mg	50
Stelazine span 10mg	70	Tertroxin tab 20mcg	152
Stelazine span 15mg	77	Tetrabid-Organon cap 250mg	28
Stelazine span 2mg	86	Tetrachel cap 250mg	49
Stelazine tab 1mg	113	Tetracycline cap 250mg	49
Stelazine tab 5mg	110	Tetracycline tab 250mg	57
Stemetil tab 25mg	88	Tetralysal cap 150mg	39
Stemetil tab 5mg	97	Tetrex cap 250mg	49
Stiboestrol tab 1mg	130	Theo-Dur tab 200mg	100
Stiboestrol tab 5mg	105	Theo-Dur tab 300mg	87
Strepsils loz	44	Theograd tab 350mg	90
Streptotriad tab	47	Thephorin tab 25mg	82
Stromba tab 5mg	76	Thiamine HCl co tab	95
Stugeron cap forte 75mg	109	Thiamine HCl co tab strong	105
Stugeron tab 15mg	121	Thiamine HCl tab 10mg	84
Sudafed tab 60mg	52	Thyroxine tab 25microgram	99
Surgam tab 200mg	117	Thyroxine tab 50microgram	118
Surgam tab 300mg	81	Thyroxine tab 100microgram	96
Surmontil cap 50mg	66	Tildiem tab 60mg	141
Surmontil tab 10mg	85	Titralac tab	156
Surmontil tab 25mg	81	Tofranil tab 10mg	108
Suscard Buccal tab 1mg	103	Tofranil tab 25mg	119
Suscard Buccal tab 2mg	114	Tolbutamide tab 500mg	131
Suscard Buccal tab 5mg	140	Topal tab	118
Sustac tab 2.6mg	308	Torecan tab 10mg	107
Sustac tab 6.4mg	128	Trancopal tab 200mg	73
Sustac tab 10mg	125	Trandate tab 100mg	125
Sustamycin cap 250mg	46	Trandate tab 200mg	135
Symmetrel cap 100mg	88	Trandate tab 400mg	132
Synadrin 60 tab	128	Trasicor tab 160mg	124
Synflex tab 275mg	69	Trasicor tab 20mg	127
Tagamet tab 200mg	122	Trasicor tab 40mg	132
Tagamet tab 400mg	76	Trasicor tab 80mg	131
Tagamet tab 800mg	46	Trasidrex tab	72
Talpen tab 250mg	28	Tremonil tab 5mg	141
Tambocor tab 100mg	108	Trental 400 tab	123
Tamoxifen tab 10mg	113	Triazolam tab 125microgram	56
Tamoxifen tab 20mg	81	Triazolam tab 250microgram	55
Tavegil tab 1mg	64	Trilisate tab 500mg	166
Tedral tab	120	Triludan tab 60mg	65
Tegretol tab 100mg	138	Trimethoprim 100mg	39
Tegretol tab 200mg	154	Trimethoprim 200mg	21
Tegretol tab 400mg	113	Trimopan tab 200mg	25
Temazepam cap 10mg	60	Triptafen tab	100
Temazepam cap 15mg	47	Triptafen-M tab	100
Temazepam cap 20mg	57	Tryptizol cap 75mg	51
Temgesic tab sublingual 0.2mg	86	Tryptizol tab 10mg	100
Tenavoid tab	69	Tryptizol tab 25mg	105
Tenoret 50 tab	57	Tryptizol tab 50mg	72

Drug	Threshold quantity	Drug	Threshold quantity
Tuinal Pulvules 100mg	104	Vibramycin cap 50mg	50
Tyrozets	48	Vibramycin cap 100mg	14
Uniphyllin Continus tab 400mg	63	Vibramycin-D tab 100mg	18
Uniphyllin paediatric Continus		Viskaldix tab	65
tab 200mg	86	Visken tab 15mg	88
Urantoin tab 100mg	45	Visken tab 5mg	116
Urantoin tab 50mg	66	Vitamin A & D cap BPC	87
Urispas tab 100mg	138	Vitamin cap BPC	89
Uticillin tab 500mg	43	Volital tab 20mg	109
Utovlan tab 5mg	84	Voltarol Retard tab 100mg	50
V-Cil-K Pulvules 250mg	35	Voltarol tab 25mg	120
V-Cil-K tab 125mg	43	Voltarol tab 50mg	107
V-Cil-K tab 250mg	34	Warfarin tab 1mg	114
Vallergan tab 10mg	65	Warfarin tab 1mg WB	114
Valoid tab 50mg	60	Warfarin tab 3mg	87
Vascardin tab 10mg	153	Warfarin tab 3mg WB	87
Vascardin tab 30mg	152	Warfarin tab 5mg	74
Vasculit tab 12.5mg	162	Warfarin tab 5mg WB	74
Velosef cap 250mg	39	Welldorm tab	75
Velosef cap 500mg	35	Zaditen cap 1mg	102
Ventolin Spandets 8mg	80	Zaditen tab 1mg	97
Ventolin tab 2mg	109	Zantac tab 150mg	79
Ventolin tab 4mg	120	Zantac tab 300mg	55
Verapamil HCl tab 40mg	152	Zarontin cap 250mg	147
Verapamil HCl tab 80mg	134	Zovirax tab 200mg	35
Verapamil HCl tab 120mg	135	Zyloric tab 100mg	113
Vermox tab 100mg	5	Zyloric-300 tab 300mg	59
Vertigon Spansule 10mg	79		

3 SPECIAL FEE (ie not paid in addition to professional fee)

	Fee per prescription p	Endorsements required by contractors
Appliances not covered by 2B (including Elastic Hosiery and Trusses not measured and fitted) and		
Dressings	60	NIL

PART IIIB

SCALE OF FEES (Appliance Contractors)
See Part II, Clause 6B(iii) (page 6)

	Fee per prescription p
1. APPLIANCES:	
ELASTIC HOSIERY (Compression Hosiery)	
Anklets, Kneecaps, Leggings	13
Below-knee, Above-knee and Thigh Stockings	18
Repairs	5
TRUSSES	
Spring .... single	50
double	78
Elastic Band .... single	23
double	30
Infants Umbilical Belt	10
Repairs	5
2. OTHER APPLIANCES	2

PART IV

CONTAINERS
See Part II Clause 6A(iii) and 6C (pages 4 and 6)

A Pharmacy Contractor shall supply in a <u>suitable container</u> any drug which he is required to supply under Part 1 of the Fourth Schedule to the Regulations.

<u>Capsules, tablets, pills, pulvules etc shall be supplied in airtight containers of glass, aluminium or rigid plastics; card containers may be used only for foil/strip packed tablets etc. For ointments, creams, pastes, card containers shall not be used.</u>

<u>Eye, ear and nasal drops shall be supplied in dropper bottes, or with a separate dropper where appropriate</u>.

<u>Payment for containers</u> is at the average rate of <u>3.80p</u> per prescription for every prescription (except a "Bulk" or oxygen prescription) supplied by contractors where or not a container is supplied.

This payment includes provision for supply of a <u>5 ml plastics measuring spoon</u> which shall comply with BS 3221:Part 6:1983 and shall be made with every oral liquid medicine except where the patient already has a spoon, or the manufacturer's pack includes one.

Payment for containers is payable to pharmacy contractors and drug store contractors only.

PART V

DEDUCTION SCALE (Pharmacy Contractors)
See Part II Clause 6A(i)(b) (page 4)

Monthly Total of Prices		Deduction Rate	Monthly Total of Prices		Deduction Rate	Monthly Total of Prices		Deduction Rate
£		%	£		%	£		%
From	To		From	To		From	To	
1	125	2.83	5126	5250	8.04	10251	10375	9.88
126	250	3.14	5251	5375	8.09	10376	10500	9.90
251	375	3.45	5376	5500	8.14	10501	10625	9.91
376	500	3.76	5501	5625	8.19	10626	10750	9.93
501	625	4.06	5626	5750	8.24	10751	10875	9.95
626	750	4.37	5751	5875	8.29	10876	11000	9.96
751	875	4.68	5876	6000	8.34	11001	11250	9.98
876	1000	4.99	6001	6125	8.39	11251	11500	10.01
1001	1125	5.30	6126	6250	8.44	11501	11750	10.03
1126	1250	5.53	6251	6375	8.49	11751	12000	10.06
1251	1375	5.74	6376	6500	8.54	12001	12250	10.08
1376	1500	5.93	6501	6625	8.59	12251	12500	10.09
1501	1625	6.09	6626	6750	8.64	12501	12750	10.11
1626	1750	6.23	6751	6875	8.69	12751	13000	10.11
1751	1875	6.34	6876	7000	8.73	13001	13250	10.12
1876	2000	6.42	7001	7125	8.78	13251	13500	10.13
2001	2125	6.50	7126	7250	8.83	13501	13750	10.13
2126	2250	6.56	7251	7375	8.88	13751	14000	10.14
2251	2375	6.62	7376	7500	8.93	14001	14250	10.16
2376	2500	6.68	7501	7625	8.97	14251	14500	10.17
2501	2625	6.75	7626	7750	9.02	14501	14750	10.18
2626	2750	6.81	7751	7875	9.06	14751	15000	10.19
2751	2875	6.87	7876	8000	9.09	15001	15250	10.19
2876	3000	6.93	8001	8125	9.14	15251	15500	10.20
3001	3125	6.99	8126	8250	9.19	15501	15750	10.22
3126	3250	7.05	8251	8375	9.24	15751	16000	10.23
3251	3375	7.12	8376	8500	9.29	16001	16250	10.24
3376	3500	7.18	8501	8625	9.34	16251	16500	10.25
3501	3625	7.24	8626	8750	9.39	16501	16750	10.27
3626	3750	7.30	8751	8875	9.44	16751	17000	10.28
3751	3875	7.36	8876	9000	9.48	17001	17250	10.29
3876	4000	7.43	9001	9125	9.53	17251	17500	10.30
4001	4125	7.49	9126	9250	9.55	17501	17750	10.32
4126	4250	7.55	9251	9375	9.61	17751	18000	10.33
4251	4375	7.61	9376	9500	9.65	18001	18250	10.34
4376	4500	7.67	9501	9625	9.70	18251	18500	10.35
4501	4625	7.73	9626	9750	9.74	18501	18750	10.35
4626	4750	7.80	9751	9875	9.77	18751	19000	10.37
4751	4875	7.86	9876	10000	9.81	19001	19250	10.38
4876	5000	7.92	10001	10125	9.83	19251	19500	10.39
5001	5125	7.98	10126	10250	9.86	19501	19750	10.40

PART V

DEDUCTION SCALE (Pharmacy Contractors) — cont
See Part II Clause 6A(i)(b) (page 4)

Monthly Total of Prices		Deduction Rate	Monthly Total of Prices		Deduction Rate
£		%	£		%
From	To		From	To	
19751	20000	10.41	30501	30750	11.00
20001	20250	10.41	30751	31000	11.03
20251	20500	10.43	31001	31250	11.07
20501	20750	10.44	31251	31500	11.11
20751	21000	10.44	31501	31750	11.14
21001	21250	10.45	31751	32000	11.18
21251	21500	10.45	32001	32250	11.22
21501	21750	10.46	32251	32500	11.24
21751	22000	10.48	32501	32750	11.28
22001	22250	10.48	32751	33000	11.32
22251	22500	10.49	33001	33250	11.35
22501	22750	10.50	33251	33500	11.38
22751	23000	10.50	33501	33750	11.42
23001	23250	10.51	33751	34000	11.44
23251	23500	10.51	34001	34250	11.48
23501	23750	10.53	34251	34500	11.50
23751	24000	10.54	34501	34750	11.54
24001	24250	10.54	34751	35000	11.56
24251	24500	10.55	35001	35250	11.60
24501	24750	10.56	35251	35500	11.63
24751	25000	10.58	35501	35750	11.65
25001	25250	10.59	35751	36000	11.69
25251	25500	10.60	36001	36250	11.71
25501	25750	10.61	36251	36500	11.74
25751	26000	10.62	36501	36750	11.76
26001	26250	10.64	36751	37000	11.80
26251	26500	10.66	37001	37250	11.82
26501	26750	10.67	37251	37500	11.85
26751	27000	10.70	37501	37750	11.87
27001	27250	10.71	37751	38000	11.90
27251	27500	10.72	38001	38250	11.92
27501	27750	10.75	38251	38500	11.95
27751	28000	10.76	38501	38750	11.97
28001	28250	10.77	38751	39000	12.00
29251	28500	10.80	39001	39250	12.02
28501	28750	10.81	39251	39500	12.05
28751	29000	10.82	39501	39750	12.07
29001	29250	10.83	39751	and over	12.10
29251	29500	10.86			
29501	29750	10.87			
29751	30000	10.88			
30001	30250	10.91			
30251	30500	10.95			

0304M/4

SCALE OF ON-COST ALLOWANCE (Pharmacy Contractors)
See Part II Clause 6A(1)(c) (page 4)

Prescriptions dispensed from 1 April 1987 shall attract an on-cost allowance of 5% of the total of the price of drugs, appliances and reagents supplied (before the subtraction of an amount set out in the Deduction Scale (Part V) (page 25-26)

PART VIB

SCALE OF ON-COST ALLOWANCE (Appliance Contractors)
See Part II Clause 6B(ii) (page 6)

Number of prescriptions dispensed during month		On-cost	Number of prescriptions dispensed during month		On-cost
From	To	%	From	To	%
1	505	25.0	1036	1048	20.3
506	515	24.9	1049	1062	20.2
516	526	24.8	1063	1076	20.1
527	537	24.7	1077	1090	20.0
538	549	24.6	1091	1105	19.9
550	561	24.5	1106	1120	19.8
562	574	24.4	1121	1136	19.7
575	588	24.3	1137	1152	19.6
589	602	24.2	1153	1169	19.5
603	617	24.1	1170	1186	19.4
618	632	24.0	1187	1203	19.3
633	649	23.9	1204	1221	19.2
650	666	23.8	1222	1240	19.1
667	684	23.7	1241	1259	19.0
685	704	23.6	1260	1279	18.9
705	724	23.5	1280	1300	18.8
725	746	23.4	1301	1321	18.7
747	756	23.3	1322	1342	18.6
757	762	23.2	1343	1365	18.5
763	770	23.1	1366	1388	18.4
771	777	23.0	1389	1413	18.3
778	785	22.9	1414	1438	18.2
786	792	22.8	1439	1463	18.1
793	800	22.7	1464	1490	18.0
801	808	22.6	1491	1518	17.9
809	816	22.5	1519	1547	17.8
817	824	22.4	1548	1577	17.7
825	833	22.3	1578	1608	17.6
834	841	22.2	1609	1641	17.5
842	850	22.1	1642	1675	17.4
851	859	22.0	1676	1710	17.3
860	868	21.9	1711	1747	17.2
869	878	21.8	1748	1785	17.1
879	887	21.7	1786	1825	17.0
888	897	21.6	1826	1867	16.9
898	907	21.5	1868	1911	16.8
908	918	21.4	1912	1957	16.7
919	928	21.3	1958	2006	16.6
929	939	21.2	2007	2056	16.5
940	950	21.1	2057	2110	16.4
951	961	21.0	2111	2166	16.3
962	973	20.9	2167	2226	16.2
974	984	20.8	2227	2288	16.1
985	996	20.7	2289	2355	16.0
997	1009	20.6	2356	2425	15.9
1010	1022	20.5	2426	2500	15.8
1023	1035	20.4			

DRUGS WITH COMMON PACK

PART VII

LIST OF DRUGS WITH A COMMONLY USED PACK SIZE
See Part II, Clause 7D (page 7)

If a drug specified in this list is supplied but the relative prescription form is not endorsed payment will be calculated on the basis of the price for the pack size listed.

Drug (1)	Common Pack (2)
Altacite Plus Suspension	500 ml
Alupent Syrup	2 litre
Antepar Elixir	500 ml
Artane Tablets, 2 mg	1,000
Asilone Suspension	500 ml
Aspellin	500 ml
Augmentin Tablets, 375 mg	100
Bactrim Drapsules	500
Balneum Bath Additive	1,000 ml
Benoral Suspension	300 ml
Betaloc Tablets, 50 mg	500
Betaloc Tablets, 100 mg	500
Betaloc – SA	300
Bricanyl Syrup	1 litre
Bricanyl Tablets	500
Brufen Tablets, 200 mg	500
Brufen 400 Tablets	250
Burinex Tablets, 1 mg	1,000
Burinex K Tablets	500
Buscopan Tablets	560
Calpol Infant Suspension	1 litre
Calpol Infant Suspension Sugar Free	1 litre
Centyl K Tablets	500
Ceporex Capsules, 250 mg	100
Ceporex Capsules, 500 mg	100
Ceporex Tablets, 250 mg	100
Ceporex Tablets, 500 mg	100
Choledyl Tablets, 200 mg	500
Cyclospasmol Tablets	250
Danol Capsules, 200 mg	100
Deteclo Tablets	500
Disipal Tablets	1,000
Distaclor Capsules	100
Diumide-K Tablets Continus	250
Dyazide Tablets	500
Elantan 20 Tablets	100
Eltroxin Tablets, 50 microgram	1,000
Eltroxin Tablets, 100 microgram	1,000
Emulsiderm	1 litre

DRUGS WITH COMMON PACK

PART VII

Drug (1)	Common Pack (2)
Epanutin Capsules, 100 mg	1,000
Erythrocin 250 Tablets	500
Franol Tablets	500
Froben Tablets, 50 mg	500
Frumil Tablets	56
Fybogel Orange Sachets	60
Galpseud Linctus	2 litre
Gaviscon Tablets	60
Hexopal Tablets	500
Hismanal Tablets	30
Hygroton Tablets, 50 mg	500
Hygroton-K Tablets	250
Imodium Capsules	250
Ismo 20 Tablets	250
Keflex Capsules, 250 mg	100
Keflex Capsules, 500 mg	100
Keflex Tablets, 250 mg	100
Keflex Tablets, 500 mg	100
Kemadrin Tablets	500
Kolanticon Gel	500 ml
Lanoxin PG Tablets	500
Lanoxin Tablets, 250 microgram	1,000
Largactil Syrup	1 litre
Lentizol Capsules, 25 mg	250
Lentizol Capsules, 50 mg	250
Lodine Capsules, 200 mg	250
Maxolon Tablets, 10 mg	84
Melleril Syrup	500 ml
Melleril Tablets, 25 mg	1,000
Melleril Tablets, 50 mg	1,000
Merbentyl Syrup	500 ml
Monit Tablets	100
Motival Tablets, 5 mg	500
Natrilix Tablets, 2.5 mg	60
Navidrex-K Tablets	500
Neo Mercazole 5 Tablets	500
Neo-Naclex-K Tablets	500
Nu-Seals Aspirin Tablets, 300 mg	500
Oilatum Emollient	1 litre
Optimax Tablets	500

DRUGS WITH COMMON PACK

PART VII

Drug (1)	Common Pack (2)
Panadol Elixir	1 litre
Penbritin Capsules, 250 mg	100
Penbritin Capsules, 500 mg	100
Persantin Tablets, 25 mg	1,000
Persantin Tablets, 100 mg	1,000
Phyllocontin Continus Tablets	1,000
Piriton Tablets	500
Polytar Emollient	1 litre
Polytar Liquid	1,000 ml
Pondocillin Tablets	500
Ponstan Capsules	500
Praxilene Capsules	100
Premarin Tablets, 625 microgram	100
Prestim Tablets	500
Priadel Tablets, 400 mg	1,000
Primolut N Tablets	500
Prothiaden Capsules	600
Prothiaden Tablets	500
Quellada Lotion	500 ml
Salazopyrin Plain Tablets	500
Savlon Liquid	500 ml
Senokot Syrup	500 ml
Septrin Tablets	500
Sorbitrate Tablets, 10 mg	500
Sparine Suspension	1 litre
Stelazine Spansule Capsules, 2 mg	250
Stugeron Tablets	1,000
Sudafed Elixir	1 litre
Sudafed Tablets	100
Tagamet Tiltab Tablets, 200 mg	120
Tagamet Tablets, 400 mg	60
Tegretol Tablets, 100 mg	500
Tegretol Tablets, 200 mg	500
Tetrabid—Organon Capsules	500
Trandate Tablets, 100 mg	250
Trandate Tablets, 200 mg	250
Triludan Tablets	60
Tryptizol Tablets, 10 mg	500
Tryptizol Tablets, 25 mg	500
Uniphyllin Continus Tablets, 400 mg	250
Velosef Capsules, 500 mg	100
Ventolin Syrup	2 litre
Ventolin Tablets, 2 mg	500
Ventolin Tablets, 4 mg	500

BASIC PRICES OF DRUGS

PART VIII

BASIC PRICES OF DRUGS
COVERED BY PART II CLAUSE 8A

The price listed in respect of a drug specified in the following list is
the basic price (see Part II, Clause 8) on which payment will be calculated
pursuant to Part II Clause 6A for the dispensing of that drug

NOTES:

1. All drugs listed in this Part have a pack size and price which has been determined by the
Secretary of State.

2. Categories A,B,C,E and S of the drugs appearing in Col.4 are as under:

(i) Category A — No endorsement is required. Broken Bulk is not allowed.

(ii) Category B — No endorsement is required other than a claim for Broken Bulk if necessary.

(iii)
Category C — Priced on the basis of a particular brand or particular manufacturer. Endorsement
of pack size is required if more than one pack size is listed in this category. Broken Bulk
may be claimed if necessary.

(iv) Category E — Extemporaneously prepared items for which the fee listed under Part III
A(a)(ii), (iii), (iv) or (v) will be claimed. No endorsement is required. Broken Bulk is not
allowed. Broken Bulk may be paid on the ingredients if they are not listed under Category A
or E.

(v) Category S — Special prices. Broken Bulk may be claimed if necessary.

3. Methylated Spirit

Industrial Methylated Spirit should be supplied or used and payment will be calculated
accordingly, where:

(i) "Methylated Spirit", "Spirit", "Spt. Vini. Meth.", "SVM", "IMS", is ordered alone or as
an ingredient of a preparation for external use, or

(ii) A liniment, lotion, etc., in the preparation of which Methylated Spirit is permitted, is
ordered and the prescriber has not indicated to the contrary.

4. Rectified Spirit

Where Alcohol (96%), or Rectified Spirit (Ethanol 90%), or any other of the dilute Ethanols is
prescribed alone or as an ingredient in a medicament for external application, payment will be
made for supply of Industrial Methylated Spirit unless the prescriber has indicated that no
alternative may be used.

Where Alcohol (96%), or Rectified Spirit (Ethanol 90%), or any other of the dilute Ethanols
is prescribed as an ingredient of a medicine for internal use, the price of the duty paid to
Customs and Excise will be allowed, unless the contractor endorses the prescription form "rebate
claimed".

BASIC PRICES OF DRUGS

PART VIII

5. Purified Water
   (Exclusive of ordinary potable water)

Payment for Purified Water will be made

   (i) where it is ordered;

   (ii) where water is included in any preparation intended for application to the eye;

   (iii)
   where, in the opinion of the pharmacist the use of ordinary potable water in a particular
   preparation would result in an undesirable change in the medicament prescribed and he endorses
   the prescription form accordingly;

   (iv) where the Family Practitioner Committee, after consultation with the Local Medical
   Committee and Local Pharmaceutical Committee, has decided with the approval of the Secretary
   of State that the water ordinarily available is unsuitable for dispensing purposes, and has
   notified the contractor accordingly.

When Purified Water is used instead of potable water, it should be freshly boiled and cooled.

6. A "bulk" prescription is an order, bearing the name of a school or institution in which at
least 20 persons normally reside, for the treatment of at least 10 of whom a particular doctor is
responsible for a drug included in the current edition of the British National Formulary (except
Controlled Drugs in Schedules 1, 2 and 3 of the Misuse of Drugs Regulations 1985 and Drugs in the
former Schedule IVA of the Poisons List).

BASIC PRICES OF DRUGS

PART VIII

Drug (1)	Quantity (2)	Basic Price (3) p	Category (4)
Acacia Powdered BP	500 g	786	B
Acetic Acid (33 per cent) BP (Syn. Acetic Acid)	500 ml	125	B
Acetic Acid Glacial BP	500 ml	160	B
Acetone BP	500 ml	181	A
Acetylcysteine BP Granules, 200 mg per sachet.........	30	575	C
Acetylsalicylic Acid Mixture BPC 1963	200 ml	27 ▽	E
(Aspirin Mixture)			
Acriflavine Emulsion — (See Proflavine Cream BPC)	–	–	–
Adrenaline Cream 1 in 5000 DTF 1982	500 g	325	B
Adrenaline Injection BP (1 ml ampoules)	10	299	A
(Syn: Adrenaline Tartrate Injection)			
Adrenaline Solution BP	25 ml	95	B
(Syn: Adrenaline Tartrate Solution)			
Alcohol 90% v/v (See Ethanol 90 per cent BP)	–	–	–
Alcohol 96% v/v (see Ethanol 96 per cent BP)	–	–	–
Alkaline Ipecacuanha Mixture BPC 1963	200 ml	16	E
(Syn. Mist. Expect Alk)			
Alkaline Phenol Mouthwash BPC 1963	200 ml	10 ▽	E
(Syn. Phenol and Alkali Mouthwash)			
Allopurinol Tablets BP 100 mg	100	252	S
Allopurinol Tablets BP 300 mg	28	400	C
	100	871	A
Almasilate Suspension 500mg/5ml......................	200 ml	76	C
Almond Oil BP	500 ml	420	B
Aloxiprin Tablets BP, 600 mg	250	620	C
Alum BP (Granular Powder)	500 g	120	B
Aluminium Hydroxide and Belladonna	200 ml	48	E
Mixture BPC			
Aluminium Hydroxide Gel	–	–	–
(See Aluminium Hydroxide Mixture BP)			
Aluminium Hydroxide Mixture BP	2 litre	366	A
(Syn: Aluminium Hydroxide Oral Suspension)			
Aluminium Hydroxide Tablets BP, 500 mg	500	726	A
Amaranth Solution BP	500 ml	205	A
Amethocaine Eye Drops BP, 0.5% w/v	10 ml	165	B
Amethocaine Eye Drops BP, 1% w/v	10 ml	146	A
Amiloride Tablets BP, 5mg	100	679	A
Aminophylline Injection BP (250 mg in 10 ml ampoules).	10	531	A
Amitriptyline Tablets BP, 10 mg	100	132	C
	500	561	C
Amitriptyline Tablets BP, 25 mg	500	205	S
Amitriptyline Tablets BP, 50 mg	100	239	A

BASIC PRICES OF DRUGS

PART VIII

Drug (1)	Quantity (2)	Basic Price (3) p	Category (4)
Ammonia Aromatic Solution BP	500 ml	183	A
(Syn. Sal. Volatile Solution)			
Ammonia Aromatic Spirit BP	500 ml	390	B
(Syn. Sal. Volatile Spirit)			
Ammonium Acetate Solution, Strong BP	500 ml	217	A
Ammonium Bicarbonate BP	500 g	178	A
Ammonium Chloride BP	500 g	172	A
Ammonium Chloride Mixture BP	200 ml	27	E
Amoxycillin Capsules BP 250 mg	100	1391 ▽	A
Amoxycillin Capsules BP 500 mg	100	2778	A
Amoxycillin Mixture BP (Syns. Amoxycillin Syrup,			
Amoxycillin Oral Suspension) 125 mg/5ml	100 ml	175	A
....250 mg/5 ml...........	100 ml	326	A
Ampicillin Capsules BP, 250 mg	500	1669	S
Ampicillin Capsules BP, 500 mg	250	1745	A
Ampicillin Mixture BP, (Syn: Ampicillin Oral Suspension)			
125 mg/5 ml,....	100 ml	76	C
250 mg/5 ml, ...	100 ml	123	C
Amyl Nitrite Vitrellae BPC, 0.2 ml	12	891	A
Anise Oil BP (Syn. Aniseed Oil)	25 ml	288	B
Anise Water, Concentrated BP	100 ml	468	A
Aqueous Cream BP	500 g	137	A
Arachis Oil BP . (Syn. Ground—nut Oil; Peanut Oil)...	500 ml	229	A
Arnica Flowers Tincture BPC 1949	100 ml	142	B
Arrowroot BPC	500 g	265	B
Ascorbic Acid BP (Syn. Vitamin C)	100 g	231	B
Ascorbic Acid Injection BPC (500 mg/5ml ampoules).....	10	651	B
Ascorbic Acid Tablets BP, 25 mg	200	61	C
Ascorbic Acid Tablets BP, 50 mg	500	155	C
Ascorbic Acid Tablets BP, 100 mg	100	114	A
Ascorbic Acid Tablets BP, 200 mg	100	118	C
Ascorbic Acid Tablets BP, 500 mg	50	145	C
Aspirin BP (Powder) (Syn. Acetylsalicylic Acid)	500 g	425	C
Aspirin Tablets BP, 300 mg	100	44	A
(Syn. Acetylsalicylic Acid Tablets)			
Aspirin Tablets, Dispersible BP 300mg	1000	446	A
(Soluble Aspirin Tablets)			
Aspirin Tablets Dispersible BP 75 mg	1000	510	B
(Soluble Paediatric Aspirin Tablets)			
Aspirin Paracetamol and Codeine Tablets DPF	50	188	C
Astemizole Tablets	30	570	C

BASIC PRICES OF DRUGS

PART VIII

Drug (1)	Quantity (2)	Basic Price (3) p	Category (4)
Atenolol Tablets BP, 50 mg	28	477	A
Atenolol Tabelts BP, 100 mg	28	674	A
Atropine Eye Drops BP, 1% w/v	10 ml	68	A
(Syn. Atropine Sulphate Eye Drops 1% w/v)			
Atropine Eye Ointment BP, 1%	3 g	101	B
Atropine Sulphate Injection BP	10	313	A
(0.6 mg in 1 ml ampoules)			
Azathioprine Tablets BP, 50 mg	100	2855 Δ	C
Baclofen Tablets BP, 10 mg	100	1231 Δ	A
Beeswax, White BP (Plates)	500 g	829	B
Beeswax, Yellow BP	500 g	841	B
Belladonna Mixture, Paediatric BPC	100 ml	14	E
Belladonna and Alkali Mixture BNF 1963	200 ml	11	E
Belladonna and Ipecacuanha Mixture, Paediatric BPC	100 ml	13	E
Belladonna Tincture BP	500 ml	295	A
Bendrofluazide Tablets BP, 2.5 mg	500	344 Δ	A
Bendrofluazide Tablets BP, 5 mg	1000	252	B
Benorylate Mixture BP,	300 ml	1147	S
(Syn: Benorylate Oral Suspension)			
Benorylate Tablets BP 750 mg	100	809	S
Bentonite BP	500 g	220	B
Benzalkonium Lozenges BPC	100	242	B
Benzalkonium Chloride Solution BP	100 ml	80	B
Benzoic Acid Ointment, Compound BPC	500 g	286	A
Benzoic Acid Solution BP	100 ml	93	B
Benzoin Tincture Compound BP (Syn. Friars' Balsam)	500 ml	280	A
Benzoin Tincture BPC	100 ml	220	B
Benzyl Benzoate BP	500 ml	295	B
Benzyl Benzoate Application BP	500 ml	190	A
Bisacodyl Suppositories BP, 5 mg	50	400	C
Bisacodyl Suppositories BP, 10 mg	12	99	B
Bisacodyl Tablets BP, 5 mg	1000	1281	B
Bismuth and Morphine Mixture BPC 1949	200 ml	27	E
(Syn. Mist. Bism. Sed)			
Bismuth Salicylate BP 1953	500 g	2800	B
Bismuth Subcarbonate BP (Syn. Bismuth Carbonate)	250 g	850	A
Bismuth Subgallate Suppositories BP 1980	12	135	B
Bismuth Subnitrate BPC	100 g	460	C
Bismuth Subnitrate and Iodoform Pasta BPC 1954	30 g	771	B
Bisoprolol Fumarate Tablets 5 mg	28	798	C
Bisoprolol Fumarate Tablets 10 mg	28	896	C
BJ6 Eye Drops	10 ml	87	A
Black Currant Syrup BP	500 ml	353	A
Boric Acid BP	50 g	18	B
Boric Acid Eye Lotion BPC 1963	200 ml	8	E
Boric Acid Ointment BPC 1963	500 g	264	B
Buckthorn Syrup BPC 1934	500 ml	667	B
Buffered Cream BP	500 g	208	B

BASIC PRICES OF DRUGS

PART VIII

Drug (1)	Quantity (2)	Basic Price (3) p	Category (4)
Cade Oil BPC	100 ml	165	B
Caffeine Citrate BPC 1959	100 g	330	B
Calamine BP (Syn. Prepared Calamine)	500 g	215	A
Calamine Aqueous Cream BP	500 g	278	C
Calamine Compound Application BPC 1973	500 g	195	B
Calamine Lotion BP	500 ml	115	B
Calamine Lotion Oily BP 1980	100 ml	35	C ⏐
Calamine & Coal Tar Ointment BP	500 g	215	B
(Syn. Compound Calamine Ointment)			
Calciferol Injection BP (300,000 u/1 ml ampoules)....	10	2576	B
(600,000 u/2 ml ampoules)....	10	3074	B
Calciferol Tablets, High-Strength BP, 250 micrograms .	100	227	A
Calciferol Tablets, Strong BP, 1.25 mg	100	296	A
Calcium Carbonate BP	1 kg	175	B
Calcium Carbonate Mixture, Compound, Paediatric BPC ..	100 ml	5	E
Calcium Gluconate Injection BP (5 ml ampoules)......	10	427	B
(10 ml ampoules).....	10	497	B
Calcium Gluconate Tablets BP, 600 mg	100	222	A
Calcium Gluconate Tablets, Effervescent BP, 1g	100	483	A
Calcium Hydroxide BP	500 g	478	B
Calcium Hydroxide Solution BP	200 ml	8	E
Calcium Lactate BP	500 g	530	B
Calcium Lactate Tablets BP, 300 mg	100	111	A
Calcium Lactate Tablets BP, 600 mg	100	200	B
Calcium Phosphate BP	500 g	880	B
Calcium Sulphate, Dried BP	2 kg	270	B
Calcium with Vitamin D Tablets BPC	500	572 Δ	A
(Syn. Compound Tablets of Calciferol)			
Camphor BP	100 g	217	A
Camphor Water Concentrated BP	100 ml	108	B
Camphor Liniment, BP 1973	100 ml	80	E
Camphor Spirit BPC 1959	100 ml	90	B
Camphorated Opium Tincture BP	500 ml	265	C
Capsicum Ointment BPC	500 g	320	B
Capsicum Tincture BPC	100 ml	115	B
Captopril Tablets, 12.5 mg	100	1886	C
Captopril Tablets, 25 mg	56	1203	C
Captopril Tablets, 50 mg	56	2050	C
Carbocisteine Capsules, 375 mg	30	320	C
Carbocisteine Syrup, 125 mg/5 ml	300 ml	350	C
Carbocisteine Syrup, 250 mg/5 ml	300 ml	450	C

BASIC PRICES OF DRUGS

PART VIII

Drug (1)	Quantity (2)	Basic Price (3) p	Category (4)
Cardamom Tincture, Aromatic BP	500 ml	531	A
Cardamom Tincture, Compound BP	500 ml	375	B
Cascara Elixir, BP	500 ml	932	B
Cascara Liquid Extract, BP 1980	500 ml	521	B
Castor Oil BP	500 ml	316	A
Catechu Tincture BP	500 ml	473	A
Caustic Pencil BP 1958	each	90	C
Cephalexin Capsules BP, 250 mg	100	1611	A
Cephalexin Capsules BP, 500 mg	100	3159	A
Cephalexin Oral Suspension BP (Syn: Cephalexin Mixture)			
125 mg/5 ml	100 ml	159	C
250 mg/5 ml	100 ml	319	C
Cephalexin Tablets BP, 250 mg	100	1613	A
Cephalexin Tablets BP, 500 mg	100	3159	A
Cetomacrogol Cream BP (Formula A)	100 g	288	A
Cetomacrogol Cream BP (Formula B)	100 g	170	B
Cetostearyl Alcohol BP	500 g	511	B
Chalk Mixture Paediatric BP	100 ml	8	E
Chalk BP (Powder) (Syn. Prepared Chalk)	1 kg	181	B
Chalk Powder, Aromatic BPC	500 g	565	B
Chalk and Catechu Mixture, Paediatric BNF 1963	100 ml	16	E
Chalk and Opium Mixture, Aromatic BP	500 ml	185	C
Charcoal BPC 1934	100 g	237	B
Chloral Hydrate BP	100 g	122	B
Chloral Elixir, Paediatric BP	500 ml	243	B
Chloral Mixture BP	200 ml	30	E
Chloral Syrup BPC 1968	500 ml	241	B
Chloramine BP (Syn. Chloramine T)	100 g	550	B
Chloramphenicol Ear Drops BP, 5% w/v	10 ml	148	A
Chloramphenicol Eye Drops BP 0.5% w/v	10 ml	67	A
Chloramphenicol Eye Ointment BP, 1% w/w	4 g	68	A
Chlordiazepoxide Capsules BP, 5mg	100	141	S
Chlordiazepoxide Capsules BP, 10 mg	100	176	S
Chlordiazepoxide Tablets BP, 5mg	100	141	S
Chlordiazepoxide Tablets BP, 10 mg	100	176	S
Chlordiazepoxide Tablets BP, 25 mg	100	355	S
Chlordiazepoxide Hydrochloride Tablets BP, 5 mg	100	100	C
Chlordiazepoxide Hydrochloride Tablets BP, 10 mg	100	112	C
Chlordiazepoxide Hydrochloride Tablets BP, 25 mg	100	220	C
Chlorinated Lime BP	500 g	226	B
Chlorinated Lime and Boric Acid Solution BPC	500 ml	71	E
(Syn. Eusol)			
Chlorinated Lime and Boric Acid Solution –			
Solution A	2 litre	285	A
Solution B	2 litre	285	A
Chloroform BP	500 ml	239	A
Chloroform Spirit BP	500 ml	250	A
Chloroform Water Concentrated BPC 1959	500 ml	161	A
Chloroform Water Double Strength BP	500 ml	16	E
Chloroform & Morphine Tincture BP	500 ml	400	A
(Syn. Chlorodyne)			

BASIC PRICES OF DRUGS

PART VIII

Drug (1)	Quantity (2)	Basic Price (3) p	Category (4)
Chloroxylenol Solution BP	2 litre	608	B
Chlorpropamide Tablets BP, 100 mg	100	90	S
Chlorpropamide Tablets BP, 250 mg	100	135	S
Cimetidine Tablets 200 mg	120	1769	A
Cimetidine Tablets 400 mg	60	1861	A
Cimetidine Tablets 800 mg	30	1772	A
Cinnamon Water Concentrated BP	25 ml	155	B
Cinnarizine Tablets 15 mg	100	550 Δ	C
Citric Acid Monohydrate BP (Powder)	500 g	311	A
Clemastine Tablets 1 mg	50	210	C
Clemastine Elixir 500 mcg/5 ml	150 ml	98	C
Clobazam Capsules 10 mg	30	241	C
Clomiphene Tablets BP 50 mg	100	3364	C
Clove Oil BP	100 ml	325	B
Coal Tar Ointment, BPC 1934	500 g	196	B
Coal Tar and Salicylic Acid Ointment BP	500 g	279	B
Coal Tar Paste BP	500 g	255	A
Coal Tar Solution BP (Methylated)	500 ml	328	A
Coal Tar Solution, Strong BP	500 ml	338	A
Co—Amilozide Tablets, 5/50	500	3350	C
Cocaine BP	5 g	3850	B
Cocaine Hydrochloride BP	1 g	758	B
Cocaine Eye Drops BPC, 4% w/v	10 ml	320	B
Co—codamol Tablets DPF, 8/500	500	710	S
(Formerly Codeine and Paracetamol Tablets)			
Co—codamol Tablets Dispersible DPF, 8/500	100	275 Δ	C
(Formerly Codeine and Paracetamol Tablets Dispersible)			
Co—codaprin, Dispersible Tablets BP,	500	780	B
(Syn: Aspirin and Codeine Tablets, Dispersible)			
Co—codaprin Tablets BP,	100	120	B
(Syn: Aspirin and Codeine Tablets BP)			
Coconut Oil BP	500 g	240	A
Coconut Oil, Fractionated BP	250 ml	495	B
(Syn. Thin Vegetable Oil)			
Codeine Linctus BP	2 litre	700	S
Codeine Linctus Diabetic BP	2 litre	1250	C
Codeine Linctus, Paediatric BP	100 ml	19	E
Codeine Phosphate BP	5 g	1205	B
Codeine Phosphate Syrup BPC	500 ml	375	A
Codeine Phosphate Tablets BP, 15 mg	250	472	A
Codeine Phosphate Tablets BP, 30 mg	250	490	S
Codeine Phosphate Tablets BP, 60 mg	100	606	A
Cod—liver Oil BP	500 ml	482	B
Co—dydramol Tablets DPF, 10/500	500	836	S
(Formerly Dihydrocodeine and Paracetamol Tablets)			
Colchicine Tablets BP, 500 microgram	100	330	B
Colchicum Tincture BP 1973	100 ml	301	B
Copper Sulphate BPC	500 g	190	B
Copper and Zinc Sulphate Lotion BPC	500 ml	22	E
Co—proxamol Tablets, 32.5/325	100	142	S
(Dextroproxyphene Hydrochloride BP, 32.5 mg and Paracetamol BP, 325 mg Tablets)			
Co—trimoxazole Oral Suspension BP	100 ml	300	C
(Syn: Co—trimoxazole Mixture BP)			

BASIC PRICES OF DRUGS

PART VIII

Drug (1)	Quantity (2)	Basic Price (3) p	Category (4)
Co-trimoxazole Oral Suspension, Paediatric, BP	100 ml	209	C
(Syn: Co-trimoxazole Mixture, Paediatric BP)			
Co-trimoxazole Tablets BP,80/400	500	2435	A
Co-trimoxazole Tablets BP, 160/800	100	1572 Δ	A
Creosote BPC 1959	100 ml	594	B
Cresol and Soap Solution BP 1968 (Syn. Lysol)	5 litre	1263	B
Cyanocobalamin Injection BP, 1.0 mg/1 ml	5	168	C
Dextropropoxyphene Capsules BP, 60 mg	100	596	C
Dextrose, Strong Injection	–	–	–
(see Glucose Intravenous Infusion BP)			
Diamorphine and Cocaine Elixir BPC	200 ml	347	E
Diamorphine Hydrochloride BP	2 g	1063	B
Diamorphine Injection BP, (5 mg ampoules)...........	5	516	B
(10 mg ampoules)	5	592	B
(30 mg ampoules)	5	709	B
(100 mg ampoules)	5	1981	B
(500 mg ampoules)	5	9413	B
Diazepam Elixir BP, 2mg/5ml	100 ml	143	S
Diazepam Tablets BP, 2 mg	1000	115	S
Diazepam Tablets BP, 5 mg	1000	120	S
Diazepam Tablets BP, 10 mg	500	130	S
Diclofenac Sodium Tablets, 25 mg (e/c)..............	100	938	C
Diclofenac Sodium Tablets, 50 mg (e/c)..............	100	1824	C
Digitalis Tablets, Prepared BP, 30 mg	1000	990	B
Digitalis Tablets, Prepared BP, 60 mg	1000	1370	B
Digoxin Tablets BP, 62.5 microgram	500	215	A
Digoxin Tablets BP, 125 microgram	1000	303	A
Digoxin Tablets BP, 250 microgram	1000	437	A
Dihydrocodeine Elixir 10mg/5 ml	150 ml	128	C
Dihydrocodeine Injection BP 50mg/1ml	5	149	C
Dihydrocodeine Tablets BP 30 mg	500	1553	S
Dill Water Concentrated BPC	100 ml	337	A
Diltiazem Hydrochloride Tablets, 60 mg	100	1500	C
Dimethicone Cream BPC	500 g	270	B
Dipyridamole Tablets BP, 25 mg	100	369	C
Dipyridamole Tablets BP, 100 mg	1000	9469	C
Disopyramide Capsules BP, 100 mg	100	793 Δ	A
Dithranol BP	25 g	2065	B
Emulsifying Ointment BP	500 g	150	S
Emulsifying Wax BP	500 g	440	B
Ephedrine Hydrochloride Elixir BP	500 ml	246	B
(Syn. Ephedrine Elixir)			
Ephedrine Hydrochloride BP	25 g	324	A
Ephedrine Hydrochloride Tablets BP, 15 mg	500	155	A
Ephedrine Hydrochloride Tablets BP, 30 mg	500	195	A
Ephedrine Hydrochloride Tablets BP, 60 mg	250	342	A
Ephedrine Nasal Drops BPC, 0.5% w/v	500 ml	169	A
Ephedrine Nasal Drops BPC, 1% w/v	10 ml	80	C
Ergometrine Tablets BP, 500 microgram	100	870 Δ	A

BASIC PRICES OF DRUGS

PART VIII

Drug (1)	Quantity (2)	Basic Price (3) p	Category (4)
Erythromycin Ethylsuccinate Mixture Paediatric, DPF 125mg/5ml	100 ml	147	A
Erythromycin Ethylsuccinate Mixture, DPF 250mg/5ml	100 ml	217	A
Erythromycin Ethylsuccinate Mixture DPF 500 mg/5ml	100 ml	359	B
Erythromycin Tablets BP, 250 mg	500	2150	S
Erythromycin Tablets BP, 500 mg	100	1005	A
Ethanol 90 per cent BP (Syn. Rectified Spirit) (Excluding rebate)	500 ml	897	A
(Including duty) (See Note 4, page 32)	500 ml	1606	A
Ethanol 96 per cent BP (Including duty)	100 ml	378	A
Ethanolamine Oleate Injection BP (2 ml ampoules)	10	701	B
(5 ml ampoules)	10	653	B
Ether Solvent BP	500 ml	335	B
Ethinyloestradiol Tablets BP, 10 microgram	100	244	B
Ethinyloestradiol Tablets BP, 20 microgram	250	750	B
Ethinyloestradiol Tablets BP, 50 microgram	100	349	B
Ethinyloestradiol Tablets BP, 1 mg	100	986	B
Ethosuximide Elixir BP	250 ml	467	C
Eucalyptus Oil BP	500 ml	576	B
Ferric Ammonium Citrate BP	500 g	475	B
Ferric Ammonium Citrate Mixture BPC	200 ml	41	E
Ferric Chloride Gargle BPC 1963	200 ml	15	E
Ferric Chloride Solution BPC	500 ml	300	A
Ferrous Gluconate Tablets BP, 300 mg	1000	586	A
Ferrous Phosphate Syrup, Compound BPC 1968	500 ml	243	B
Ferrous Sulphate BP	500 g	205	B
Ferrous Sulphate, Mixture, Paediatric BP	100 ml	9	E
(Syn: Ferrous Sulphate Oral Solution Paediatric)			
Ferrous Sulphate Tablets BP, 200 mg	1000	373	A
Ferrous Sulphate Tablets Compound BPC	1000	466 ▽	A
Flexible Collodion BP (Methylated)	500 ml	613	A
Flucloxacillin Capsules BP 250 mg	100	1350	C
Flucloxacillin Capsules BP 500 mg	100	2800	C
Flucloxacillin Oral Solution BP, 125 mg/5 ml	100 ml	322 Δ	A
(Syn: Flucloxacillin Elixir; Flucloxacillin Syrup)			
Flucloxacillin Oral Suspension BP, 125 mg/5 ml	100 ml	332	C
250 mg/5 ml	100 ml	664	C
Fluorescein Sodium BP	25 g	190	B
Folic Acid Tablets BP, 5 mg	500	160	A
Formaldehyde Solution BP	500 ml	132	A
Framycetin Sulphate Eye Drops BNF	5 ml	127	C
Framycetin Sulphate Eye Ointment BNF	3.5 g tube	61	C
Frusemide Tablets BP, 20 mg	100	143	A
Frusemide Tablets BP, 40 mg	1000	400	S
Frusemide Tablets BP, 500 mg	100	2996	C

BASIC PRICES OF DRUGS

PART VIII

Drug (1)	Quantity (2)	Basic Price (3) p	Category (4)
Gelatin BP (Powder)	500 g	531	B
Gelsemium Tincture BPC 1973	100 ml	333	B
Gentamicin Ear Drops 0.3% w/v	10 ml	194 Δ	C
Gentamicin Eye Drops BP 0.3% w/v	10 ml	194 Δ	C
Gentian Acid Mixture BPC	200 ml	21 ▽	E
Gentian, Alkaline Mixture BP	200 ml	20	E |
Gentian, Alkaline with Phenobarbitone Mixture BPC	200 ml	37	E
Gentian, Infusion, Compound Concentrated BP	500 ml	390 ▽	C |
Ginger, Powdered BP	500 g	484	B
Ginger Syrup BPC 1973	500 ml	120	E
Ginger Tincture, Strong BP (Syn. Ginger Essence)	100 ml	199	B
Glibenclamide Tablets BP 2.5 mg	100	320	A
Glibenclamide Tablets BP 5 mg	100	340	A
Glucose For Oral Use BP 1980	2 kg	365	B
Glucose Intravenous Infusion BP, 25% w/v (25 ml ampoules)	10	2008	B
50% w/v (25 ml ampoules)	10	2824	B
50% w/v (50 ml ampoules)	10	2660	B
Glucose Liquid BPC 1963	450 g	119	B
Glycerol BP (Syn. Glycerin)	500 ml	273	A
Glycerol Suppositories BP (Syn. Glycerin)			
Infant's size, mould size, 1 g wrapped	12	42	A
Child's size, mould size, 2 g wrapped	12	47	A
Adult's size, mould size, 4 g wrapped	12	54	A
*Glyceryl Trinitrate Tablets BP, 500 microgram	100	44	A
*Glyceryl Trinitrate Tablets BP, 600 microgram	100	65	A
Green S & Tartrazine Solution BP 1980	25 ml	271	B
Hamamelis with Zinc Oxide Suppositories BPC	12	235	B
Hamamelis Water BPC	500 ml	195	B
Homatropine Eye Drops BP, 1% w/v	10 ml	168	A
Homatropine Eye Drops BP, 2% w/v	10 ml	179	A
Hydralazine Hydrochloride Tablets BP 25 mg	100	135	C
Hydralazine Hydrochloride Tablets BP 50 mg	100	275	C
Hydrochloric Acid BP	500 ml	212	B
Hydrochloric Acid, Dilute BP	500 ml	132	A
Hydrocortisone BP	1 g	265	B
Hydrocortisone Acetate BP	1 g	488	B
Hydrocortisone Acetate Cream, 1% w/w	–	–	–
(See Hydrocortisone Cream, 1% w/w)			
Hydrocortisone Cream BP, 0.5% w/v	15 g	38	A
	30 g	60	C
Hydrocortisone Cream BP, 1% w/w	15 g	47	A
Hydrocortisone Eye Ointment BPC, 0.5% w/w	3 g	85	B
Hydrocortisone Eye Ointment BPC, 1% w/w	3 g	100	B
Hydrocortisone Eye Ointment BPC, 2.5% w/w	3 g	75	B
Hydrocortisone Ointment BP, 0.5% w/w	15 g	39	A
	30 g	60	C

*Special containers — see Clause 10 B(ii)(page 8)

BASIC PRICES OF DRUGS

PART VIII

Drug (1)	Quantity (2)	Basic Price (3) p	Category (4)
Hydrocortisone Ointment BP, 1% w/w	15 g	49	A
Hydrocortisone Suppositories BPC, 25 mg	12	431	A
Hydrocortisone Sodium Succinate Injection BP (100 mg vial)	1	67	C
Hydrogen Peroxide Ear Drops BP 1980...................	10 ml	1	E
Hydrogen Peroxide Solution BP (6 per cent)	200 ml	39	B
Hydrotalcite Suspension, 500 mg/5 ml	500 ml	196	C
Hydrotalcite Tablets BP, 500 mg	56	81	C
Hydrous Ointment BP (Syn. Oily Cream)	500 g	176	A
Hydrous Wool Fat Ointment, BPC 1973	500 g	324	A
Hydroxocobalamin Injection BP 1 mg/1 ml	5	180	C
Hyoscine Eye Drops BP, 0.25% w/v	10 ml	84	A
Hyoscine Injection BP, (400 microgram/1 ml ampoules)	10	1113	B
Hyoscyamus Tincture BP 1980	500 ml	316	A
Hypromellose Eye Drops BPC	10 ml	75	A
Ibuprofen Tablets BP, 200 mg	500	642	S
Ibuprofen Tablets BP, 400 mg	250	642	S
Ibuprofen Tablets BP, 600 mg	100	678	S
Ichthammol BP	100 g	315	B
Ichthammol Glycerin BPC	500 ml	377 ▽	A
Ichthammol Ointment BP 1980	500 g	342	A
Imipramine Tablets BP, 10 mg	250	183	A
Imipramine Tablets BP, 25 mg	500	343	A
Indomethacin Capsules BP, 25 mg	500	440	S
Indomethacin Capsules BP, 50 mg	100	275	B
Indomethacin Suppositories BP, 100 mg	10	183	A
Industrial Methylated Spirit BP	2 litre	291	A
Iodine BP	100 g	400	B
Iodine Aqueous Solution BP	100 ml	143	A
(Syns: Lugol's Solution, Iodine Aqueous Oral Solution)			
Iodine Solution, Decolourised BPC 1934 (Methylated)....	100 ml	27	E
Iodine Solution, Strong BP 1958	500 ml	515	B
Iodine Paint, Compound BPC 1968	500 ml	629	B
Ipecacuanha Mixture BPC 1963 (See Alk. Ipecac Mixture)	-	-	-
Ipecacuanha Mixture, Paediatric, BPC	100 ml	11	E
Ipecacuanha and Ammonia Mixture Paediatric BPC	100 ml	8	E
Ipecacuanha, Opiate Mixture, Paediatric BPC	100 ml	13	E
Ipecacuanha Tincture BP...............................	500 ml	610	A
Isoniazid Tablets BP, 50 mg	250	350	B
Isoniazid Tablets BP, 100 mg	100	164	A
Isosorbide Mononitrate Tablets, 20 mg	100	700	C

BASIC PRICES OF DRUGS

PART VIII

Drug (1)	Quantity (2)	Basic Price (3) p	Category (4)
Kaolin Light BP	1 kg	222	A
Kaolin Mixture BP	2 litre	321	A
Kaolin Mixture, Paediatric BP 1980	500 ml	141	A
Kaolin and Morphine Mixture BP	2 litre	288	A
Kaolin Powder, Compound BPC 1963	500 g	139	E
Kaolin Poultice BP	200 g	127	A
	500 g	213	A
(To be supplied in lever-lidded tins, or approved polypropylene jars)			
Labetolol Tablets BP, 100 mg	250	1785 Δ	A
Labetolol Tablets BP, 200 mg	250	2841 Δ	A
Labetolol Tablets BP, 400 mg	250	4481	A
Lachesine Eye Drops BPC, 1% w/v	10 ml	360	B
Lactic Acid BP	500 ml	490	B
Lactic Acid Pessaries BP	12	700	B
Lactose BP (Syn. Milk Sugar)	500 g	175	B
Lactulose Solution BP 3.35 g/5 ml	1 litre	773	S
Lemon Oil BP	100 ml	220	B
Lemon Spirit BP	100 ml	465	A
Levodopa Tablets BP, 500 mg	200	1339	C
(Syn. L-Dopa Tablets 500 mg)			
Linseed Oil BP 1964	500 ml	367	B
Liquefied Phenol BP	500 ml	570 ∇	C	
Liquid Paraffin Emulsion BP (Syns: Liquid Paraffin ... Mixture, Liquid Paraffin Oral Emulsion)	2 litre	398	A
Liquorice Liquid Extract BP	500 ml	419	A
Liquorice Lozenges BPC, (Syn. Brompton Cough Lozenges)	500 g	805	B
Lisinopril Dihydrate Tablets 10 mg	28	1213	C

BASIC PRICES OF DRUGS

PART VIII

Drug (1)	Quantity (2)	Basic Price (3) p	Category (4)
Lobelia Simple Tincture, BPC 1949	100 ml	443	B
Loprazolam Mesylate Tablets, 1 mg	28	168	C
Lorazepam Tablets BP, 1 mg	100	115	A
Lorazepam Tablets BP, 2.5 mg	100	183	A
Lormetazepam Tablets, 0.5 mg	100	422	C
Lormetazepam Tablets, 1 mg	100	546	C
Lysol (See Cresol and Soap Solution BP 1968)	–	–	–
Magnesium Carbonate, Heavy BP	500 g	226	A
Magnesium Carbonate, Light BP	500 g	243	A
Magnesium Carbonate Mixture BPC	2 litre	385	C
Magnesium Carbonate Aromatic Mixture BP	2 litre	304	A
Magnesium Carbonate Powder, Compound BPC	500 g	141	B
Magnesium Oxide, Heavy BP	500 g	620	B
Magnesium Sulphate BP	2 kg	173	A
Magnesium Sulphate, Dried BP (Powder)	500 g	175	B
Magnesium Sulphate Mixture BP	200 ml	18	E
Magnesium Sulphate Paste BP. (Syn. Morison's Paste)	500 g	364	A
Magnesium Trisilicate BP	500 g	309	A
Magnesium Trisilicate Mixture BP	2 litre	226 ∇	A
Magnesium Trisilicate Powder Compound BP	100 g	79	B
Magnesium Trisilicate and Belladonna Mixture BPC	200 ml	27 ∇	E
Magnesium Trisilicate Tablets, Compound BP	500	505	A
Maize Oil BP 1980 (Syn. Corn Oil)	2 litre	745	B
Malt Liquid Extract BPC 1954	500 ml	430	B
Medroxyprogesterone Acetate Tablets 100 mg	100	4162	C
Menthol BP	100 g	678	A
Menthol & Eucalyptus Inhalation BP 1980..............	500 ml	193	A
Meprobamate Tablets BP 1980, 200 mg	250	186	C
Meprobamate Tablets BP 1980, 400 mg	250	281	C
Metformin Tablets BP, 500 mg	100	239	B
Metformin Tablets BP, 850 mg	60	240	A
Metipranolol Eye Drops 0.1% w/v	5 ml	403	C

BASIC PRICES OF DRUGS

PART VIII

Drug (1)	Quantity (2)	Basic Price (3) p	Category (4)
Methadone Linctus BP	500 ml	471	B
Methadone Mixture, 1 mg/1ml BNF	200 ml	111	E
Methadone Hydrochloride BP	5 g	2180	B
Methylcellulose 20 BP	100 g	205	B
Methyldopa Tablets BP 125 mg	250	542	A
Methyldopa Tablets BP, 250 mg	1000	3415	S
Methyldopa Tablets BP, 500 mg	500	3438	S
Methyl Salicylate BP	500 ml	435	A
Methyl Salicylate Liniment BP	500 ml	246	A
Methyl Salicylate Ointment BP	500 g	479	A
Metoclopramide Tablets BP 10 mg	100	230	C
	500	1134	C
Metoprolol Tablets 50 mg	100	471	C
Metoprolol Tablets 100 mg	100	875	C
Metronidazole Tablets BP, 200 mg	250	725	C
Metronidazole Tablets BP, 400 mg	100	725	C
Mianserin Hydrochloride Tablets BP, 10 mg	100	667	A
Mianserin Hydrochloride Tablets BP, 20 mg	100	1338	A
Mianserin Hydrochloride Tablets BP, 30 mg	100	2000	A
Morphine and Cocaine Elixir BPC	200 ml	335	E
Morphine Hydrochloride BP	2 g	948	B
Morphine Hydrochloride Solution BPC	100 ml	449	B
Morphine Hydrochloride Suppositories BPC, 15 mg	12	345	B
Morphine Sulphate BP	2 g	948	B
Morphine Sulphate Injection BP (10 mg/1 ml ampoules)	5	183	B
(15 mg/1 ml ampoules)	5	189	B
(30 mg/1 ml ampoules)	5	206	B
Morphine Sulphate Suppositories BPC, 15 mg	12	351	B
Morphine Sulphate Suppositories BPC, 30 mg	12	551	B
Myrrh Tincture BPC	100 ml	210	B
Naproxen Tablets BP, 250 mg	250	2058	A
Naproxen Tablets BP, 500 mg	100	1648	A
Neomycin Cream BPC	15 g	52	A
Neomycin Eye Ointment BP, 0.5%	3 g	64	B
Neomycin Sulphate Eye Drops BP, 0.5% w/v	10 ml	153	A
(Syn. Neomycin Eye Drops 0.5% w/v)			
Nicotinic Acid Tablets BP, 50 mg	500	325	A
Nifedipine Capsules 5 mg	100	796 Δ	A
Nifedipine Capsules 10 mg	100	1144	A
Nitrazepam Mixture, 2.5 mg/5 ml	150 ml	336	S
Nitrazepam Tablets BP,5 mg	500	170	S
Nitric Acid BP	500 ml	283	B
Nitrous Ether Spirit BPC 1959	100 ml	135	B
Nux Vomica Tincture BP 1980	500 ml	238	A
Nystatin Oral Suspension BP 100,000 u/ml	30 ml	250	C

BASIC PRICES OF DRUGS

PART VIII

Drug (1)	Quantity (2)	Basic Price (3) p	Category (4)
Oily Cream, (See Hydrous Ointment BP)	–	–	–
Oleic Acid BP	500 ml	190	B
Olive Oil BP	250 ml	135	C
Opium Tincture BP	100 ml	235	C
Opium Camphorated Compound Mixture BPC	200 ml	20	E
Orange Spirit, Compound BP	25 ml	207	B
Orange Syrup BP	500 ml	276	A
Orange Tincture BP	100 ml	556	B
Oxazepam Tablets BP, 10 mg	100	122	S
Oxazepam Tablets BP, 15 mg	100	136	S
Oxazepam Tablets BP, 30 mg	100	165	S
Oxprenolol Tablets BP, 20 mg	100	148	S
Oxprenolol Tablets BP, 40 mg	100	214	S
Oxprenolol Tablets BP, 80 mg	100	356	S
Oxprenolol Tablets BP, 160 mg	100	690	S
Oxytetracycline Tablets BP, 250 mg	1000	1182	S
Paracetamol, Elixir, Paediatric BP	500 ml	229	A
(Syn: Paracetamol Oral Solution Paediatric)			
Paracetamol Oral Suspension BP, 120 mg/5 ml (Paediatric)	500 ml	216	C
Paracetamol Oral Suspension BP, 250 mg/5 ml	100 ml	116	C
Paracetamol Soluble Tablets 500 mg	60	130	C
(Syns: Paracetamol Dispersible Tablets			
Paracetamol Effervescent Tablets.)			
Paracetamol Tablets BP, 500 mg	5000	2096	A
Paraffin, Hard BP	500 g	145	B
Paraffin, Hard BP (MP 43–46oC)	500 g	250	B
Paraffin, Liquid BP	2 litre	355	A
Paraffin Liquid Light BP	500 ml	161	B
Paraffin Ointment BP	200 g	79	E
Paraffin Soft, White BP (Syn. White Petroleum Jelly)....	500 g	167	A
Paraffin Soft, Yellow BP (Syn. Yellow Petroleum Jelly)..	500 g	185	A
Pentazocine Lactate Injection BP, (30mg/1 ml)	10	699	C
Pentazocine Lactate Injection BP, (60mg/2 ml)	10	1341	C
Pentazocine Suppositories 50 mg	20	830	C
Pentazocine Tablets BP, 25 mg	100	823	S
Peppermint Emulsion, Concentrated BP	100 ml	80	B
Peppermint Oil BP	100 ml	591	A
Peppermint Water Concentrated BP 1973	100 ml	333	A
Pethidine Injection BP (50 mg in 1 ml)	10	111	C
(100 mg in 2 ml)	10	140	C
Pethidine Tablets BP, 50 mg	50	97	C

BASIC PRICES OF DRUGS

PART VIII

Drug (1)	Quantity (2)	Basic Price (3) p	Category (4)
Phenobarbitone Elixir BP	500 ml	265	A
Phenobarbitone Sodium BP	25 g	200	A
Phenobarbitone Tablets BP, 15 mg	1000	280	A
Phenobarbitone Tablets BP, 30 mg	1000	332	A
Phenobarbitone Tablets BP, 60 mg	1000	514 Δ	A
Phenobarbitone Tablets BP, 100 mg	250	220	B
Phenol BP (Crystals)	100 g	253	B
Phenol Ear Drops BPC	10 ml	7	E
Phenol Gargle BPC	200 ml	10	E
Phenol Glycerin BP	500 ml	472	B
Phenolphthalein BP	25 g	440	B
Phenoxymethylpenicillin Capsules BP, 250 mg	100	254	C
(syns: Phenoxymethylpenicillin Potassium capsules Penicillin VK Capsules)			
Phenoxymethylpenicillin Oral Solution BP			
125 mg/5 ml	100 ml	53	A
250 mg/5 ml	100 ml	82	A
(Syns. Phenoxymethylpenicillin Elixir Phenoxymethylpenicillin Syrup)			
Phenoxymethylpenicillin Tablets BP 250 mg	1000	1650	S
(Syn: Phenoxymethylpenicillin Tablets)			
Phenylephrine Eye Drops BPC	10 ml	175	A
Phenytoin Tablets BP, 50 mg	500	349	A
Phenytoin Tablets BP, 100 mg	1000	694	A
Pholcodine Linctus BP	500 ml	144	S
Pholcodine Linctus, Strong BP	500 ml	234	A
Physostigmine Eye Drops BP, 0.25% w/v	10 ml	190	A
(Syn. Eserine Eye Drops 0.25% w/v)			
Physostigmine Eye Drops BP, 0.5 w/v	10 ml	190	A
(Syn. Eserine Eye Drops 0.5% w/v)			
Phytomenadione Injection BP (10 mg/1 ml)	10	410	C
Phytomenadione Injection BP (1 mg/0.5 ml)	10	219	C
Phytomenadione Tablets BP 10 mg	25	420	C
Pilocarpine Eye Drops BP, 0.5% w/v	10 ml	111	A
Pilocarpine Eye Drops BP, 1% w/v	10 ml	111	A
Pilocarpine Eye Drops BP, 2% w/v	10 ml	120	A
Pilocarpine Eye Drops BP, 3% w/v	10 ml	136	A
Pilocarpine Eye Drops BP, 4% w/v	10 ml	151	A
Piroxicam Capsules BP, 10 mg	60	869	A
Piroxicam Capsules BP, 20 mg	30	869	A
Podophyllin Paint BPC 1954	10 ml	37	E
Podophyllin Paint, Compound BP	100 ml	336	B
Podophyllum Resin BP	25 g	349	B
Potassium Bicarbonate BPC	500 g	258	A

BASIC PRICES OF DRUGS

PART VIII

Drug (1)	Quantity (2)	Basic Price (3) p	Category (4)
Potassium Bromide BP	500 g	315	A
Potassium Bromide Mixture BPC 1963	200 ml	31	E
Potassium Bromide and Chloral Mixture BPC 1963	200 ml	30	E
Potassium Bromide and Valerian Mixture, BPC 1963	200 ml	34	E
Potassium Chlorate BPC	500 g	327	A
Potassium Chloride BP	500 g	195	B
Potassium Chloride Tablets, Slow BNF 1976-78, 600 mg...	500	254	C
Potassium Citrate BP	500 g	263	A
Potassium Citrate Mixture BP 5 in 4	2 litre	708	B
Potassium Citrate Mixture BPC	200 ml	57	E
Potassium Citrate & Belladonna Mixture, Paediatric BNF 1963	100 ml	20	E
Potassium Citrate and Hyoscyamus Mixture BPC..........	200 ml	79	E
*Potassium Effervescent Tablets BPC 1968	100	271	A
Potassium Hydroxide BP .... (Syn. Caustic Potash)(Pellets)	500 g	532	B
Potassium Hydroxide Solution BP	500 ml	190	A
Potassium Iodide BP	100 g	338	B
Potassium Iodide Mixture Ammoniated BPC .... (Syn. Potassium Iodide and Ammonia Mixture)	200 ml	31	E
Potassium Nitrate BP	500 g	340	B
Potassium Permanganate BP	500 g	365	B
Potassium Permangante Solution BNF	100 ml	1	E
Prednisolone Tablets BP, 1 mg	500	182	C
Prednisolone Tablets 2.5 mg e/c	56	62	C
Prednisolone Tablets BP, 5 mg	500	384	C
	1000	767	C
Prednisone Tablets BP, 1 mg	500	245	A
Prednisone Tablets BP, 5 mg	500	384	C
	1000	767	C
Procyclidine Tablets BP, 5 mg	100	502 Δ	A
Proflavine Cream BPC (Syns: Flavine Cream, ... Proflavine Emulsion)	500 ml	166	B
Proflavine Hemisulphate BPC	5 g	278	B
Proflavine Solution BPC 1949	100 ml	8	E
Propranolol Tablets BP, 10 mg	500	125	S
Propranolol Tablets BP, 40 mg	1000	400	S
Propranolol Tablets BP, 80 mg	500	375	S
Propranolol Tablets BP, 160 mg	100	130	S
Propylene Glycol BP	500 ml	175	A
Propylthiouracil Tablets BP, 50 mg	100	750	C
Protamine Sulphate Injection BP, (50 mg/5 ml).........	10	980	B

*Special container — see Clause 10.B(ii)(page 8)

0306M/18

BASIC PRICES OF DRUGS

PART VIII

Drug (1)	Quantity (2)	Basic Price (3) p	Category (4)
Pumilio Pine Oil BP 1980.............................	100 ml	175	B
Purified Talc BP (Sterile)	500 g	160	B
Purified Talc BP	500 g	143	A
Purified Water BP	5 litre	145	A
Pyridoxine Hydrochloride Tablets BP, 10 mg	100	159	B
Pyridoxine Hydrochloride Tablets BP, 20 mg	100	141	C
Pyridoxine Hydrochloride Tablets BP, 50 mg	100	255	A
Quillaia Tincture BP	100 ml	139	B
Quinidine Sulphate Tablets BP, 200 mg	250	1636	A
Quinidine Sulphate Tablets BP, 300 mg	250	2195	A
Quinine Bisulphate Tablets BP, 300 mg	100	390	A
Quinine Dihydrochloride Tablets BPC, 300 mg	100	1005	B
Quinine Sulphate Tablets BP, 125 mg	100	251	B
Quinine Sulphate Tablets BP, 200 mg	250	928	A
Quinine Sulphate Tablets BP, 300 mg	500	1800	S
Raspberry Syrup BP	500 ml	302	A
Rectified Spirit BP (See Ethanol 90 per cent)	–	–	–
Resorcinol BP	100 g	295	B
Rifampicin Capsules BP, 150 mg	100	1720	C
Rifampicin Capsules BP, 300 mg	100	3440	C
Rosemary Oil BPC	100 ml	418	B
Saccharin Sodium BP	25 g	131	B
Salbutamol Aerosol Inhalation BPC 100 microgram per actuation	200 dose	208	A
Salbutamol Injection BP 50 mcg/ml (5 ml ampoules)	10	570	C
Salbutamol Respirator Solution 5 mg/ml	1	271	C
Salbutamol Syrup, 2 mg/5 ml	150 ml	71	C
	2 litre	896	C
Salbutamol Tablets BP 2 mg	500	415	C
Salbutamol Tablets BP 4 mg	120	200	C
Salicylic Acid Collodion BP	500 ml	591	A
Salicylic Acid Lotion BP	500 ml	84	E
Salicylic Acid Ointment BP	500 g	357	A
Salicylic Acid & Sulphur Ointment BPC	500 g	423	A
Salicylic Acid BP (Powder)	500 g	438	A
Senega Infusion Concentrated BP 1980.................	500 ml	1500	B

BASIC PRICES OF DRUGS

PART VIII

Drug (1)	Quantity (2)	Basic Price (3) p	Category (4)
Senna Tablets BP, 7.5 mg	500	700	S
Silver Nitrate BP	25 g	2169	C |
Silver Nitrate Lotion BNF	50 ml	23	E
Silver Protein, Mild BPC 1968	25 g	1402	B
Simple Linctus BP	2 litre	324	A
Simple Linctus, Paediatric BP	2 litre	335	A
Simple Ointment BP (White)	500 g	170	B
Soap, Soft BP	500 g	205	B
Soap, Liniment BPC (Methylated)	500 ml	245	A
Soap Spirit BP (Methylated)	500 ml	269	B
Sodium Acid Phosphate BP	500 g	326	A
Sodium Benzoate BP	500 g	265	B
Sodium Bicarbonate BP (Powder)	2 kg	190	C
Sodium Bicarbonate Ear Drops BP	10 ml	2	E
Sodium Bicarbonate Intravenous Infusion BP, 5% w/v (Syn. Sodium Bicarbonate Injection)			
(20 ml ampoules)	10	1548	B
(50 ml ampoules)	10	2777	B
Sodium Bicarbonate Mixture, Paediatric BPC	100 ml	15	E
Sodium Bicarbonate Tablets, Compound BP	1000	350	B
(Syn. Soda Mint Tablets)			
Sodium Chloride BP	500 g	130	B
Sodium Chloride Intravenous Infusion BP, 0.9% w/v (Syn. Sodium Chloride Injection 0.9% w/v)			
(2 ml ampoules)	10	230	B
(5 ml ampoules)	10	295	B
(10 ml ampoules)	10	336	B
(20 ml ampoules)	10	623	B
(50 ml ampoules)	10	1523	B
(100 ml ampoule)	1	120	B
Sodium Chloride Mixture, Compound BPC	200 ml	5	E
Sodium Chloride Mouthwash, Compound BP	200 ml	8	E
Sodium Chloride Solution BP	100 ml	3	E
Sodium Chloride Tablets BP, 300 mg	100	97	B
Sodium Citrate BP	500 g	331	A
Sodium Citrate Mixture BPC	200 ml	63	E
Sodium Hydroxide BP (Pellets)	500 g	600	C |
Sodium Iodide BP	100 g	625	B
Sodium Metabisulphite BP	100 g	116	B
Sodium Perborate BP	500 g	484	B
Sodium Phosphate BP	500 g	341	B
Sodium Potassium Tartrate BPC	500 g	213	B
Sodium Salicylate BP (Crystals)	500 g	405	A
Sodium Salicylate Mixture, Strong BP	200 ml	24	E
Sorbitol Solution (70 per cent) (Non—Crystalising)BP ..	1 litre	300	C

BASIC PRICES OF DRUGS

PART VIII

Drug (1)	Quantity (2)	Basic Price (3) p	Category (4)
Spironolactone Tablets BP, 25 mg	500	1350	S
Spironolactone Tablets BP, 50 mg	100	1200	C
Spironolactone Tablets BP, 100 mg	100	1100	S
Squill Oxymel BP	2 litre	811	B
Squill Tincture BP 1980	500 ml	368	B
Starch Maize BP (Powder)	500 g	130	A
Stearic Acid BPC	500 g	245	B
Stilboestrol Tablets BP, 1 mg	100	433 Δ	A
Stilboestrol Tablets BP, 5 mg	100	816 Δ	A
Stramonium Tincture BP 1980	500 ml	298	B
Stramonium and Potassium Iodide Mixture BPC	200 ml	32	E
Strychnine Hydrochloride Solution BPC 1963	100 ml	177	A
Sucrose BP	1 kg	52	C
Sulphacetamide Sodium Eye Drops BP, 10% w/v	10 ml	144	A
Sulphacetamide Sodium Eye Ointment BP, 6% w/w	4 g tube	111	A
Sulphasalazine Tablets 500 mg	100	680	A
Sulphur Lotion, Compound BPC	200 ml	15	E
Sulphur Ointment BP 1980	500 g	195	B
Sulphur, Precipitated BP	500 g	146	A
Sulphur, Sublimed BPC	500 g	125	B
Sulphuric Acid BP	500 ml	215	B
Sulphuric Acid, Dilute BP	500 ml	140	B
Surgical Spirit BP	2 litre	341	A
Syrup BP	2 litre	294	A
Syrup BP (unpreserved)	2 litre	285	C
Tamoxifen Citrate Tablets BP, 10 mg	30	664	A
Tamoxifen Citrate Tablets BP, 20 mg	30	961	A
Tamoxifen Tablets BP 40 mg	30	2200	C
(Syn: Tamoxifen Citrate Tablets)			
Tannic Acid BP 1973	500 g	1600	B
Tartaric Acid BP	500 g	299	B
Tartrazine Solution, Compound BP 1980	100 ml	154	B
Temazepam Capsules 10 mg (Soft Gelatin Gel filled)	500	1206	C
Temazepam Capsules 15 mg (Soft Gelatin Gel filled)	60	186	C
Temazepam Capsules 20 mg (Soft Gelatin Gel filled)	250	1052	C
Temazepam Capsules 30 mg (Soft Gelatin Gel filled)	60	372	C
Temazepam Elixir 10 mg/5 ml	300 ml	795	C
Temazepam Tablets 10 mg	500	1206	C
Temazepam Tablets 20 mg	250 ml	1052	C

BASIC PRICES OF DRUGS

PART VIII

Drug (1)	Quantity (2)	Basic Price (3) p	Category (4)
Tetracycline Tablets BP, 250 mg	500	748	A
Thiamine Hydrochloride Tablets BP, 25 mg	100	61	S
Thiamine Hydrochloride Tablets BP, 50 mg	100	102	S
Thiamine Hydrochloride Tablets BP, 100 mg	100	176	S
Thiamine Hydrochloride Tablets BP, 300 mg	100	287	S
Thiamine Tablets, Compound BPC	-	-	-
(See Vitamin B Tablets Compound BPC)			
Thiamine Tablets, Compound, Strong BPC	-	-	-
(See Vitamin B Tablets, Compound, Strong)			
Thymol BP	100 g	270	B
Thymol Glycerin, Compound BP (Methylated)	2 litre	322	A
Thyroxine Tablets BP, (Syn Thyroxine Sodium Tablets)			
50 microgram	1000	221	A
100 microgram	1000	239	A
Tolbutamide Tablets BP, 500 mg	500	725	S
Tragacanth Mucilage BPC	500 g	220	B
Tragacanth, Powdered BP	100 g	1203	A
Tragacanth Powder, Compound BP 1980...................	100 g	318	A
Triazolam Tablets 125 microgram	30	172	C
Triazolam Tablets 250 microgram	30	232	C
Triclofos Elixir BP (Syn: Triclofos Oral Solution).....	100 ml	435	A
Trimethoprim Tablets BP 100 mg	100	311 Δ	A
Trimethoprim Tablets BP 200 mg	100	453	A
Turpentine Liniment BP	500 ml	217	B
Turpentine Oil BP	500 ml	214	B
Valerian Infusion, Concentrated BPC 1963	500 ml	517	A
Valerian Tincture, Simple BPC 1949	500 ml	720	B
Verapamil Hydrochloride Tablets BP, 40 mg	100	446	C
Verapamil Hydrochloride Tablets BP, 80 mg	100	890	C
Verapamil Hydrochloride Tablets BP, 120 mg	100	1362	C
Verapamil Hydrochloride Tablets BP, 160 mg	100	1638	C
Vitamins Capsules BPC	500	458	A
Vitamin A Capsules, Strong BNF 1957)50,000 Units)	100	254	B
Vitamin B Tablets, Compound BPC	500	165	C
(Syns: Compound Aneurine Tablets,			
Compound Thiamine Tablets)			
Vitamin B Tablets, Compound, Strong BPC	500	315	A
(Syns: Strong Compound Aneurine Tablets,			
Strong Compound Thiamine Tablets)			

BASIC PRICES OF DRUGS

PART VIII

Drug (1)	Quantity (2)	Basic Price (3) p	Category (4)
Vitamins B & C Injection BPC (IM weak/4 ml)	3	119	C
	12	476	C
(IM strong/7 ml)	3	128	C
	12	512	C
(IV strong/10 ml)	3	128	C
	12	512	C
Vitamin B12 Injection (See Hydroxocobalamin Injection BP)	–	–	–
Warfarin Tablets BP, 1 mg	500	221	C
Warfarin Tablets BP, 3 mg	500	255	C
Warfarin Tablets BP, 5 mg	500	400	C
Water for Injections BP (1 ml ampoules)	10	120	B
(2 ml ampoules)	10	114	A
(5 ml ampoules)	10	168	A
(10 ml ampoules)	10	212	A
(20 ml ampoules)	10	491	A
(50 ml ampoules)	10	1031	B
Wheat–germ Oil BPC 1954	25 ml	177	B
White Liniment BP (Syn. White Embrocation)	2 litre	437	A
Wild Cherry Syrup BP 1980...........................	500 ml	286	B
Wool Alcohols Ointment BP	500 g	483	B
Wool Fat BP (Syn. Anhydrous Lanolin)	500 g	256	A
Wool Fat, Hydrous BP (Syn. Lanolin)...................	500 g	345	A
Xylometazoline Hydrochloride Nasal Drops BP,.0.05% w/v.	10 ml	78	C
Xylometazoline Hydrochloride Nasal Drops BP, 0.1% w/v .	10 ml	78	C
Yeast Tablets, Dried BPC, 300 mg	1000	185	B
Zinc & Castor Oil Ointment BP .... (Syn. Zinc & Castor Oil Cream)	500 g	265	A
Zinc & Coal Tar Paste BP	500 g	446	B
Zinc Paste, Compound BP	500 g	180	B
Zinc Cream BP	500 g	441	B
Zinc Ointment BP	500 g	399	B
Zinc Oxide BP	500 g	191	A
Zinc & Salicylic Acid Paste BP (Syn. Lassar's Paste) ..	500 g	296	A
Zinc Sulphate BP	500 g	416	A
Zinc Sulphate Eye Drops BP	10 ml	164	A
Zinc Sulphate Lotion BP	200 ml	2	E

BASIC PRICES OF DRUGS

PART VIII

BASIC PRICES OF DRUGS

PART VIII

APPROVED LIST OF APPLIANCES
See Part II, Clause 8A (page 7)

The price listed in respect of an appliance specified in the following list is
the basic price (see Part II, Clause 8 on which payment will be calculated
pursuant to Part II, Clause 6 in respect of the dispensing of appliances.

NOTES

1. Definition - The appliances that may be supplied against orders on Forms FP10 are listed below
and must conform with the specifications shown. See Part 1, Clause 2 (page 3). These
specifications include published official standards ie BP, BPC or relevant British Standard or the
Drug Tariff Technical Specification. It should be emphasized that any appliance must conform with
the entry in this part of the Tariff as well as with the official standard or technical
specification quoted therein. Other dressings and appliances which may be necessary will normally
be provided through the Hospital Services.

2. Sealed Packets - These are those which are sealed with an easily detachable device that
prevents removal of the contents without the seal being broken. Additionally in the case of
sterile products: once a sealed package has been opened it should not be possible to re-seal it
easily. Where an appliance, other than a bandage, required by the Tariff to be supplied in a
sealed packet is ordered of a quantity or weight not listed in the Tariff, the quantity ordered
should be made up as nearly as possible with the smallest numbers of sealed packets available for
the purpose. Where the quantity ordered is less than the smallest quantity/ weight, supply the
smallest pack. The quantity of material in each packet supplied should be recorded on the
prescription form.

3. Weights - All weights specified in the Tariff in respect of appliances are exclusive of
wrappings and packing material.

4. Invoice price - This is the price chargeable for the appliance to the contractor by the
manufacturer, wholesaler or supplier.

5. Technical Specifications - Numbered Technical Specifications for the items in Part IXA/B/C
were published separately in 1981 in loose leaf volume and a revised list was published in 1983.
The Specifications will not be reprinted annually but individual specifications will be amended
and reprinted, or withdrawn, as necessary. A list of the Technical specifications is given on
pages 57a/b.

0307M/1

PART IX
LIST OF TECHNICAL SPECIFICATIONS

	Spec. No.	Date of last revision
Absorbent Cotton, Hospital Quality	1	1981
Bandages		
Elastic Web with Foot Loop	2a	1983
Elastic Web without Foot Loop	2b	1981
Flexible Adhesive, Porous	3	1981
Knitted Polyamide & Cellulose Contour	45	1989
Zinc Paste and Calamine	5	1981
Catheters		
Nelaton	38a	1987
Scott Female	38b	1987
Foley	38a	1987
Chemical Reagents		
Blood Glucose Testing Strips (BGTS) Colorimetric	44	9/1989
Biosensor	48	9/1989
Chiropy Appliances		
Metataral Pads	6	1981
Contraceptive Devices		
Intrauterine Contraceptive Devices	7	5/1990
Vaginal Contraceptive Caps (Pessaries)	8	1981
Dressings		
Calcium Alginate	41	1988
Dextranomer Paste Pad	49	6/1990
Hydrocolloid	42	4/1990
Hydrogel	50	5/1990
Povidone Iodine Fabric	43	1988
Sterile Dressing Pack	10	1981
Sterile Dressing Pack with NW Pads	35	1983
Elastic Hosiery		
Graduated Compression	40	1988
Suspender Belt	13	1981
Gauze Tissues		
Gauze and Cotton Tissue	14	1983

PART IX
LIST OF TECHNICAL SPECIFICATIONS (CONT)

	Spec. No.	Date of last revision
Hypodermic Equipment		
Non-Sterile		
Hypodermic Needles (Luer Fitting)	15	1981
Hypodermic Syringes (Luer Fitting)	16	1981
Hypodermic Insulin Syringe Carrying Case	17a	1983
Screw-cap for above when used with pre-set Syringe	17b	1983
Pre-set Insulin Syringe 1ml.U100	36a	1983
Click-count Insulin Syringe 1ml.U100	36b	1983
Sterile		
Insulin Syringe with Needle	39a	2/1990
Hypodermic Needles	39b	1988
Laryngectomy Protectors	18	1981
Latex Foam Adhesive	19	1981
Pessaries	20	1981
Protectives		
EMA Film Gloves, Disposable	21	1981
Rectal Dilators ., ...	22	1981
Stockinette		
Elasticated Surgical Tubular, Foam Padded	25	1983
Elasticated Viscose	46	1989
Elastic Net Surgical Tubular	26	1983
Swabs		
Non-woven Fabric	28	9/1989
Non-woven Fabric, Filmated	29	1981
Trusses		
Spring	31a	1981
Elastic Band	31b	1981

PART IXA - APPLIANCES

Appliance (1)	Size or Weight (2)	Basic Price (3) p

ABSORBENT COTTONS
To be supplied in sealed packets (film wrapped cartons)
as received from the manufacturer or wholesaler.
(See Note 2 page 57).

each

Absorbent Cotton BP	25 g	43
	100 g	99
	500 g	343

Where no quantity is stated on the prescription the
25g pack is to be supplied.

Absorbent Cotton, Hospital Quality	100 g	69
Specification 1	500 g	231
To be supplied only where specifically ordered.		

APPLICATORS - VAGINAL
Plastics syringe-type applicator with transparent or
translucent barrel and opaque or translucent plunger.
The end of the barrel has an internal screw thread.
(Length not less than 11 cm and capacity not less
than 5 ml)

Type 1. (Ortho)		75
Type 2. (Durex)		75

NB:
1. To be supplied suitably wrapped as received
   from the manufacturer or wholesaler.
2. Where an Ortho pack ordered by the prescriber
   does not include an applicator, and the contractor
   considers that one is required, an Ortho Vaginal
   Applicator should be supplied and the
   prescription form endorsed accordingly.
3. Where Duracreme or Duragel Spermicide Jelly
   is ordered by the prescriber without an
   applicator and the contractor considers that
   one is required, a Durex Vaginal Applicator
   should be supplied and the prescription form
   endorsed accordingly.
4. For details of prescription charges payable,
   See Part XVI, page 350.

ARM SLINGS		118
Web, Adjustable.		

PART IXA – APPLIANCES

Appliance (1)	Size or Weight (2)	Basic Price (3) p

each

ATOMIZERS, HAND OPERATED

Nebulizers
(a) Inhalers
All-glass, plastics or plastics and glass with a rubber
or plastics bulb, for use with any liquid intended for
administration by inhalation and capable of producing
an extremely fine mist.

(i)   Type specified by the prescriber:
         Brovon Midget Inhaler   514
         Riddell Minor   530
         Pocket Riddopag Inhaler (without mask)   967
         Rybar Standard Inhaler No 1 (without mask) ..   929
         Rybar Standard Inhaler No 2 (without mask) ..   929

         Other inhalers conforming to this specification
         may be supplied if specifically ordered and
         endorsed providing the *invoice price does not
         exceed   967

(ii)   Type not specified by the prescriber:
         The invoice price must not exceed   514

                  Where an atomizer or spray is ordered by the
                  prescriber without specification and where
                  the contractor considers an appliance for
                  the administration of a liquid medicament by
                  inhalation is required, a nebulizer should be
                  supplied and the prescription form endorsed
                  with the net cost and type or brand supplied.
                  The basic price must not exceed that given
                  for (ii) above.

Spare Parts for above ....   *Invoice price

*For invoice price see note 4 (page 57)

Appliance (1)	Size or Weight (2)	Basic Price (3) p
Nebulizers - cont		
(b) Devices for use with Pressurised Aerosols. Pressurised aerosols are generally regarded as drugs for prescribing purposes, even when supplied in a plastic container incorporating a spring mechanism operated by intake of breath, or with a collapsible 'spacer' device. However other devices are regarded as appliances.		
Large Volume Reservoir Chamber Device incorporating one-way valve and mouthpiece. The device is reusable and should last for an extended period.		each
Plastic cone-shaped 750 ml capacity:		
Type 1 - One piece, to take aerosol cannister without actuator (Astra)		475
Type 2 - In two detachable parts, to take aerosol with actuator (Allen and Hanbury)		275
Plastic spherical, 250 ml capacity:		
Type 3 - In two detachable parts, to take aerosol with actuator (Tillotts)		275

BANDAGES

1. The term "bandage" used in a prescription form without qualification is to be interpreted to mean an Open-Wove Bandage, Type 1 BP 5 cm x 5 m. All bandages supplied are to be of the lengths and widths specified in the Tariff. Where a bandage longer than those specified in the Tariff is ordered, the number of bandages which will, in total, provide the length nearest to that ordered should be supplied. Where a bandage in a width other than those specified is ordered, the next wider specified width should be supplied.

2. Except for Elastic Web, all bandages to be supplied completely wrapped as received from the manufacturer or wholesaler. Elastic Adhesive Bandages and Plaster of Paris Bandages to be supplied sealed in containers as received from the manufacturer or wholesaler. Except where otherwise stated all bandages possessing elasticity to be not less than 4.5 m in length when fully stretched.

PART IXA - APPLIANCES

Appliance (1)	Size or Weight (2)	Basic Price (3) p
BANDAGES (cont)		each
Cotton Conforming Bandage BP		
- Type A		
Crinx	5 cm x 3.5 m	42
	7.5 cm x 3.5 m	54
	10 cm x 3.5 m	66
	15 cm x 3.5 m	90
- Type B		
Kling	5 cm x 3.5 m	42
	7.5 cm x 3.5 m	54
	10 cm x 3.5 m	66
	15 cm x 3.5 m	88
Cotton Elastic Heavy Bandage - See Heavy Cotton and Rubber Elastic Bandage BP, (Below).		
Cotton Crepe Bandage BP	7.5 cm x 4.5 m	189
	10 cm x 4.5 m	244
Crepe Bandage BP	5 cm	64
	7.5 cm	88
	10 cm	116
	15 cm	166
Elastic Adhesive Bandage BP	5 cm	221
	7.5 cm	323
	10 cm	430
Where no size is stated by the prescriber the 7.5 cm size should be supplied.		
Elastic Diachylon Bandage, Ventilated BPC .... (Lestreflex, Ventilated)	7.5 cm x 4.5 m stretched	262
Elasticated Tubular Bandage - see Stockinettes page 96-8		
		Per me
Elastic Web Bandage BP Blue/Line	7.5 cm	61
	10 cm	85
		each
Elastic Web Bandage with Foot Loop Blue/line .... Specification 2a	7.5 cm	321
Elastic Web Bandage Without Foot Loop .... Red/Line (Scott-Curwen) Specification 2b	7.5 cm x 2.75 m 2.5 m approx. unstretched length	285
	7.5 cm x 3.75 m 3.5 m approx. unstretched length	345
To be supplied wrapped with instruction folder and bandage fastener.		
Heavy Cotton and Rubber Elastic Bandage BP	7.5 cm	812

Appliance (1)	Size or Weight (2)	Basic Price (3) P
BANDAGES (cont)		each
Knitted Polyamide and Cellulose Contour Bandage Specification No 45 ("K band")		
For dressing retention 　　　　length 4 m stretched:..	5　cm	13
	7　cm	17
	10　cm	20
	15　cm	35
Open—Wove Bandage, Type 1 BP	2.5 cm x 5 m	22
(Syn. White Open—Wove Bandage)	5　cm x 5 m	37
	7.5 cm x 5 m	53
	10　cm x 5 m	68
Plaster of Paris Bandage BP	7.5 cm x 2.7 m	107
(Gypsona)	10　cm x 2.7 m	143

Polyamide and Cellulose Contour Bandage, BP (formerly: Nylon and viscose stretch Bandage.)		each Easifix	each Slinky	each Stayform
length 4 m stretched:	5　cm	23	31	25
	7.5 cm	29	43	32
	10　cm	33	52	36
	15　cm	55	73	62
Porous Flexible Adhesive Bandage BP (Poroplast) (Syn. Titanium Dioxide Elastic Adhesive Bandage) To be supplied only where specifically ordered.	7.5 cm			299

Appliance (1)	Size or Weight (2)	Basic Price (3) p
BANDAGES (cont)		each
Suspensory Bandage, Cotton		
Type 1. Cotton net bag with draw tapes and webbing waistband (Each in a carton or envelope)	Small	107
	Medium	107
	Large	107
	Ex. Large	111
Type 2. Cotton net bag with elastic edge and webbing waistband (Each in a carton or envelope).	Small	117
	Medium	121
	Large	125
	Ex. Large	131
Type 3. Cotton net bag with elastic edge and webbing waistband with insertion of elastic centre-front (Each in a carton or envelope). Note: Type supplied to be endorsed.	Small	127
	Medium	127
	Large	127
	Ex. Large	131
Triangular Calico Bandage BP .... (Individually wrapped)	Sides - 90 cm Base - 127 cm	83
Tubular Bandage - See Stockinette, page 96. White Open-Wove Bandage - See Open-Wove Bandage, Type 1		
ZINC PASTE BANDAGES - To be supplied enclosed in sealed packages, which prevent the passage of moisture, as received from the manufacturer or wholesaler. Zinc Paste Bandage BP		each
Viscopaste PB7	7.5 cm x 6 m	211
Zincaband	7.5 cm x 6 m	199
Zinc Paste and Coal Tar Bandage BP	7.5 cm x 6 m	215
Zinc Paste and Ichthammol Bandage BP	7.5 cm x 6 m	212
Zinc Paste, Calamine and Clioquinol Bandage BP (Quinaband)	7.5 cm x 6 m	223
Zinc Paste and Calamine Bandage .... (Calaband) Specification 5(ii)	7.5 cm x 6 m	223
BREAST RELIEVER .... Plasticised PVC polymer bulb with glass or polycarbonate receiver	60 ml approx	332
BREAST SHIELDS .... Plastics circular - each shield made in two sections with an opening in the concave section (one pair in box). (Not to be confused with Nipple Shields page 94)		per pair 344

PART IXA — APPLIANCES

Appliance (1)	Size or Weight (2)	Basic Price (3) p

BRUSHES   each

Iodine Brush — (Formerly Camel Hair) Goose Quill   19

> For details of prescription charges payable,
> See Part XVI, page 347.

CATHETERS, URETHRAL STERILE

1.   Catheter sizes are designated by the Charrière
(Ch) gauge system — even numbers only. (The equivalent
metric sizes for Charrière gauges 8–30 are 2.7 mm–10 mm,
rising in 0.66 mm). Where size is not stated by
the prescriber, size 14 or 16 should be supplied.

2.   If a balloon size is not stated by the prescriber
when ordering a Foley catheter, a 10 ml balloon catheter
should be supplied — a 5 ml balloon in the case of a
paediatric catheter. (These are the minimum sizes available)

NB BS 1695:1986 now defines the balloon size as that amount
of fluid required to fully inflate the volume of the
lumen. Care should be taken to distinguish between
an adult Catheter formerly labelled as "5 ml" but
requiring 10 ml for full inflation, and a paediatric
catheter labelled "5 ml" in accordance with the BS.

3.   Each sealed unit pack (ie. one or five units for
Nelaton packs; five units only for Scott packs;
one unit only for Foley packs) to be supplied in an
outer protective pack as received from the
manufacturer or wholesaler.

4.   Where the brand is not stated by the prescriber, the basic price of each listed
catheter supplied must not exceed:
> Nelaton   87
> Nelaton (Female)   90
> Foley   166
> Foley (female)   227
> Foley (paediatric)   294

PART IXA - APPLIANCES

Appliance (1)	Size or Weight (2)	Basic Price (3) p

(a) Nelaton Catheter ('ordinary' cylindrical catheter)

Specification: 38A

	Gauge (Ch) (see Note 1) (Above)	each	Per 5 * pack
EMS PVC Nelaton (Male)	8–14	87	360
EMS PVC Nelaton (Female)	8–14	90	390
Lofric Nelaton (Male) (DT 9000 – 5)	8–24	–	584
Lofric Nelaton (Female) (DT9400 – 5)	8–18	–	584
Lofric Nelaton (Paediatric) (DT9200 – 5)	8–10	–	584
ψ Bard Reliacath teflon coated Latex Nelaton (0159C)	14	–	594
ψ Bard Reliacath Plastic Nelaton (Male) (DT 5030)	12–18	–	475
ψ Bard Reliacath Plastic Nelaton (Female) (DT 5031)	12–18	–	475
ψ Bard Reliacath Plastic Nelaton (Paediatric) (DT 5032) ..	8–10	–	475
Simcare PVC Nelaton (Male) (WS 850/8–14)	8–14	–	615
Simcare PVC Nelaton (Female) (WS 5854/8–14)	8–14	–	591
Portex PVC Nelaton (Male) (300/111)	8–14	–	615
Portex PVC Nelaton (Female)	8–14	–	591
Warne PVC Jacques/Nelaton (DTS6115) – 1/5)	8–30	128	550
Warne PVC Jacques/Nelaton (Female) (DT6114) – 1/5)	8–18	118	500
Warne Soft Red Rubber Jacques/Nelaton (DT5143–1/5)	8–24	116	485

(b) Scott Catheter (Short curved tubular catheter for women and girls)
Specification: 38B

Simcare Polyethylene Scott (WS852/8–14)	8–14	–	993

* 5–units of plastic catheters, for example, represents on average one month's supply for patients practising intermittent catheterisation.

ψ Previously called Uriplan.

See pages 154–155 for names and addresses of suppliers

PART IXA - APPLIANCES

Appliance (1)	Size or Weight (2)	Basic Price (3) p

(c) **Foley Catheter** (indwelling Nelaton catheter with balloon
2 way)

Specification: 38A

	Balloon Size (ml) (see Note 2) (page 64)	Guage (Ch) (see Note 1) (page 64)	

(i) For Short/Medium Term Use: | | | each

Bard Uriplan Teflon-coated Latex Foley

(1265 LV)	10	12-26	168
(1266 LV)	30	16-28	168

Bard Uriplan Teflon-coated Latex Foley
- female (0169-LV) .... | 10 | 12-26 | 271

\# Bard Uriplan Teflon-coated Latex Foley
(1265 AL) .... | 10 | 12-26 | 191

Eschmann Folatex Latex Foley .... | 10 | 12-26 | 161
| | 30 | 16-28 | 161

Eschmann Folatex Latex Foley - female .... | 10 | 12-26 | 283
| | 30 | 16-28 | 283

Franklin Simplastic PVC Foley (5312) .... | 10 | 12-26 | 363
(5316) .... | 30 | 16-26 | 363

Franklin Soft Simplastic PVC Foley (5412) | 10 | 12-26 | 363
(5416) | 30 | 16-26 | 363

Franklin Soft Simplastic PVC Foley - female (5410) | 10 | 12-26 | 398
(5311) | 30 | 16-26 | 398

Warne 100 plus TM Latex Foley with Teflon coating
(DT 71002-1)................... | 10 | 12-26 | 166
(DT 73002-1)................... | 30 | 16-26 | 166

Warne 100 plus TM Female Latex Foley with Teflon
Coating
(DT 81002-1)................... | 10 | 12-22 | 227
(DT 83002-1) .... | 30 | 16-22 | 227

\# Pre-filled with sterile water

See pages 154-155 for names and addresses of suppliers

PART IXA - APPLIANCES

Appliance (1)	Size or Weight (2)	Basic Price (3) p

CATHETERS, URETHRAL, STERILE - cont.

	Balloon Size (ml) (see Note 2) (page 64)	Gauge (Ch) (see Note 1) (page 64)	
(ii) For Short/Medium Term Use - Paediatric:			each
Bard Uriplan Teflon-coated Latex Foley (0165PV) ...	5	8-10	485
Eschmann Folatex Latex Foley	5	8-10	294
Warne 100 plus TM Teflon-coated Latex Foley (DT 7052-1)	5	8-10	425
(iii) For Long Term Use:			
Bard Biocath 2-way Hydrogel coated Foley (Male) (DT 2265)	10	12-26	523
(DT 2266)	30	12-26	523
Bard Biocath 2-way Hydrogel coated Foley (Female) (DT 2269)	10	12-26	523
# Bard Biocath 2-way Hydrogel coated Foley (Male) (DT 2264)	10	12-26	545
# Bard Biocath 2-way Hydrogel coated Foley (Female) (DT 2268)	10	12-26	545
Bard Uriplan 2-Way Silicone Elastomer-coated Latex Foley (DT 1657)	10	12-26	580
(DT 1667)	30	16-28	580
Bard Uriplan 2-Way Silicone Elastomer-coated Latex Foley-female (DT 1647)	30	16-26	580
# Bard Uriplan 2-Way Silicone Elastomer Coated Latex Foley (DT 1657AL)	10	12-26	627
# Bard Uriplan 2-Way Silicone Elastomer Coated Latex Foley-female (DT 1637AL)	10	12-26	627
Bard Uriplan 2-Way All Silicone Foley (DT 1658)	10	12-24	598
(DT 1668)	30	16-24	598
Dow Corning Silastic Silicone Coated Foley			
336	10	12-24	626
334	30	16-28	626
Eschmann Folatex-S All Silicone Foley (male).......	10	12-26	659
	20	18	659
	30	20-26	659
(female) ...	10	12-26	602
	20	18	602
	30	20-26	602
Franklin Silikon 100 Foley (5492)	10	12-26	556
(5493)	20	18-20	556
(5493)	30	22-26	556

Pre-filled with sterile water

See pages 154-155 for names and addresses of suppliers

PART IXA - APPLIANCES

Appliance (1).	Size or Weight (2)		Basic Price (3) p
CATHETERS, URETHRAL, STERILE - cont.	Balloon Size (ml) (see Note 2)	Gauge (Ch) (see Note 1)	
(c) Foley Catheter - cont.	(page 64)	(page 64)	each

(iii) For Long Term Use - cont.

† Kendal Curity All Silicone Foley	10	14-24	500
	30	18-24	530
Sherwood Argyle All Silicone Foley	10	12-26	520
	30	16-26	520
Sherwood Argyle All Silicone Foley - Female	10	12-18	520
Simpla All Silicone Foley	10	12-26	615
	20	16-28	615
	30	20-26	615
Simpla All Silicone Foley - female	10	12-18	610
	30	20-26	610

(iv) For Long Term use - Paediatric:

Bard Biocath 2-way Hydrogel coated Foley (DT 2263)	5	8-10	523
Dow Corning Silastic Silicone Coated Foley 338 ..	5	8-10	596
Franklin Silikon 100 Foley	5	8-10	556
Sherwood Argyle All Silicone Foley	5	8-10	629
Simpla All Silicone Foley	5	8-10	645

See pages 154-155 for names and addresses of suppliers.

† to be deleted, October 1990

PART IXA – APPLIANCES

Appliance (1)	Size or Weight (2)	Basic Price (3)

PART IXA - APPLIANCES

Appliance (1)	Size or Weight (2)	Basic Price (3) p
		each

CELLULOSE TISSUE - see Gauze Tissues page 88

| CELLULOSE WADDING BP .... | 500 g | 179 |

May be supplied in stout polythene bag with clip
closure as received from the manufacturer or
wholesaler

| CHIROPODY APPLIANCES | | each |

| Adhesive Zinc Oxide Felt .... | 10 cm x 7.5 cm x 7 mm thick | 71 |

Adhesive, spread on semi-compressed all-wool
felt (Each in envelope)

| All-wool Felt .... | 10.5 cm x 8.3 cm x 7 mm thick | 63 |

Semi-compressed (Each in envelope)

| Animal Wool for Chiropody BP .... | 25 g | 68 |

(Syn. Animal Wool; Long Strand Lamb's wool
for chiropody)

| | | per box |
| Bunion Rings .... | | 48 |

Self-adhesive, semi-compressed felt
(in box of 4 pieces)

Corn Plasters
Salicylic Acid Adhesive Plaster BP
(Syn. Salicylic Acid Self-Adhesive Plaster;
Salicylic Acid Plaster)   each
Plaster containing 20% w/w salicylic acid in

| the plaster mass (each in envelope) .... | 7.5 cm x 4.5 cm | 19 |

Plaster containing 40% w/w salicylic acid in

| the plaster mass (each in envelope) .... | 7.5 cm x 4.5 cm | 23 |

When the strength of the plaster is not specified
by the prescriber a plaster containing 20% w/w
salicylic acid in the plaster mass should be
supplied.

| | | per box |
| Corn Rings .... | 5 mm thick | 48 |

Self-adhesive, semi-compressed felt in a box
of 9 pieces

| | | per pair |
| Metatarsal Pads .... | | 360 |

Specification 6   (Price of single
article is half
that of a pair)

| | | per piece |
| Sponge Rubber .... | 9 cm x 15 cm 10 mm thick | 51 |

Soft, non adhesive (in a box of 3 pieces)

PART IXA - APPLIANCES

Appliance (1)	Size or Weight (2)	Basic Price (3) p

CONTRACEPTIVE DEVICES

each

Fertility (Ovulation) Thermometer   140
    A mercury-in-glass thermometer, conforming to British
    Standard 691: 1979 - "Clinical maximum thermometers.
    Section three. Ovulation thermometers" Range 35^0
    to 39^0 Celsius subdivided in 0.1^0C with a minimum
    scale length of 32 mm and an accuracy of $+ 0.1^0C$.
    Figured at each degree. Each thermometer shall bear
    the BSI certification mark indicating approval under
    the BSI certification mark scheme, or be supplied with
    an individual certificate of examination by the BSI.

    To be supplied in a re-usable screw capped
    plastics protective case.

        NB: TEMPERATURE CHARTS (Form FP 1004)
            and advice on their use are given by the
            prescribing doctor.

Intrauterine Contraceptive Device

† Type 3 (Gravigard) Specification 7   845
    To be supplied in the individual sealed carton
    containing the sealed and sterilised pack as
    received from the manufacturer or wholesaler.

Type 4a (Ortho Gyne-T) Specification 7   899
    To be supplied in the individual sealed carton
    containing the sealed and sterilised pack as
    received from the manufacturer or wholesaler.

Type 4b (Ortho Gyne-T380S) Specification 7   940
    To be supplied in the individual sealed carton
    containing the sealed and sterilised pack as
    received from the manufacturer or wholesaler.

Type 5a (Multiload CU 250) Specification 7   675
    To be supplied in the individual sealed carton
    containing the sealed and sterilised pack as
    received from the manufacturer or wholesaler.

Type 5b (Multiload CU 250/Short) Specification 7   675
    To be supplied in the individual sealed carton
    containing the sealed and sterilised pack as
    received from the manufacturer or wholesaler.

† To be deleted 1 March 1991

0307M/17

Appliance (1)	Size or Weight (2)	Basic Price (3) p

CONTRACEPTIVE DEVICES — cont   each

Type 5c (Multiload CU 375) Specification 7   875
    To be supplied in the individual sealed carton
    containing the sealed and sterilised pack as
    received from the manufacturer or wholesaler.

    (Note: Prescribers have been advised that pain
    during and after insertion of Multiload Cu250,
    Multiload Cu250 Short or Multiload Cu375
    is more likely to occur in nulliparous than
    in parous women.)

Type 6 (Novagard; Nova — T) Specification 7   990
    To be supplied in the individual sealed carton
    containing the sealed and sterilised pack as
    received from the manufacturer or wholesaler.

    The type of the device and the size (where more
    than one is listed above) must be specified
    by the prescriber.

Vaginal Contraceptive Caps (Pessaries)
    Specification 8

Type A (Dumas Vault Cap) ....   No 1)
        Translucent rubber pessary   2)
        The size designation is moulded onto the rim   3)   472
                                           4)
                                         5)
    To be supplied in the individual pack as received
    from the manufacturer or wholesaler (plus postage 50p)

Type B (Prentif Cavity Rim Cervical Cap) ....   22 mm)
    Opaque rubber pessary   25 mm)   567
    The normal internal diameter of the rim is   28 mm)
    moulded onto the rim ....   31 mm)
    To be supplied in the individual pack as received
    from the manufacturer or wholesaler (plus postage 50p)

Type C (Vimule Cap) ....   No 1)
    Translucent rubber pessary   2)   472
    The size designation is moulded onto the rim   3)
    To be supplied in the individual pack as received from
    the manufacturer or wholesaler (plus postage 50p).

    The size of the pessary and the type must be
    specified by the prescriber.

Appliance (1)	Size or Weight (2)	Basic Price (3) p

CONTRACEPTIVE DEVICES – cont   each

Vaginal Contraceptive Diaphragm
    Complies with British Standard 4028:1966
    A dome-shaped occlusive diaphragm of good quality
    natural or synthetic rubber. The periphery is
    reinforced by an enclosed metal spring.

Type A ....   55–95 mm   549
    Rubber diaphragm with a flat metal spring.   (rising in 5 mm)
    The diaphragm is marked in the centre with
    the size.

Type B ....   55–95 mm   553
    Opaque rubber Diaphram with a coiled metal rim. The   (rising in 5 mm)
    diaphragm is marked on the periphery with the size.

    The diaphragm is enclosed in a strong plastics case,
    and cardboard box. A booklet of instruction to the
    patient regarding care and use may be included.

    The size of the diaphragm, and the type must be
    specified by the prescriber.

Cotton Wools – See Absorbent Cottons – page 58.

DOUCHES
    with Rectal and Vaginal fittings
Plastics Douche – Rigid plastics container, with 2m   1 litre   460
    approx. flexible plastics tubing, a tap and   approx.
    vulcanite or rigid plastics rectal pipe and plastics
    vaginal pipe.
    Spare Plastics Tubing ....   2 m approx.   75

    Where type not specified by the prescriber, plastics
    tubing to be supplied.

DRESSINGS   per pack
Boil Dressings   49

    To be supplied in the original pack as received
    from the manufacturer or wholesaler.
    Each pack contains three dressings, two boil
    dressings and one healing dressing. The boil
    dressing may be unmedicated or medicated with 1%
    Mercury and 0.2% Chlorocresol or, 0.75%
    Hexachlorophane.

PART IXA — APPLIANCES

Appliance (1)	Size or Weight (2)	Basic Price (3) p

DRESSINGS — cont each

Multiple Pack Dressing No 1 253
    To be supplied in sealed cartons as received
    from the manufacturer or wholesaler.
    Carton containing:
    Absorbent Cotton BP (interleaved) 25 g
    Absorbent Cotton Gauze. Type 13 Light BP, sterile 90 cm x 1 m
    Open—Wove Bandages BP (banded) 3 x 5 cm x 5 m

Multiple Pack Dressing No. 2 426
    To be supplied in sealed cartons as received from
    the manufacturer or wholesaler. To be supplied
    only where specifically ordered.
    Carton containing:
    Absorbent Cotton BP 100 g
    Absorbent Cotton Gauze, Type 13 Light BP sterile 3 x 90 cm x 1 m
    Open—Wove Bandages, BP (banded) 2 x 5 cm x 5 m
    1 x 7.55 cm x 5 m

Perforated Film Absorbent Dressing BP, Type 1 .... 5 cm x 5 cm 8
    (Melolin) (Syn.P.F.A. Dressing) 10 cm x 10 cm 17
    20 cm x 10 cm 31

    To be supplied in the individual pack, sealed and
    sterilised as received from the manufacturer or
    wholesaler.
    Where not specified by prescriber, the 5 cm size
    to be supplied.

Povidone Iodine Fabric Dressing Sterile
(Inadine)
Specification 43 .... 5 cm x 5 cm 17
    9.5 cm x 9.5 cm 31
Knitted Viscose Primary Dressing BP impregnated with a
polyethyleneglycol/water-based ointment complying with
Povidone Iodine Ointment USP 10% w/w

Sterile one piece pack consisting of a sealed impermeable
peelable pouch containing a single piece of the impregnated
fabric between two protective layers. The product shall
comply with the general requirements of the British
Pharmacopoeia for sterile surgical dressings.

The labelling of each pack shall include:

The title.
"Contents sterile if pack is undamaged or unopened".
Note. The exact number of packs, ie pieces, ordered by the
prescriber are to be dispensed. Where not specified by the
prescriber, the 5 cm size is to be supplied.

PART IXA – APPLIANCES

Appliance (1)	Size or Weight (2)	Basic Price (3) p

DRESSINGS – cont

each

Semipermeable Adhesive Film BP

Type 1 (Opsite Dressing)	10 cm x 12 cm	99

    To be supplied in the individual pack sealed
and sterilised as received from the
manufacturer or wholesaler.

Type 2 (Tegaderm Dressing)	10 cm x 12 cm	94

    To be supplied in the individual pack sealed
and sterilised as received from the
manufacture or wholesaler.

Type 3 (Bioclusive Dressing)	10.2 cm x 12.7 cm	93

    To be supplied in the individual pack sealed
and sterilised as received from the
manufacturer or wholesaler.

Semipermeable Waterproof Plastic Wound

Dressing BP sterile	8.5 cm x 6 cm	23

(Syn. Microporous Waterproof Plastic Wound
Dressing: Semi-permeable Plastic Dressing:
WMP Wound Dressing)
(Elastoplast Airstrip in which the pad consists of
Perforated Film Absorbent Dressing)
To be supplied in the individual pack sealed and
sterilised as received from the manufacturer or
wholesaler.

Standard Dressings
    To be supplied in sealed packets as received
    from the manufacturer or wholesaler.
No 4 Medium Elastic Adhesive Wound Dressing

per packet

BPC 1963	packet of 3	40

each

No.16 Eye Pad with Bandage BPC, sterile		39

PART IXA – APPLIANCES

Appliance (1)	Size or Weight (2)	Basic Price (3) p

DRESSINGS – cont

Sterile Dressing Packs

These packs contain a selection of sterile dressings
required in special nursing procedures (usually for
post–operative re–dressing of wounds) when
performed in the home. Prescribers have been
advised to order this dressing only for an individual
patient for whom such a sterile dressing operation is
essential and to restrict their orders to the number
of packs considered to be required for that patient.
The exact number of packs ordered by the prescriber
to be dispensed. A pack is to be used for each ·
sterile dressing operation.

each

Sterile Dressing Pack		55
Specification 10		
Sterile Pack containing:		
Gauze and Cotton Tissue Pad	8.5 cm x 20 cm	
Gauze Swabs 12 ply	4 x 10 cm x 10 cm	
Absorbent Cotton Balls, large	4 x 0.9g approx	
Absorbent Paper Towel	45 cm x 50 cm	
Water Repellent Inner Wrapper opens out	50 cm x 50 cm	

as a sterile working field

To be supplied in the individual pack, sealed and
sterilised as received from the manufacturer or
wholesaler.

Sterile Dressing Pack with   54
Non–Woven Pads (Patient Ready)

Specification 35		
Sterile Pack containing:		
Non–woven Fabric Covered Dressing Pad (Surgipad)	10 cm x 20 cm	
Non–woven Fabric Swabs (Topper 8)	4 x 10 cm x 10 cm	
Absorbent Cotton Wool Balls	4 x 0.8g approx	
Absorbent Paper Towel	45 cm x 51 cm	
Water Repellent Inner Wrapper opens out	50 cm x 50 cm	

as a sterile working field.

Sterile Knitted Viscose Dressing
Knitted Viscose Primary Dressing BP

To be supplied in the individual pack sealed and sterilised
as received from the manufacturer or wholesaler.

N–A Dressing	9.5 cm x 9.5 cm	23
Tricotex	9.5 cm x 9.5 cm	18

0307M/22

PART IXA – APPLIANCES

Appliance (1)	Size or Weight (2)	Basic Price (3) p

WOUND MANAGEMENT DRESSINGS

CALCIUM ALGINATE DRESSINGS

Indications: Medium to heavily exuding portion of wounds.

Precautions: Not the dressing of choice for infected wounds; not suitable for those which are very dry or covered with hard necrotic tissue.

DEXTRANOMER PASTE PAD DRESSING

For further information see Data Sheet.

Indications: Sloughy and infected, medium to heavily exudating wounds.

Precautions: Not suitable for dry wounds. Transient pain which can occur in the wound area can be avoided by wetting the wound before pad application.

HYDROCOLLOID DRESSINGS

Indications: Light to medium exudating wounds.

Precautions: Not suitable for infected wounds. Heavy exudate leads to too frequent changes of dressing. Dressing should seal round the borders of a wound.

HYDROGEL DRESSING

Indications: Dry "sloughy" or necrotic wounds; lightly exudating wounds; granulating wounds.

Precautions: Not suitable for infected or heavily – exudating wounds. Care should be taken to choose the appropriate secondary dressing.

POLYURETHANE FOAM DRESSING

Indications: Light to medium exudating wounds.

Precautions: Not recommended for dry superficial wounds. Dresssings should be secured at the edge by adhesive tape. Dressing should not be covered by occlusive tape or film. Secondary absorbent dressing is not required.

Appliance (1)	Size or Weight (2)	Basic Price (3) p

DRESSINGS

CALCIUM ALGINATE DRESSING - STERILE

Specification 41

		each
Type 1 (Sorbsan) .... 5 cm x 5 cm		77
Type 2 (Kaltostat) .... 5 cm x 5 cm		50
7.5 cm x 12 cm		122

Sterile one-piece pack consisting of:

A sealed peelable unit container or pouch containing a single piece of flat, evenly laid non-woven dressing which may be enclosed between two pieces of film or paper. Packed in an outer container not exceeding ten units.

The labelling of each pack shall include:

The title, and "Drug Tariff Specification" and the type. "Contents guaranteed sterile if pack is undamaged or unopened."

Note: The exact number of pieces, ie packs, ordered by the prescriber is to be dispensed.

DEXTRANOMER PASTE PAD DRESSING - STERILE

Specification 49   Sachet

("Debrisan Absorbent Pad") 3g   236
(Syn: dextranomer absorbent pad-sterile)

One-piece pack consisting of a sealed impermeable sachet containing a paste of dextranomer 90% with polyethylene glycol and water enclosed within a polyamide net pouch.

The dressing shall comply with the British Pharmacopoeia (BP) general requirements for sterile surgical dressings.

The labelling of each pack shall include:

The Title
Drug Tariff Specifications
Contents Sterile if pack is undamaged or unopened.

Note: The exact number of sachets, each containing one dressing, ie packs, ordered by the prescriber is to be dispensed.

Appliance (1)	Size or Weight (2)	Basic Price (3) p

HYDROCOLLOID DRESSING - SEMI-PERMEABLE - STERILE

Specification 42

Sterile one-piece pack consisting of: each

    Type 1. ("Granuflex")................... 10 cm x 10 cm   177
    Type 2. ("Comfeel") (Bevelled edge)....... 10 cm x 10 cm   164

A sealed peelable outer pouch containing a single piece of flat dressing
consisting of an adhesive hydrocolloid wound contact layer bonded to a
plastics foam layer, with an outer semi-permeable plastics film. The exposed
adhesive surface is covered with a suitable protective release paper.

The labelling of each pack shall include:

      The title
      "Drug Tariff Specification"
      "Contents sterile if pack is undamaged or unopened" - or similar

Note. The exact number of packs, ie pieces, ordered by the prescriber is to be dispensed.

HYDROGEL DRESSING - STARCH CO-POLYMER - STERILE   each

Specification 50

("Scherisorb")   15g   140

Sterile one-piece foil-laminate sachet pack incorporating a tear notch.

The labelling of each pack shall include:

    The title
    "Drug Tariff Specification"
    "Contents sterile if pack is undamaged or unopened"

Note: The exact number of packs, ie sachets, ordered by the prescriber is
to be dispensed.

POLYURETHANE FOAM DRESSING BP - STERILE

(Lyofoam)   7.5 cm x 7.5 cm   63
                                            10 cm x 10 cm   75

Sterile one piece pack consisting of:

    A sealed peelable unit container or pouch containing a single piece of flat
    dressing which may be enclosed between two pieces of film or paper packed
    in an outer container not exceeding 10 units.

Note: The exact number of pieces, ie packs, ordered by the prescriber is
to be dispensed.

0307M/25

each

DROPPERS   23

    - Glass, with bull-nose or curved flat end and fitted   (each in box)
with good quality rubber teat
Where appropriate, a dropper should be supplied
with eye, ear and nasal drops (See Part IV, containers,
(page 24) and Part XVI (page 340) for details of
prescription charges payable).

ELASTIC HOSIERY

GRADUATED COMPRESSION HOSIERY

Specification 40

Explanation of garments available

Class I

    Light (Mild) Support
    Compression at ankle   14mm Hg - 17mm Hg

    Indications - Superficial or early Varices. Varicosis during pregnancy

    Styles   - Thigh length or Below knee with knitted in heel (reciprocated)

Class II

    Medium (Moderate) Support
    Compression at ankle   18mm Hg - 24mm Hg

    Indications - Varices of medium severity
            - Ulcer Treatment and prevention of recurrence. Mild Oedema
            - Varicosis during pregnancy
            - Anklets and Kneecaps: for soft tissue support

    Styles   - Thigh length or Below knee with knitted in heel (reciprocated)

Class III

    Strong Support
    Compression at ankle   25mm Hg - 35mm Hg

    Indications - Gross Varices
            - Post Thrombotic Venous Insufficiency
            - Gross Oedema
            - Ulcer Treatment and prevention of Recurrence
            - Anklets and Kneecaps: for soft tissue support

    Styles   - Thigh length or Below knee open or knitted in heel (reciprocated)

NB.   The "Class" can be expressed either with roman or arabic numerals.

PART IXA – APPLIANCES

GENERAL NOTES

PRESCRIBING

Before the prescription can be dispensed the following details must be given by the prescriber.

1. Quantity – Single or Pair

2. Article including any accessories (see pages 83 & 84 for knit, style and price.)

3. Compression Class I, II or III

Constructional Specification

The Complete Structural Specification, as well as performance requirements are contained in the Drug Tariff Technical Specification Publication.

Specially Made Garments

1.   In cases where stock sizes are not suitable for patients owing to irregular limb dimesions, surgical stockings in the prescribed compression class, to be made to the patients' individual measurements, should be specified.

2.   All such garments are specially shaped during manufacture and may have a knitted–in or open heel and open or knitted in toe.

0307M/27

Diagrams of the Hosiery available:

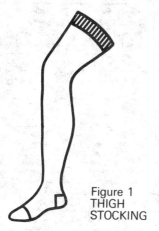

Figure 1
THIGH
STOCKING

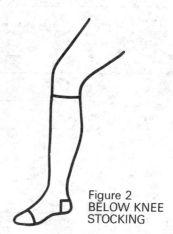

Figure 2
BELOW KNEE
STOCKING

Figs. 1 and 2 are available in a range of stock sizes or may be made to measure.

<u>ACCESSORIES</u> Any thigh length garment for men may be supplied with suspenders which are also available separately. **Suspender belts are also available.**

Figure 3

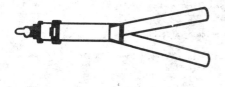

Figure 4

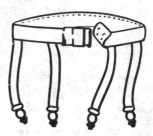

<u>SIZING</u>

All articles must conform to BS 6612:1985 with regard to size designation.

<u>LABELLING</u>

All articles must state clearly on the packaging that they conform with Drug Tariff Technical Specification No 40. The packaging should also provide clear washing instructions in conformity with handwashing at 40°C as defined in BS 2747 and washing instructions should be durably and clearly marked on each garment. the packaging should clearly define the garments percentage fibre content.

<u>ANKLETS AND KNEECAPS</u> (see page 84)

PART IXA – APPLIANCES

DESCRIPTION OF ARTICLES AVAILABLE			PRICE PER PAIR IN PENCE	
Compression Class (See page 79)	Type of Garment		Standard + Stock Sized Garments Supplied	Made-to-measure Garments Supplied
	Knit	Style		
I	Circular	Thigh	550	
		B. Knee	500	
	Lt. Wt Elastic Net	Thigh		1270
		B.Knee		990
II	Circular	Thigh	820	2400
		B.Knee	730	1500
	Net	Thigh		1270
		B. Knee		990
	Flat Bed	Thigh		2400
		B Knee		1500
III	Circular	Thigh	970	2400
		B Knee	830	1500
	One Way Stretch	Thigh		2400
		B Knee		1500

		PRICE PER ITEM IN PENCE
Accessories	Additional Price for fitted suspender	42
	Spare suspender for thigh stockings (Fig 3)	42
	Suspender Belt Drug Tariff Specification No 13 (Fig 4)	318

NB The reimbursible price for one item is half the price of a pair.

+ All such garments are specially shaped during manufacture and many have a knitted in or open heel and open or knitted in toe with the following exceptions:

   Class II   Flat Bed Knit can only be supplied with closed heel and open toe.

   Class III   One Way Stretch can only be supplied with open heel and open toe..

Note: Prescriptions should be endorsed with the style, ie, fabric or knit supplied.

For Above Knee Stockings – see Thigh Length.

ANKLETS AND KNEECAPS

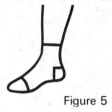

Figure 5

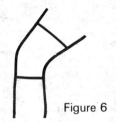

Figure 6

COMPRESSION CLASS	DESCRIPTION OF ARTICLES AVAILABLE		PRICE PER PAIR IN PENCE	
	KNIT	TYPE OF GARMENT	STANDARD STOCK SIZED GARMENTS	MADE TO MEASURE GARMENTS
CLASS II	Circular Knit	Anklet	420	420
		Kneecap	420	420
	Flat Bed	Anklet	880	880
		Kneecap	880	880
	Net	Anklet		816
		Kneecap		678
CLASS III	Circular	Anklet	584	584
		Kneecap	562	562
	One Way Stretch	Anklet	584	584
		Kneecap	562	562

APPENDIX

NOTES TO CONTRACTORS

Garments <u>previously</u> supplied against the discontinued Specification No's 11 and 12 and which <u>also</u> meet the performance standards in Specification No 40 are listed below.

Supplier – Credenhill Ltd
        Credalast Supreme Flatbed   – Class II

Supplier – STD Hereford
        Flatbed   – Class II

Supplier – Lastonet

        Lastolita Superfine   – Class I
        Lastoyarn Nylon   – Class II
        Lastoyarn Cotton   – Class II

Supplier – E Sallis Ltd

        Nyfine   – Class I
        Nyfine Lycra   – Class I
        Circular Standard   – Class II
        Eesiness Flat Bed   – Class II
        Sheerine Flat Bed   – Class II
        Below Knee Stout Thread   – Class III

Supplier – Scholl

        Nyalastik Thigh   – Class I
        Superlastik Thigh   – Class II
        Superlastik Below Knee   – Class II
        Soft Grip Thigh Cotton   – Class II
        Soft Grip below Knee   – Class II
        Seamless Fine One–Way stretch
        Below knee   – Class III

NB Size charts for these garments may differ from others in a manufacturer's range.

PART IXA - APPLIANCES

Appliance (1)	Size or Weight (2)	Basic Price (3) p
		Each
EYE BATHS .... Squat shape, with finger grips, rigid plastics, smooth inner surface and base, rounded rim.		23
EYE SHADES .... Plastics, semi-rigid, non flam., perforation along top for ventilation, to fit either eye (each in box)		20
		per box
FINGER COTS Seamless latex	box of 10	26 Δ
FINGER STALLS		per pkt
Polythene, Disposable - with apron	packet of 25 packet of 50	156 259 Δ
To be supplied in a sealed polythene envelope as received from the manufacturer or wholesaler		
		each
Simulated Leather .... On a knitted fabric base, with adjustable elastic wrist band	small,) medium, large,) extra-large)	29
GAUZES To be supplied in sealed packets* as received from the manufacturer or wholesaler		
Absorbent Cotton Gauze, Type 13 Light BP, sterile (Syn. Absorbent Gauze)	90 cm x 1 m 90 cm x 3 m 90 cm x 5 m 90 cm x 10 m	70 146 228 441
(*ie. an inner sealed paper wrapper, in a film wrapped carton) Where no quantity is stated by the prescriber the 1 m packet should be supplied.		
Absorbent Cotton Gauze, Type 13 Light BP not sterilised .... (Syn. Absorbent Gauze) (*ie. sealed paper wrapper)	25 m roll	977
Absorbent Cotton and Viscose Ribbon Gauze BP Sterile (*ie. an inner sealed paper wrapper, in an outer paper wrapper)	1.25 cm x 5 m 2.5 cm x 5 m	49 56

0307M/32

PART IXA – APPLIANCES

Appliance (1)	Size or Weight (2)	Basic Price (3) p

GAUZE DRESSINGS (IMPREGNATED)
.   To be supplied in a sealed packet or double sealed
    box as received from the manufacturer or wholesaler

		per pack

Chlorhexidine Acetate Gauze Dressing BP

| Sterile one–piece pack consisting of .... | 5 cm x 5 cm | 17 |
| A sealed peelable pouch containing a single piece | 10 cm x 10 cm | 35 |

of impregnated gauze between 2 leaves of paper or
plastics film of the size.

The labelling of each pack shall include:
"Sterile"; the size of its contents, "5 cm x 5 cm" or
"10 cm x 10 cm"; and "The dressing shall not be
issued nor the contents used if the wrapper or seal is
broken".

Note: The exact number of pieces ordered by the
prescriber are to be dispensed.
Where not specified by the prescriber, the 5 cm size
to be supplied.

Framycetin Sulphate Gauze Dressing BP
    (Sofra Tulle)

		each
Sterile one–piece pack consisting of:	10 cm x 10 cm	24

A sealed peelable foil laminate wrap containing a
single piece of impregnated gauze between two
layers of parchment.
The labelling of each pack shall include:

"Sterile" "10 cm x 10 cm".
"This package shall not be issued nor the contents
used if the wrapper is broken".
Each pack bears instructions for cutting to smaller
sizes.

Note: The exact number of pieces ordered by the
prescriber are to be dispensed.

PART IXA - APPLIANCES

Appliance (1)	Size or Weight (2)	Basic Price (3) p

GAUZE DRESSINGS (IMPREGNATED) - cont

Paraffin Gauze Dressing BP Sterile
    (Syn. Tulle Gras Dressing)
                  each

Sterile one-piece pack consisting of: ....   10 cm x 10 cm   23
    A peelable outer wrap containing a single piece of
    impregnated gauze each piece separately enclosed
    between two pieces of film or paper.

                  per pack
Sterile pack of ten pieces ....   10 cm x 10 cm   162
    Note: Packs to be supplied against orders for:
    1-7 pieces - the exact number of one-piece packs
    respectively.
    8-15 pieces - 1 x 10 piece pack
    16-25 pieces - 2 x 10 piece pack.
    Over 25 pieces - Supply to the nearest 10 below
    (1-5) or above (6-10)

    The labelling of each pack shall include:
    "Sterile" "10 cm x 10 cm"
    "This package shall not be issued nor the contents
    used if the wrapper is broken"

Povidone Iodine "Gauze" Dressing - see page 74

Sodium Fusidate Gauze Dressing Sterile, BP
    (Fucidin Intertulle)
    Cotton gauze of leno weave impregnated with
    Sodium Fusidate ointment BP 2% w/w
                  each

Sterile one-piece pack consisting of: ....   10 cm x 10 cm   22
    A sealed peelable foil laminate wrap containing a
    single piece of impregnated gauze between two
    layers of paper.
    The labelling of each pack shall include:
    "Sterile" "10 cm x 10 cm".
    "This package shall not be issued nor the contents
    used if the wrapper is broken".
    Note: The exact number of pieces (ie packs) ordered
    by the prescriber to be dispensed.

Gauze Pads - See SWABS page 104
Gauze Swabs - See SWABS page 104

PART IXA — APPLIANCES

Appliance (1)	Size or Weight (2)	Basic Price (3) p

GAUZE TISSUES   each
   To be supplied in sealed packets* as received from
   the manufacturer or wholesaler. (See Note 2 page 57).

Gauze and Capsicum Cotton Tissue BPC ....   Size 1   126
   (Thermogene)   approx. 28g
   (Syn. Capsicum Tissue)   Size 2   202
   (*ie. film wrapped cartons)   approx. 56g
   Where the size or weight is not specified by the
   prescriber the approx. 28 g carton should be
   supplied.

Gauze and Cellulose Wadding Tissue BP 500g   219
   (Syn. Cellulose Tissue)
   (*ie. sealed paper wrapper or heat—sealed stout
   plastics bag)

Gauze and Cotton Tissue BP ....   500 g   457
   (Syn. Absorbent Gauze Tissue, Gauze Tissue)
   (*ie. sealed paper wrapper or heat—sealed stout
   plastics bag).

Gauze and Cotton Tissue (Drug Tariff) ....   500 g   342
   Specification 14
   (*ie. sealed paper wrapper or heat—sealed stout
   plastics bag)
   To be supplied only where specifically ordered.

HYPODERMIC EQUIPMENT

A.   Hypodermic Needles   22
      Specification 15
      British Standard 3522 Luer mount needles

      NB: The appropriate British Standard Needles
      must be supplied if the old "Hypo" sizes are
      ordered.

B.   Hypodermic Syringes
        Glass barrels with Luer taper conical fittings.

(i)   Syringes for use with U100 insulin
      Both 0.5 and 1 ml syringes are marked in units
      and are numbered every 10 units. Each
      graduation between the numbered calibrations
      represents one unit of insulin on the 0.5 ml syringe
      and two units of insulin on the 1 ml syringe.

      a.   U100 Insulin Syringe ....   0.5 ml   972
      British Standard 1619/2 1982 Luer mount   1 ml   972
      syringe bearing the BSI Certification mark
      supplied with a dosage chart in a strong
      box.

0307M/35

PART IXA – APPLIANCES

Appliance (1)	Size or Weight (2)	Basic Price (3) p
HYPODERMIC EQUIPMENT – cont.		each

Where the size is not specified by the prescriber the 0.5 ml syringe should normally be supplied unless the patient is known to take more than 50 units of insulin per injection.

b. Pre-Set U100 Insulin Syringe, ... Specification 36. For use by blind patients. Supplied with a dosage chart in a strong box.	1 ml	1581
c. Click/Count U100 Insulin Syringe .... (Hypoguard) Specification 36. For blind patients who have been trained in the use of this syringe and for whom the Pre-Set syringe is unsuitable. Supplied with a dosage chart in a strong box.	1 ml	1450

(ii) Syringes for use with drugs other than insulin Ordinary Purpose Syringe .... Specification 16. British Standard 1263 Luer mount Syringe. Supplied with two Luer needles in a strong box.	1 ml 2 ml	533 533

C. (i) Hypodermic Syringe Carrying Case .... Specification 17a (revised 1983) May be prescribed for patients who need to use their syringe away from home. Suitable for use with all Drug Tariff insulin syringes in paragraph B above except the Pre-Set U100 insulin syringefor which a special, deeper cap must be fitted.		193
(ii) Screw-Cap to convert Hypodermic Syringe Carrying Case for use with Pre-Set U100 insulin syringe. Specification 17b.		63

PART IXA — APPLIANCES

Appliance (1)	Size or Weight (2)	Basic Price (3) p

HYPODERMIC EQUIPMENT — cont

D. (i) U100 INSULIN SYRINGES WITH NEEDLE — STERILE, SINGLE-USE OR SINGLE PATIENT-USE
Specification 39A

Sterile: intended for single use, or single patient-use, for the injection of U100 insulin by diabetics in the community.

NB. Intended for use immediately after filling, and not for containing insulin over extended periods of time.

The syringe may have permanently fixed needles, or detachable needles fitted ready for use. Alternatively syringes with a separate needle may be supplied.
The sterility of the fluid pathway and functional surfaces shall be protected by either end caps or suitable unit containers. These shall be tamper-evident.

Needles shall be not less than 12mm long and the range of needle diameters shall be as follows:

0.5mm (25G), 0.45mm (26G), 0.4mm (27G) and 0.36mm (28G).

COLOUR CODING: The colour orange is used to distinguish U100 insulin syringes.

INSTRUCTIONS FOR DISPOSAL — These are given on the multiple (sales) packs and may be given on the unit or multiple unit pack. (A leaflet containing guidance may be supplied at the time of issue).

Note: Each scale graduation represents one unit on the 0.5ml syringe and two units on the 1.0ml syringe. The graduations on the syringes are clearly numbered at every 5 or 10 units. When the size is not specified by the prescriber the 0.5ml syringe with needle should be supplied. If the patient is known to inject more than 50 units of insulin per injection the 1.0 ml syringe shall be supplied.

Size	each
0.5ml syringe and needle	9
1.0ml syringe and needle	9

PART IXA – APPLIANCES

Appliance (1)	Quantity (2)	Basic Price (3) P

(ii) HYPODERMIC NEEDLES–STERILE, SINGLE–USE
         Specification 39B
      For use with the re–usable glass syringes listed in this Tarriff
      on pages 88 and 89. The sterility of the fluid pathway and
      functional surfaces shall be protected by a suitable unit
      container, which shall be tamper–evident.

      The needles shall be of length not less than 12mm and the
      following diameters may be supplied:

              0.5 mm (25G)
              0.45 mm (26G)
              0.4 mm (27G)

              Size   Each

              0.5 mm   100   220
              0.45 mm   100   220
              0.4 mm   100   220

(iii) NEEDLE CLIPPING (CHOPPING) DEVICE   104

      Consisting of a clipper to remove the needle from its hub, and
      incorporating a suitable receptacle from which the cut–off
      needles cannot be retrieved. Sufficiently robust to accommodate
      needles of diameter 0.45 mm (26 G) or finer; length: 16 mm or
      shorter. Not generally suitable for use with lancets. Designed
      to hold approximately 1,200 such needles.

E.   LANCETS – STERILE, SINGLE–USE

Manufactured in accordance with the DHSS Guide to GMP.

Point moulded in plastic –

Type A – Mount fluted longitudinally   100   305
           (Owen Mumford "General Purpose" ... 200   578
           Sherwoods "Monolet") ...   200   550

Type B – Mount with concentric ribs ...   100   305
           (Owen Mumford "Unilet")   200   578

Type C – Mount: flat and oblong ...   100   290
           (B D "Micro-fine")

Disposal: Please see guidance in para 4 of the Appendix to Part IXR page 278.

PART IXA – APPLIANCES

Appliance (1)	Quantity (2)	Basic Price (3) p

Appliances (1)	Size or Weight (2)	Basic Price (3) p
INHALERS		each
Earthenware (Nelson) with mouthpiece	500 ml approx.	1025
Spare Tops - mouthpiece and cork .... See also Nebulizers page 59		115

INSUFFLATORS

Plastics - For inhalation of fine powders

    Type 2 (Intal Spinhaler). For inspiratory operation; plastics body with detachable mouthpiece, containing a propeller, with integral capsule piercing device of stainless steel; to hold unit dose capsules of microfine powdered medicament.

                    180

    Type 3 (Rynacrom). For nasal inspiratory operation; tubular plastics body with a nose-piece which is removable to insert unit dose capsule of microfine powdered medicament, enclosed by plastics dust cover; fitted with a rubber bulb incorporating a needle device for piercing the capsule.

                    166

    Type 4 (Becotide Rotahaler, Ventolin Rotahaler, Ventide Rotahaler). For inspiratory operation; plastics body with detachable mouthpiece, containing capsule opening device; to hold unit dose capsules of microfine powder medicament.

                    78

LARYNGECTOMY PROTECTORS

Type 1 (Buchanan) ....
   Specification 18
   A bib containing plastics foam, which is tied around the neck, for covering the stoma, and helping to filter and humidify the air.

                    223

Type 2 (Laryngofoam) ....
   Specification 18
   A piece of plastics foam with an adhesive strip (each individually wrapped in sealed plastics envelope).

   5.1 cm x 6.2 cm   24
   4 mm thick

PART IXA - APPLIANCES

Appliances (1)	Size or Weight (2)	Basic Price (3) p
		per piece
LATEX FOAM, ADHESIVE, raised cotton backed	22.5 cm x 45 cm	324
Specification 19	7 mm thick	
	box of 4	
Adhesive, Latex Foam, is for use with Cervical Collars		
LINT		
To be supplied in sealed packets (film wrapped cartons) as received from the manufacturer or wholesaler.		
		each
Absorbent Lint BPC	25 g	56
(Syn. Absorbent Cotton Lint; Cotton Lint; Plain Lint	100 g	175
White Lint)	500 g	737
Where no quantity is stated on the prescription form the 25g pack is to be supplied.		
Boric Acid Lint BPC 1963	100 g	194
(Syn. Boric Lint; Boracic Acid Lint)		
NIPPLE SHIELDS PLASTICS		38
Semi-rigid polypropylene base with latex teat (Each in carton). (Not to be confused with Breast Shields page 63)		
PESSARIES		
Hodges		
Perspex	8 mm thick	
Specification 20(1)	55-108 mm	
	sizes	
	1-2	219
Perspex Hodges Pessaries to be supplied against any	3	234
orders for Vulcanite and Celluloid Hodges Pessaries	4-6	236
Shaped pessaries (eg. Hodges) may revert to a	7	244
circular shape if boiled	8-9	276
	10-12	280
Ring		
Fluid Ring	15 mm thick	
Filled with combination fluid	1-12	525
	other sizes	Invoice price (see note 4) (page 57)

PART IXA - APPLIANCES

Appliances (1)	Size or Weight (2)	Basic Price (3) p

PESSARIES - cont

each

Ring - cont

Polythene .... 7.5 mm thick)
    Specification 20(ii)

       50-80 mm)
       rising in 3 mm))   125
       85-100 mm)
Note: (rising in 5 mm))
Antiseptics containing phenols or cresols should be   110 mm)
avoided as these may be absorbed causing severe
irritation in use. The rings may be washed in soapy
water or boiled.

PVC .... 1.25 cm thick)
    Specification 20(iii)   50-80 mm)
       (rising in 3 mm))   135
       85-100 mm)
       (rising in 5 mm))
       110 mm)

Antiseptics containing phenols or cresols should be
avoided as these may be absorbed causing irritation
in use.

Watch-Spring .... Thin   1.25 cm thick
    Covered with india-rubber   Sizes 1-12   334
                       Medium   1.4 cm thick
         Sizes 1-12   363
         All other sizes   Invoice price (see note 4) (page 57)

each

With Perforated Rubber Diaphragm ....   1.3 cm thick
    (Syn. Diaphragm Pessary)   Sizes 1-12   283
         51 mm to 86 mm
         All other sizes   Invoice price (see note 4) (page 57)

PLASTERS

each

Belladonna Adhesive Plaster BP ....   medium   45
    (Syn. Belladonna Self-Adhesive Plaster; Belladonna   19 cm x 12.5 cm
    Plaster)   large   86
         28 cm x 17.5 cm

Salicylic Acid Adhesive Plaster BP

    See Chiropody Appliances page 70.

Spool-Plasters - See Surgical Adhesive Tapes; page 101.

0307M/42

PART IXA – APPLIANCES

Appliances (1)	Size or Weight (2)	Basic Price (3) p

PROTECTIVES

EMA Film Gloves–Disposable ....   small   per pkt
(Dispos-A-Gloves) Specification 21   medium   149
For use as a barrier during manual evacuation of   large
the bowel.   (packet of 30)

Polythene Occlusive Dressings, Disposable
    For use as occlusive dressings with medicated
    creams.

                                                          per pkt
    Gloves – Polythene, 100 gauge ....   packet of 25   50
    To be supplied in sealed packets as received from
    the manufacturer or wholesaler. "The sizes given are
    lay-flat width x length."   per pkt of 10

	Size or Weight	Basic Price p
Arm Sleeve – Polythene, 150 guage	small 20 cm x 30 cm	69
	large 20 cm x 60 cm	69
Leg Sleeve – Polythene, 150 gauge	small 25 cm x 45 cm	75
	medium 32.5 cm x 45 cm	75
	large 32.5 cm x 75 cm	75
Foot Bag – Polythene, 150 gauge	32.5 cm x 50 cm	69
Shorts – Polythene, 150 gauge	medium	200
	large	230
Torso Vest – Polythene, 150 gauge	60 cm x 60 cm	230
Trousers – Polythene, 150 gauge	large	395

    Note: Packets of 10 articles containing the number
    nearest to the number ordered by the prescriber
    are to be supplied.
    ie. for:
    Up to 15 articles, 1 packet of 10,
    16–25 articles, 2 packets of 10.

RECTAL DILATORS

    Specification 22
Perspex non-boilable   each
    (a) Cone 19 mm diam. tapering to 12.5 mm ....   small   346 Δ
       Base 2.5 cm diam. – Length 8.6 cm
    (b) Cone 19 mm diam. tapering to 15 mm ....   large   346 Δ
       Base 2.5 cm diam. Length 8.6 cm

    The dilators may be washed in hot soapy water.

STOCKINETTE
    To be supplied in sealed packets as received from the
    manufacturer or wholesaler.

    When Elasticated Stockinette is ordered or prescribed
    without qualification, the term is to be interpreted
    as Elasticated Surgical Tubular Stockinette.

PART IXA – APPLIANCES

Appliances (1)	Size or Weight (2)	Basic Price (3) p

STOCKINETTE – cont   each

Cotton Surgical Tubular Stockinette BP	2.5 cm x 1 m	18
Heavyweight.	5 cm x 1 m	28
(Syn. Plain Cotton Stockinette)	7.5 cm x 1 m	35
	10 cm x 6 m	240

    NB. 1 m in length for use as a basic for Plaster of
        Paris or other bandages. 6 m length for use
        as a compression bandage.

Elasticated Surgical Tubular Stockinette BP.
    (Syn: Elasticated Tubular Bandage: ESTS; Formerly, Elasticated Stockinette)

Size or Weight (2)   Basic Price (3) p each

Size or Weight		(Lastogrip)	(Rediform)	(Tensogrip)	(Texagrip)	(Tubigrip)
6.25 cm x 0.5m		45	51	51	39	60
6.25 cm x 1.0m	'B'	82	92	95	76	109
6.75 cm x 0.5m		48	55	55	41	65
6.75 cm x 1.0m	'C'	86	98	100	78	116
7.5 cm x 0.5m		48	56	55	41	65
7.5 cm x 1.0m	'D'	86	100	100	78	116
8.75 cm x 0.5m		54	62	62	43	73
8.75 cm x 1.0m	'E'	93	105	108	83	124
10.0 cm x 0.5m		54	63	62	43	73
10.0 cm x 1.0m	'F'	93	105	108	83	124
12.0 cm x 0.5m		57	64	65	50	76
12.0 cm x 1.0m	'G'	107	121	125	94	143

NB 1:   Where the brand is not stated by the prescriber the basic price of this stockinette
      must not exceed:

	each (p)		each (p)
6.25 cm x 0.5 m	39	6.75 cm x 0.5 m	41
6.25 cm x 1.0 m	76	6.75 cm x 1.0 m	78
7.5 cm x 0.5 m	41	8.75 cm x 0.5 m	43
7.5 cm x 1.0 m	78	8.75 cm x 1.0 m	83
10.00 cm x 0.5 m	43	12.00 cm x 0.5 m	50
10.00 cm x 1.0 m	83	12.00 cm x 1.0 m	94

PART IXA – APPLIANCES

Appliances (1)		Size or Weight (2)	Basic Price (3) p
STOCKINETTE – cont			each
Elasticated Surgical Tubular Stockinette Foam Padded (Tubipad) Specification 25			
Heel, Elbow, Knee	small	6.5 cm x 60 cm	181
	medium	7.5 cm x 60 cm	195
	large	10.0 cm x 60 cm	210
Sacral	small	22 cm x 27 cm)	
	medium	28 cm x 27 cm)	929
	large	35 cm x 27 cm)	

Elasticated Viscose Stockinette

(Syn: Lightweight Elasticated Viscose Tubular Bandage)
(Tubifast)
    Specification 46
A lightweight plain-knitted elasticated tubular fabric
for dressing retention; washable for reuse.

Medium Limb	5.0 cm x 1 m (Green Line)	59
Large Limb	7.5 cm x 1 m (Blue Line)	77
Limbs O.S., Heads		
Trunks (Child)	10.75 cm x 1 m (Yellow Line)	124
Trunks (Adult)	17.5 cm x 1 m (Beige Line)	156

Appliances (1)	Size or Weight (2)	Basic Price (3) p

STOCKINETTE - cont

Elastic Net Surgical Tubular Stockinette
Specification 26
A lightweight, elastic, openwork net tubular fabric for
retaining dressings, particularly on awkward sites; for
long-term re-use.

		each
Type A. (Netelast)		
Arm/leg	1.8 cm (Size C) x 40 cm	32
Thigh/head	2.5 cm (Size E) x 60 cm	58
Trunk (adult)	4.5 cm (Size F) x 60 cm	85
Trunk (OS adult)	5.4 cm (Size G) x 60 cm	114
Type B. (Setonet) - Now withdrawn		
Type C. (Macrofix)		
Arm/leg	1.8 cm (Size C) x 40 cm	25
Thigh/head	2.7 cm (Size E) x 60 cm	48
Trunk (adult)	5.5 cm (Size F) x 60 cm	67
Trunk (OS adult)	6.0 cm (Size G) x 60 cm	85

NB. Both size and type must be specified by the
prescriber.

Ribbed Cotton and Viscose Surgical Tubular
Stockinette BP
(Syn. Ribbed Cotton and Viscose Stockinette)
For use as protective dressings with tar-based and
other non-steroid ointments.

Type A. Lightweight (Seton)		
Arm/leg (child); arm (adult)	5 cm x 5 m	158
Arm (OS adult); leg (adult)	7.5 cm x 5 m	205
Leg (OS adult)	10 cm x 5 m	272
Trunk (child)	15 cm x 5 m	392
Trunk (adult)	20 cm x 5 m	452
Trunk (OS adult)	25 cm x 5 m	542

Type B. Heavyweight (Eesiban)		
Arm/leg (child); arm (adult)	5 cm x 5 m	147
Arm (OS adult); leg (adult)	7.5 cm x 5 m	192
Leg (OS adult)	10 cm x 5 m	253
Trunk (child)	15 cm x 5 m	365
Trunk (adult)	20 cm x 5 m	420
Trunk (OS adult)	25 cm x 5 m	504

NB. One 5 m length of the relevant width is sufficient to provide two sets of dressing for a pair
of limbs or a trunk.
Two full suits for an OS adult are provided from one pack each of the 7.5 cm, 10 cm and 25 cm
widths.
Two full suits for a standard sized adult are provided from one pack each of the 5 cm, 7.5 cm
and 20 cm widths.
Two full suits for a young child are provided from one pack each of the 5 cm and 15 cm widths.

PART IXA - APPLIANCES

Appliances (1)	Size or Weight (2)	Basic Price (3) p

SUPRAPUBIC BELTS: Replacements only

List Price
(See Clause 8B(ii))

NB. 1.   Original Belts are supplied by the Hospital Service

2.   Prescription ordering replacement of a complete Belt or Outfit may
only be accepted by a pharmacy or appliance contractor who will carry
out the actual measurement, fitting and supply of the belt.

3.   Orders for replacement of "a belt" are to be taken as being for the
belt alone and the prescription referred back to the prescriber to specify
orders for a Complete Belt or Outfit where such appears to be required.

Parts may include the following:

Rubber Flaps
Rubber Shields
Rubber Understraps
Rubber Urinal, single or double-chambered
    (See Incontinence Appliances - page 108)
Belt, webbing
Night Drainage Bag, Plastics (See Incontinence Appliances - page 107)
Night Tube and Glass or Plastics Connector

SUPRAPUBIC CATHETERS:

Invoice Price
(see note 4)
(page 57)

Catheters, Suprapubic, Self-retaining
eg. de Pezzer, Malecot's, Dowse's

NB: For prescribable Urethral Catheters including 2 way Foley
      Catheters see under Catheters, Urethral.

Introducers ordered for use with self-retaining catheters.

PART IXA – APPLIANCES

Appliances (1)	Size or Weight (2)	Basic Price (3) p

SURGICAL ADHESIVE TAPES

To be supplied on spools, suitably protected, or in tins or cartons as received from the manufacturer or wholesaler.

each

Elastic Surgical Adhesive Tape BP .... (Syn. Elastic Adhesive Plaster, Zinc Oxide Elastic Adhesive Plaster; Zinc Oxide Elastic Self-Adhesive Plaster)	2.5 cm x 1.5 m stretched 2.5 cm x 4.5 m stretched 5 cm x 4.5 m (See Elastic Adhesive Bandage page 61.)	53 102
Impermeable Plastic Surgical Adhesive Tape BP (Syn. Water proof Plastic Surgical Adhesive Tape; Water proof Plastic Self-Adhesive Plaster; Plastic Adhesive Strapping; Water proof Strapping)	2.5 cm x 3 m 2.5 cm x 5 m 5 cm x 5 m 7.5 cm x 5 m	79 118 152 219
Impermeable Plastic Surgical Synthetic Adhesive Tape BP (Syn. Waterproof Plastic Surgical Synthetic Adhesive Tape) (Blenderm Surgical Tape)	2.5 cm x 5 m 5 cm x 5 m	109 207

† Permeable Woven Synthetic Adhesive Tape BP (Syn. Permeable Woven Synthetic Adhesive Tape)

	Basic Price	
Size or weight	Dermicel	Leukosilk
1.25 cm x 5 m	63	55
2.5 cm x 5 m	91	80
5 cm x 5 m	160	140

† Where no brand is stated by the prescriber the basic price of the tape must not exceed that of the cheaper listed brand.

PART IXA – APPLIANCES

Appliances (1)	Size or Weight (2)	Basic Price (3) p

SURGICAL ADHESIVE TAPES – cont

each

Permeable Non-Woven Surgical Synthetic Adhesive
   Tape BP (Syn. Permeable Non-Woven Synthetic
   Adhesive Tape)

Size or Weight (2)	Basic Price (3) p each

	Dermilite	Hypal 2	Leukopor	Micropore	Scanpor
1.25cm x 5m	46	46	39	43	34
2.5 cm x 5m	72	71	61	67	54
5.0 cm x 5m	128	129	107	119	96

Where no brand is stated by the prescriber, the basic
price of the tape supplied must not exceed.

1.25 cm x 5 m	34
2.5 cm x 5 m	54
5 cm x 5 m	96

Zinc Oxide Surgical Adhesive Tape BP ....
   (Syn. Zinc Oxide Self Adhesive Plaster;
   Zinc Oxide Plaster; Adhesive Plaster)

1.25 cm x 1 m	20
1.25 cm x 3 m	41
1.25 cm x 5 m	57
2.5 cm x 1 m	27
2.5 cm x 3 m	62
2.5 cm x 5 m	84
5 cm x 5 m	142
7.5 cm x 5 m	201

Where no size or quantity is stated by the prescriber
2.5 cm x 1 m should be supplied.

PART IXA – APPLIANCES

Appliances (1)				Size or Weight (2)	Basic Price (3) p

SURGICAL SUTURES

ABSORBABLE SUTURES
Sterile Catgut Chromic BP

per pack
of 12

Ethicon Code No	Metric Gauge	Length	Needle	
W480	2	75 cm	16 mm Curved Cutting	1266
W548	2	75 cm	16 mm Curved round bodied	1266
W565	3.5	75 cm (extra chromic)	25 mm Tapercut half circle heavy	1464
W488	3.5	75 cm	35 mm Tapercut half circle	1428
W492	3.5	75 cm	45 mm Tapercut half circle heavy	1464

NON ABSORBABLE SUTURES

Sterile Polyamide 6 Suture, Monofilament BP

	Ethicon Code No	Metric Gauge	Length	Needle	
†	W506	0.7	35 cm (black)	16 mm curved cutting	1027
	W507	0.7	45 cm (black)	15 mm slim blade curved cutting	1271
	W319	1.5	45 cm (blue)	19 mm curved reverse cutting	845
	W539	1.5	45 cm (blue)	25 mm slim blade curved cutting	1413
	W320	2.0	45 cm (blue)	26 mm curved reverse	900

Sterile Polyamide 66 Suture, Braided BP

Ethicon Code No	Metric Gauge	Length	Needle	
W 5414	3.5	1 m (black)	50 mm Tapercut half circle heavy	1210

Sterile Braided Silk Suture BP

	Ethicon Code No.	Metric Gauge	Length	Needle	
	W 501	1.5	75 cm (black)	16 mm curved cutting	870
	W 533	2	45 cm (black)	25 mm super cutting curve	1118
	W 321	3	45 cm (black)	26 mm curved reverse cutting	870
†	W 667	3	75 cm (black)	35 mm curved reverse cutting	870

SKIN CLOSURE STRIPS, STERILE (Steri-strip)

per pack of
12 envelopes

3M Code No.

GP 41	6 mm x 75 mm	3 strips per envelope	574

Note: These items are specifically for personal administration by the prescriber.

† To be deleted 1 December 1990

0307M/50

PART IXA – APPLIANCES

Appliances (1)	Size or Weight (2)	Basic Price (3) p

SWABS (See note * below on sterile swabs)

Gauze Swabs   per pkt
    Gauze Swab, Type 13 Light BP Non Sterile | 10 cm sq | 425
       Swabs of folded 8-ply undyed gauze | 100 pads per pkt |

    Gauze Swab, Type 13 Light BP, sterile* .... | 7.5 cm sq | 25
       Sterile swabs of folded 8-ply undyed gauze | 5 pads per pkt |

    Filmated Gauze Swab BP Non Sterile............... | 10 cm sq |
       A thin layer of Absorbent Cotton enclosed | 100 pads per pkt | 525
       Absorbent Cotton Gauze Type 13 Light | |

Non-Woven Fabric Swabs
    Non-Woven Fabric Swab (Topper 8)
    Non Sterile .... | 10 cm sq | 269
       Specification 28 | 100 pads per pkt |
       Swabs of folded 4 ply non-woven viscose fabric
       These swabs are an alternative to Gauze Swabs,
       Type 13 Light BP, for general swabbing and
       cleansing purposes.

    Non-Woven Fabric Swab, Sterile*
    (Topper 8) .... | 7.5 cm sq | 21
       Specification 28 | 5 pads per pkt |
       Sterile swabs of folded 4-ply non-woven
       viscose fabric. These swabs are an
       alternative to Gauze swabs, Type 13 Light
       BP sterile.

    Filmated Non-Woven Fabric Swab (Regal) Non Sterile | 10 cm sq | 367
    Specification 29 | 100 pads per pkt |
    Swabs of folded 8-ply non-woven viscose fabric
    containing a film of viscose fibres to increase
    absorbency.
    These swabs are an alternative to Filmated
    Gauze Swabs BP for general swabbing and
    cleansing purposes.

    *NB. Sterile Swabs – These sterile dressings are to
be supplied in packs of 5 swabs 7.5 cm square in a
sealed pack as received from the manufacturer, supplier
or wholesaler. They should not be confused with the
10 cm size in packets of 100 swabs used for general
swabbing purposes.

The exact number of sterile swabs ordered are to be supplied
except for orders not in multiples of 5 (See note 2 page 57).
A packet to be used for each sterile dressing operation; unused
swabs to be discarded as unsterile.

PART IXA — APPLIANCES

Appliances (1)	Size or Weight (2)	Basic Price (3) p
SYRINGES		each
Bladder/Irrigating .... Polypropylene with catheter nozzle graduated from 0 to 100 ml in 5 ml graduation marks, clearly numbered in multiples of 10.	100 ml	299
Ear .... Plastics—plasticised PVC polymer, moulded in one piece, fine pointed.	60 ml approx	84
Enema .... Higginson's: Plastics — plasticised PVC polymer or rubber bulb, with inverted flutter valve moulded in the tube, or with metal valve, (duralumin or pewter), inserted in the tube; full length tubes; polypropylene rectal pipe; PVC polymer or rubber vaginal pipe; PVC polymer shield.		460
Spare Vaginal Pipes — Plastics or rubber, straight	15 cm	36
TEST TUBES	12.5 cm x 16 mm	4

PART IXA — APPLIANCES

TRUSSES

The price listed in respect of a truss specified in the following list is the basic price [see Part II, Clause 8] on which payment will be calculated pursuant to Part II, Clause 6 A and B for the supply of such a truss. PROVIDED it is so supplied on an order by the prescriber and complies fully with the specification, included in this Part [see Note 5] and in the Drug Tariff Technical Specifications.

Before the prescription can be dispensed three details must be given by the prescriber:
   (i)   Single, or double, and the side, if single
   (ii)   Position   — eg. Inguinal,
                          Scrotal
   (iii) Type   — eg. Spring truss
                          Elastic band truss.

In the event of a dispute between the patient and the pharmacy or the appliance contractor about whether the truss supplied is satisfactory, the doctor's decision shall be binding.

Appliances (1)	Size or Weight (2)		Basic Price (3) p
TRUSSES [See Part 1, Clause 2 page 3]			
Spring Truss			
Specification 31(a)			
Spring Trusses shall conform to the British Standard 2930 : 1970 for Surgical Spring Trusses			each
Inguinal	Single		1841
	Double		2568
Inguinal Rat-tail	Single		2267
	Double		3388
Femoral	Single		2033
	Double		3146
Scrotal	Single		2267
	Double		3388
Double Inguinal/Scrotal			3440
Back Pad, fixed or sliding (if ordered)		extra	523
Slotted, polished Spring Ends (if ordered)	Single	extra	280
	Double	extra	565
"Special Trusses	Single	extra	586
— conforming to the requirements in	Double	extra	1157
Specification 31b			
NB: Requirement for a "Special" Truss should normally be confirmed by the prescriber.			
Replacements and repairs:-			
Understrap for Inguinal or Femoral Trusses			162

PART IXA - APPLIANCES

Appliances (1)	Size or Weight (2)	Basic Price (3) p

TRUSSES - cont

Elastic Band Truss
    Specification 31(b)
    Elastic Band Trusses shall conform to the British
    Standard 3271: 1970 for Surgical Elastic Band Trusses.   each

Inguinal	Single	1306
	Double	2175
Scrotal	Single	1359
	Double	2213

Umbilical, Single belt		1483
Double belt where specified by prescriber		2131
"Special" Trusses	Single extra	384
- conforming to the requirements in	Double extra	556
Specification 31b		
NB: Requirement for a "Special" Truss should		
normally be confirmed by the prescriber		

Umbilical "Belts" - Infants	25 cm - 56 cm	526
India-rubber, porous, with stud-fastenings		

URINALS, PORTABLE - See Incontinence Appliances - page 108

URINALS, PORTABLE - See Incontinence Appliances - page 108

		each
URINE SUGAR ANALYSIS SET (Clinitest)		267

Test tube, dropper, colour chart, instruction sheet
and analysis record, with one bottle of 36 Diagnostic
Solution-Tablets of Copper, in a suitable container.

Replacement Test Tubes, hard glass		26
Replacement Droppers, glass with fine pointed		
rubber teat		26
Replacement Diagnostic Solution Tablets of Copper (See page 274)		

INCONTINENCE APPLIANCES

1. Prescribers and suppliers should note that products not included in the list are <u>not</u> prescribable (See Part 1 Clause 2). Attention is drawn particularly to the information on the average life-in-use of each type of product which, together with the pack size, should enable prescribers to calculate their patients' requirements with reasonable accuracy.

2. Only basic information on each product has been provided and prescribers may on occasions wish to seek further information about certain products eg when assessing a patient for the first time. If so, this is always available from the manufacturers (addresses and telephone numbers are given at the end of the entry). Information may also be sought from community nurses and community pharmacists. Where possible manufacturers'/suppliers' order code numbers have been shown but prescribers should note that the order numbers shown are not necessarily the full codes for the appliances they wish to order. This is particularly true of urinal systems where additional code numbers are usually necessary to denote variations from the basic design and individual sizes.

3. Prescribers are reminded that incontinence pads (including products not necessarily described as such but using the absorption principle), incontinence garments, skin wipes and occlusive devices such as female vaginal devices and male penile clamps are not prescribable under the Drug Tariff provisions.

List of components and accessories:

Drainable Dribbling Appliances (page 109)

Incontinence Belts (page 110)

Incontinence Sheaths (page 111)

Incontinence Sheath Fixing Strips and Adhesives (page 118)

Leg Bags (page 119)

Night Drainage Bags (page 125)

Suspensory Systems (page 127)

Tubing and Accessories (page 128)

Urinal Systems (page 132)

PART IXB – INCONTINENCE APPLIANCES

DRAINABLE DRIBBLING APPLIANCES

Bags or pouches which use absorptive material to soak up urine are not prescribable.

With the exception of the Alexa bags the appliances listed below may be re-used, on average, for at least a month.

Manufacturer (1)	Appliance (2)	Order No (3)	Quantity (4)	List Price (5) p
CS Bullen Ltd	Dribblet bag	LU–15	10	1844
	Dribblet sheath bag	LU–20	10	4137
Henleys Medical Supplies Ltd	Alexa dribbler bag – Plain bag with draw strings	DB–A	100	422 Δ
As above with non return valve		DB–B	100	1188 Δ
Kinpax & F T Mitchell Group Ltd	Dribbling bag with loops and tapes	Fig 18	1	1300
	Drip Male Urinal with tap	M 100	1	3480
	Replacement belt for M100	JB/100	1	860
Leyland Medical Ltd (Peoplecare)	Peoplecare drip male urinal	755300	1	3797
Thackraycare (C F Thackray Ltd)	Aquadry male incontinence pouch – short tube	78–0375	1	565
	– long tube	78–0367	1	565
	Aquadry drip type urinal	57–1016	1	4300
Ward Surgical Appliance Co	Male Dribbling bag with diaphragm and belt	WM60	1	2113
	Plastic dribbling bag	WM61	1	1052

PART IXB - INCONTINENCE APPLIANCES

INCONTINENCE BELTS

Average Life In Use - 6 Months

Manufacturer (1)	Appliance (2)	Order No (3)	Quantity (4)	List Price (5) p
Downs Surgical Ltd - see Simcare				
GU Manufacturing Ltd - see S G & P Payne - page 139				
Kinpax & F T Mitchell Group Ltd	Waist belt for Kipper bags	KBWB	1	430
	1 1/2 webbing band	WB	1	430
Leyland Medical Ltd (Peoplecare)	Waist and support strap for Kipper bag	886103	1	510
	Rubber belt	810029	1	281
Simcare	Rubber belt	WS-101-61A	1	432
	Elastic support			
	Medium	WS-102-01K	1	924
	Small	WS-103-01P	1	924
	Large	WS-103-04V	1	924
	Web Belt	WS-105-91C	1	895
		WS-106-01C	1	895
		WS-107-01G	1	895
Ward Surgical Appliance Co	Waist belt for black kipper bag	WM62	1	387
	Rubber belt for PP Urinal	WM63	1	335
S R Willis & Sons Ltd	Waist band 2" white	SP/6/532/38"	1	409
	web with looped	SP/6/532/46"	1	409
	strap to support bag	SP/6/532/larger	1	438

INCONTINENCE SHEATHS

The incontinence sheaths (also known as penile sheaths and external catheters) listed below, are, except where indicated, of the soft, flexible, latex type. Sheaths are available with and without fixing devices which may be applied externally (around the outside of the sheath) or internally (around the penis between the skin and the sheath). A list of fixing devices and other adhesion products is included at page 118.

Each Sheath may be left in place for 1 to 3 days between changes.

Manufacturer (1)	Appliance (2)	Order No (3)	Quantity (4)	List Price (5) p
Aldington Laboratories Ltd	Dryaid penile sheath (including adhesive strip)			
	Small	834001	20	2236
	Medium	834002	20	2236
	Large	834003	20	2236
	Ex Large	834004	20	2236
	Dryaid penile sheath (without strip)			
	Small	861001	20	1294
	Medium	861002	20	1294
	Large	861003	20	1294
	Ex Large	861004	20	1294
	Polymed penile sheath (including adhesive strip)			
	Small	835001	20	2236
	Medium	835002	20	2236
	Large	835003	20	2236
	Ex Large	835004	20	2236
	Polymed penile sheath (without strip)			
	Small	863001	20	1294
	Medium	863002	20	1294
	Large	863003	20	1294
	Ex Large	863004	20	1294
Bard Ltd	Uriplan Penile sheath (including crixiline strip) 20mm, 25mm, 30mm, 35mm, 40mm	C52	30	2700
	Uriplan Penile sheath 20mm, 25mm, 30mm, 35mm, 40mm	U52	30	1920

INCONTINENCE SHEATHS - cont

Manufacturer (1)	Appliance (2)	Order No (3)	Quantity (4)	List Price (5) p
Bard Ltd - contd	Uriplan Uro sheath (washable - may be re-used many times) small, (25mm) medium (35mm) large (40mm)	1502	1	400
Camp Ltd	Posey incontinence sheath A	6551	10	435
	Posey 'Fast Flow' Incontinence			
	Sheath 25mm	6557	10	540
	30mm	6557	10	540
	35mm	6557	10	540
Coloplast Ltd	Conveen Sheath with Anti-Kink Device (including Uriliner adhesive strip)			
	paediatric	5117	30	3330
	very small	5120	30	3330
	small	5125	30	3330
	medium	5130	30	3330
	large	5135	30	3330
	Ex-large	5140	30	3330
	Conveen self-sealing Urisheath			
	small	5200	30	3270
	medium	5205	30	3270
	large	5210	30	3270
ConvaTec Ltd	Accuseal penile sheath			
	20mm diameter	S400	10	699
	25mm "	S401	10	699
	30mm "	S402	10	699
	35mm "	S403	10	699
	40mm "	S404	10	699
Downs Surgical Ltd - see Simcare				
EMS Medical Ltd	Incontinence sheath			
	20mm	T110/S	100	3900
	25mm	T110/M	100	3900
	30mm	T110/L	100	3900
	35mm	T110/EL	100	3900
	Incontinence sheath with liner			
	25mm	T25/S	30	2600
	30mm	T30/M	30	2600
	35mm	T35/L	30	2600
	40mm	T40/XL	30	2600

0308M/5

PART IXB — INCONTINENCE APPLIANCES

INCONTINENCE SHEATHS — cont

Manufacturer (1)	Appliance (2)		Order No (3)	Quantity (4)	List Price (5) p
Eschmann Bros and Walsh Ltd — see Simcare					
Fry Surgical International Ltd	Uridom (including adhesive strip		476–413–130	30	2610
Hospital Management and Supplies Ltd	Macrodom (including adhesive strip) with 2" tube			30	1825
	with 5" tube			25	1917
	Macrodom Plus (including adhesive strip)				
	Small		GS7656	30	2300
	Medium		GS7657	30	2300
	Large		GS7658	30	2300
Incare Medical, Products	Male Incontinence sheath Self Adhesive	22mm	9806	15	1970
		26mm	9807	15	1970
		30mm	9809	15	1970
		34mm	9808	15	1970
Mediplus Ltd	Medimates incontinance sheath with single sided adhesive strip (Straight)	20mm	S20S	30	2670
		25mm	S25S	30	2670
		30mm	S30S	30	2670
		35mm	S35S	30	2670
		40mm	S40S	30	2670
	(bulb)	25mm	B25S	30	2670
		30mm	B30S	30	2670
		35mm	B35S	30	2670
	Medimates incontinence sheath with double sided adhesive strip (straight)	20mm	S20D	30	2850
		25mm	S25D	30	2850
		30mm	S30D	30	2850
		35mm	S45D	30	2850
		40mm	S40D	30	2850
	(bulb)	25mm	B25D	30	2850
		30mm	B30D	30	2850
		35mm	B35D	30	2850

0308M/6

PART IXB - INCONTINENCE APPLIANCES

INCONTINENCE SHEATHS - cont

Manufacturer (1)	Appliance (2)		Order No (3)	Quantity (4)	List Price (5) p
North West Medical Supplies Ltd	Uridrop incontinence sheath				
	Size 1	(70mm)	30/80	30	1120
	" 2	(80mm)	30/81	30	1120
	" 3	(100mm)	30/82	30	1120
	" 4	(107mm)	30/83	30	1120
	" Paed	42mm	30/60	30	1120
	" Paed	55mm	30/61	30	1120
	Uridrop incontinence sheath and uristrip adhesive strip				
	Size 1	(70mm)	8480	30	2160
	" 2	(80mm)	8481	30	2160
	" 3	(100mm)	8482	30	2160
	" 4	(107mm)	8483	30	2160
	Size Paed 42mm		8460	30	2160
	" Paed 55mm		8461	30	2160
S G & P Payne	Incontiaid penile and Adhesive Strips available in 5 sizes 0-4 with instruction			10	1075
	Incontiaid penile sheath available in 5 sizes 0-4			1	70
	Incontiaid Adhesive strips			10	350
Rehab Products - see Camp Ltd					
Salt & Son Ltd	Heritage Cohesive/Sheath Pack	17mm	ZL0023	30	2741
		22mm	ZL0024	30	2741
		25mm	ZL0025	30	2741
		32mm	ZL0026	30	2741
		34mm	ZL0027	30	2741
	Male Continence Sheath				
		17mm	ZL0028	10	619
		22mm	ZL0029	10	619
		25mm	ZL0030	10	619
		32mm	ZL0031	10	619
		34mm	ZL0032	10	619

PART IXB - INCONTINENCE APPLIANCES

INCONTINENCE SHEATHS - cont

Manufacturer (1)	Appliance (2)	Order No (3)	Quantity (4)	List Price (5) p
Seton Products Ltd	Seton incontinence sheath			
	Small	7625	30	2599
	Medium	7626	30	2599
	Large	7627	30	2599
	Ex Large	7628	30	2599
	Seton male incontinence Sheath with Self Adhesive Liner			
	Small	7630	30	3096
	Medium	7631	30	3096
	Large	7632	30	3096
	Ex Large	7633	30	3096
Sherwood	Texas Catheter (including adhesive strip)	8884-731300	12	759
	Uri Drain Sheath double sided adhesive strap			
	small(25mm)	1814-736600	10	700
	medium(30mm)	1814-736700	10	700
	large(35mm)	1814-736800	10	700
Simcare	Incontinence Sheath			
	very small	WS165-00-D	1	105
	small	WS165-01-F	1	111
	medium	WS165-03-K	1	111
	large	WS165-05-P	1	111
	extra large	WS165-07-T	1	111
	Uro Flo sheath (including adhesive strip)			
	small	WS166-01-K	30	3380
	medium	WS166-02-M	30	3380
	large	WS166-03-P	30	3380
	Uro Flow sheath Mk 2			
	small	WR166-01-N	30	3380
	medium	WR166-02-Q	30	3380
	large	WR166-03-S	30	3380
	Male incontinence sheath	48-232-14	100	5390

PART IXB – INCONTINENCE APPLIANCES

INCONTINENCE SHEATHS – cont

Manufacturer (1)	Appliance (2)	Order No (3)	Quantity (4)	List Price (5) p
Simpla Plastics Ltd	Bubble U Sheath (with adhesive foam strip)			
	Small	380820	30	2184
	Medium	380821	30	2184
	Large	380822	30	2184
	Ex Large	380823	30	2184
	Bubble U Sheath with Self Adhesive Uriseal liner			
	Small	380910	30	3140
	Medium	380911	30	3140
	Large	380912	30	3140
	Ex Large	380913	30	3140
Smith &, Nephew Medical, Ltd	Regard, Sheath and liners			
	Small	6131	30	3000
	Medium	6132	30	3000
	Large	6133	30	3000
	Ex Large	6134	30	3000
Squibb Surgicare Ltd – see ConvaTec Ltd				
Thackraycare (C F Thackray Ltd)	Aquadry Penile sheath			
	Small (dia 22mm)	57-0508	10	878
	Medium (dia 26mm)	57-0516	10	878
	Large (dia 28mm)	57-0524	10	878
	Ex Large (dia 32mm)	57-0532	10	878
	Aquadry Penile Sheath (Bulbous End)			
	Small	78-74-18	30	2532
	Medium	78-74-26	30	2532
	Large	78-74-34	30	2532
	Aquadry Freedom sheath (Self-adhesive)			
	Small	78-6268	30	3560
	Medium	78-6276	30	3560
	Large	78-6284	30	3560

PART IXB – INCONTINENCE APPLIANCES

INCONTINENCE SHEATHS – cont

Manufacturer (1)	Appliance (2)	Order No (3)	Quantity (4)	List Price (5) p
Thackray Care (CF Thackray) Contd	Aquadry Freedom plus sheath (Self-adhesive)			
	Small	78-6292	30	3560
	Medium	78-6306	30	3560
	Large	78-6314	30	3560
Vygon (UK) Ltd	Peniflow penile sheath	477	40	3840
Warne Franklin Medical Ltd	Portasheath 25mm	800046	25	1955
	30mm	800047	25	1955
	35mm	800048	25	1955
	Secure external catheter kit (including adhesive strip)			
	25mm diameter	4000-025	10	749
	30mm "	4000-030	10	749
	35mm "	4000-035	10	749

PART IXB - INCONTINENCE APPLIANCES

INCONTINENCE SHEATH FIXING STRIPS & ADHESIVES
(Available separately from sheaths)

Manufacturer (1)	Appliance (2)	Order No (3)	Quantity (4)	List Price (5) p
Aldington Laboratories Ltd	Dryaid strip	832005	20	942
	Polymed strip	832004	20	942
Associated Hospital Supply see Bio Diagnostics				
Bio Diagnostics	Urifix Tape 5m	SU1	1	490
Camp Ltd	Posey Sheath holder Adult	6550	12	1200
	Paediatric	6555	12	1020
ConvaTec Ltd	Urihesive strips	S120	15	514
Dow Corning Ltd	Adhesive B (Silicone adhesive aerosol)	895-6	207g	897
	355 Medical Adhesive (brush-on silicone adhesive)	DC355	1	272
EMS Medical	Urifix Tape 5 m	T115	1	490
North West Medical Supplies Ltd	Uristrip Adhesive strip	30/84B	30	1040
Rehab Products - see Camp Ltd				
Salt & Son Ltd	Heritage Sheath Collar Pack	ZL0022	30	315
Squibb Surgicare Ltd - See ConvaTec Ltd				
Thackraycare (C F Thackray Ltd)	Aquadry medical adhesive (brush-on)	470651	1	300
	Aquadry Penile liners	781649	20	750

LEG BAGS

The leg bags listed are suitable for collection of urine from indwelling catheters or incontinence sheaths. They are intended for daytime use although the larger bags may have adequate capacity for overnight use by some patients. The bags may be worn in different positions on the leg and the intended position (eg thigh, knee or calf) will determine the length of the inlet tube. The bags are attached to the leg by means of straps (included with each pack) which are generally either latex or foam with velcro fasteners.

Plastic leg bags identified in the list with an asterisk* may on average be used for 5-7 days, sometimes longer. With proper care and cleansing rubber leg bags are re-usable for 4-6 months.

Manufacturer (1)	Appliance (2)	Order No (3)	Quantity (4)	List Price (5) p
Aldington Laboratories Ltd	*350ml long tube leg bag	240003	10	1236
	*350ml short tube leg bag	240002	10	1152
	*500ml long tube leg bag	240005	10	1236
	*500ml short tube leg bag	240004	10	1152
Argyle	*350ml leg bag	8887-601121	20	3680
	*500ml leg bag	8887-601139	20	3680
Bard Ltd	*Uriplan Range:- shaped leg bags with tap outlet and elastic velcro straps			
	*350 ml, direct inlet	DT3S	10	2080
	*350 ml, 12" inlet tube	DT3L	10	2050
	*500 ml, direct inlet	DT5S	10	2100
	*500 ml, 4" inlet tube	DT5M	10	2109
	*500 ml, 12" inlet tube	DT5L	10	2109
	*750 ml, direct inlet	DT7S	10	2120
	*750 ml, 4" inlet tube	DT75	10	2120
	*750 ml, 12" inlet tube	DT7L	10	2120
	*Seton leg bags Long tube	7671	10	930
	Short tube	7679	10	900
	*Seton Urisac leg bag			
	*350 ml Long tube	7660	10	1050
	*350 ml Short Tube	7661	10	1020
	*500 ml Long tube	7662	10	1140
	*500 ml Short tube	7663	10	1110
	*750 ml Long tube	7664	10	1220
	*750 ml Short tube	7665	10	1170

* Plastics

PART IXB - INCONTINENCE APPLIANCES

LEG BAGS - cont

Manufacturer (1)	Appliance (2)	Order No (3)	Quantity (4)	List Price (5) p
Bradgate Unitech Ltd	Careline Log Bag			
	350 ml short tube	45-01SVC	10	1800 |
	350 ml long tube	45-02SVL	10	1800 |
	500 ml short tube	45-05SVC	10	1850 |
	500 ml long tube	45-06SVL	10	1850 |
	750 ml short tube	45-09SVC	10	1900 |
	750 ml long tube	45-10SVL	10	1900 |
Camp Ltd	Leg bag - thigh	6552	10	530
	- calf	6553	10	530
Coloplast Ltd	*Conveen leg bag 500 ml			
	10cm tube	5150	10	1670
	40cm tube	5151	10	1670
	*Conveen Contour 600ml			
	leg bag (adjustable tube)	5170	10	2100
	5cm inlet tube	5172	10	2100
	30cm inlet tube	5173	10	2100
	*Conveen Contour 800 ml			
	leg bag 45cm tube	5175	10	2100
ConvaTec Ltd	*350ml Accuseal leg bag	S435	10	1326
	*500ml Accuseal leg bag	S450	10	1464
	*750ml Accuseal leg bag	S475	10	1464
Downs Surgical Ltd - see Simcare				
EMS Medical Ltd	*Leg drainage bag (long tube)	T120	10	1180
	*Leg drainage bag (short tube)	T122	10	1180
GU Manufacturing Ltd - see S G & P Payne				
Incare Medical Products	*Urinary Leg Bag 540 ml with 37 cm extension tube	9820	10	2110
	*Urinary Leg Bag 540 ml with direct inlet connector	9814	10	1999

* Plastics

PART IXB - INCONTINENCE APPLIANCES

LEG BAGS - cont

Manufacturer (1)	Appliance (2)	Order No (3)	Quantity (4)	List Price (5) p
Kinpax & F T Mitchell Group Ltd	Kipper bag, black white or trans	KB	1	1970
	*Leg Drainage bag with tap outlet (350ml) plastic	LBWT/350	10	1690
	*Leg Drainage bag with tap outlet (500ml) plastic	LBWT/500	10	1690
	*Leg Drainage bag with tap outlet (750ml) plastic	LBWT/750	10	1765
Leyland Medical Ltd (Peoplecare)	Kipper bag, trans/white without strap and buckle	886000	1	1748
	Kipper bag, trans/white	886001	1	2132
	All black rubber	886002	1	2132
	Plastic	886003	1	2132
LIC Ltd	*Tribag (various tube lengths)		1	95
SG & Payne	*Incontaid leg bag		1	210
	Single chambered rubber bag with box outlet tap	GU532/879/LT	1	3920
	Single chambered rubber bag for night use	GU532/879/40	1	4280
	Single chambered bag for females	GU532/879/F	1	3180
	Single-chambered rubber bag, Kipper style	GU532/879	1	3180
	Single-chambered rubber bag, Ross type	GU532/879/R	1	3630

Redland Medical Ltd - see Bard Ltd
Rehab Products - see Camp Ltd

* Plastics

PART IXB - INCONTINENCE APPLIANCES

		LEG BAGS - cont		

Manufacturer (1)	Appliance (2)	Order No (3)	Quantity (4)	List Price (5) p
Salt & Son Ltd	*Heritage leg bag pack	ZL0020	5	814
†	*350ml - short tube	ZL2320	1	95
†	*500ml - short tube	ZL2322	1	105
†	*500ml - long tube	ZL2323	1	107
†	*750ml - short tube	ZL2324	1	117
†	*750ml - long tube	ZL2325	1	120
	*350ml - short tube	ZL0405	10	1020
	*500ml - short tube	ZL0407	10	1130
	*500ml - long tube	ZL0408	10	1150
	*750ml - short tube	ZL0409	10	1260
	*750ml - long tube	ZL0410	10	1290
Seton Products Ltd - See Bard Ltd				
Simcare	*Catheter drainage bag -			
	large	WP-205-01-S	1	305
	small	WP-205-05-B		305
	Rubber bag with leg strap	WS111-05-U	1	2822
	Uro-flo			
	Leg Bags			
	*350ml short tube	WS 167-20-T	10	1190
	*350ml long tube	WS 167-21-V	10	1190
	*500ml short tube	WS 167-22-X	10	1190
	*500ml long tube	WS 167-23-A	10	1190
	*750ml short tube	WS 167-24-C	10	1190
	*750ml long tube	WS 167-25-E	10	1190
	Uro-flo X Tend Leg Bag			
	short tube 500 ml	WS 167-51-B	10	2110
	long tube 500 ml	WS 167-54-E	10	2110
Simpla Plastics Ltd	Trident			
	*350ml short tube	370802	10	2087
	*500ml long tube	370817	10	2109
	*500ml short tube	370807	10	2109
	*750ml long tube	370819	10	2119
	*750ml short tube	370809	10	2119
	*750ml adjustable long tube	370904	10	2119
Smith & Nephew Medical LTD	Regard			
	*350ml bag, short tube	6137	10	2087
	*500ml bag, short tube	6138	10	2109
	*500ml bag, adjustable long tube	6139	10	2109
	*750ml bag, adjustable long tube	6141	10	2119

* Plastics
† to be deleted 1 October 1990

PART IXB - INCONTINENCE APPLIANCES

LEG BAGS - cont

Manufacturer (1)	Appliance (2)	Order No (3)	Quantity (4)	List Price (5) p
Squibb Surgicare Ltd - See ConvaTec Ltd				
Thackraycare	*Aquadry catheter drainage			
	bag, small	78-6438	10	2065
	large	78-6411	10	2120
	*Aquadry leg bag			
	*350ml short tube	78-3463	10	1850
	*350ml long tube	78-3501	10	1850
	*500ml short tube	78-3471	10	1850
	*500ml long tube	78-3528	10	1850
	*750ml short tube	78-3498	10	1850
	*750ml long tube	78-3536	10	1850
Universal Hospital	Unicorn leg bag			
Supplies	*350 ml short tube	UN222V	10	1760
	*500 ml short tube	UN333V	10	1780
	*500 ml long tube	UN333VL	10	1780
	*750 ml short tube	UN444V	10	1800
	*750 ml long tube	UN444VL	10	1800
H G Wallace Ltd	Leg bag with rubber cap outlet			
(Medical Assist Ltd)	and natural latex straps			
	*350 ml short tube	350	10	1862
	*500 ml short tube	500	10	1919
	Leg bag with valve outlet and			
	natural latex straps			
	*350 ml short tube	350 EM-TY	10	2022
	*350 ml long tube	350 V 30	10	2078
	*500 ml short tube	500 EM-TY	10	2065
	*500 ml long tube	500 V 30	10	2118
	*750 ml short tube	750 EM-TY	10	2096
	*750 ml long tube	750 V 30	10	2108

* Plastics

LEG BAGS — cont

Manufacturer (1)	Appliance (2)	Order No (3)	Quantity (4)	List Price (5) p
Wallace H G Ltd (cont) (Medical Assist Ltd)	Leg bag with twist tap and elastic straps			
	*350 ml short tube	E 350 V	10	2031
	*350 ml long tube (30cm)	E 350 V 30	10	2084
	*500 ml short tube	E 500 V	10	2052
	*500 ml long tube (30cm)	E 500 V 30	10	2111
	*500 ml medium tube	E 500 V M	10	2084
	*750 ml short tube	E 750 V	10	2096
	*750 ml long tube (30cm)	E 750 V 30	10	2108
	Tri-Form leg bag			
	*500 ml short tube	TF 500	10	2052
	*500 ml medium tube	TF 500 M	10	2084
	*500 ml long tube	TF 500 L	10	2111
Ward Surgical Appliance Co	Kipper bag, black trans or white rubber	WM64	1	1763
	*Leg drainage bag 350ml	WM65	10	851
	500ml	WM66	10	877
	750ml	WM67	10	929
	Ward's Comfort Range			
	*Leg drainage bag 350ml	WM68	10	855
	500ml	WM69	10	879
	750ml	WM70	10	925
Warne-Franklin Medical	*750ml leg bag	800100	10	860
S R Willis & Sons Ltd	Rubber bag for catheter drainage, short neck leg strap	SP/1	1	2418
	As above with 2" web belt and bag support strap	SP/1a	1	2829
	Female rubber drainage bag with conical mount	SP/5	1	2295
	As above with web belt and looped support strap	SP/5a	1	2706
	Rubber single chambered bag with olive mount	SP/6/532	1	2430
	As above with web belt and support strap	SP/6a/532	1	2829

* Plastics

PART IXB – INCONTINENCE APPLIANCES

NIGHT DRAINAGE BAGS

These bags are suitable for night-time use for the collection of urine from indwelling catheters or incontinence sheaths. They are generally used in conjunction with a bag hanger which, being a nursing aid, is not prescribable. Supply arrangements for bag hangers tend to vary throughout the country but they are normally supplied through the community nursing service.

The Drainage Bags listed below have a life in use of, on average 5-7 days

Manufacturer (1)	Appliance (2)	Order No (3)	Quantity (4)	List Price (5) p
Aldington Laboratories Ltd	2 litre urine drainage bags	C	10	901
		CV	10	1005
		CVT	10	1042
	2 litre urine drainage bag	DVT	10	937
Bard Ltd	Uriplan drainage bag	DT81-3131	10	860
Bradgate Unitech	Careline E1, 2 litre urine drainage bag with 90 cm inlet tube	45-30-LBC	10	156
	Careline E2, 2 litre urine drainage bag with 90 cm inlet tube and non return valve	45-40-LBC	10	165
	Careline E4, 2 litre urine drainage bag with 90 cm inlet tube and non return valve and tap outlet	45-20-IDC	5	410
Coloplast Ltd	Conveen drainage bag 1.5 Litre	5062	10	1050
ConvaTec Ltd	Accuseal drainage bag	S500	5	637
	Night drainage bag	S320	5	637
Downs Surgical Ltd – see Simcare				
EMS Medical Ltd	2 litre urine drainage bag	T200	100	9800
Hospital Management and Supplies Ltd	Macpak 3		5	386
	Macpak 1 Non drainable bag		10	147
	Macpak 5 Non drainable bag		10	146
Kinpax & F T Mitchell Group Ltd	2 litre drainage bag with tap outlet	2LNB	1	115
Rand Rocket Ltd	Non drainable urine drainage bag			
	Short tube	9778	25	375
	Long tube	9777	25	375

0308M/18

PART IXB — INCONTINENCE APPLIANCES

NIGHT DRAINAGE BAGS — cont

Manufacturer (1)	Appliance (2)		Order No (3)	Quantity (4)	List Price (5) p
Redland Medical Ltd — See Bard Ltd					
Salt and Son	2 litre urine drainage bag †		ZL2310	1	88
	2 litre urine drainage bag		ZL0400	10	925
Seton Products Ltd — See Bard Ltd					
Simcare ††	Uro-flo night drainage bag	A	WS-167-44-J	1	116
		B	WS-167-46-N	1	116
	Uro-flo night drainage bag	male	WS-167-45-K	10	1160
		female	WS-167-47-Q	10	1160
Simpla Plastics Ltd	S4 Urine drainage bag — long tube		340805	10	933
	S1 Non drainable urine drainage bag		311102	10	177
	S2 Non drainable urine drainage bag with non-return valve		320902	10	188
	Night Drainage Bag with short tube		340801	10	878
Smith & Nephew Medical LTD	Regard Overnight drainage bag		6145	10	868
Squibb Surgicare Ltd — See ConvaTec Ltd					
Thackraycare (C F Thackray Ltd)	Urine drainage bag		47-0600	1	115
	Aqua 4 urine drainage bag, 2 litre		78-3560	10	790
	Aqua 2 urine drainage bage 2 litre		78-3552	10	175
H G Wallace Ltd (Medical Assist Ltd)	Community INBEDS Night Bag		IB2000C	10	1140
Ward Surgical Appliance Co	2 litre drainage bag push/pull outlet		WM71	10	925

† to be deleted 1 October 1990
†† to be deleted 1 November 1990

PART IXB — INCONTINENCE APPLIANCES

SUSPENSORY SYSTEMS

These appliances should not be confused with leg bag garments which are not prescribable. Each system comprises a drainage bag with its means of support.

The bags may be used for 5-7 days, sometimes longer, but the support systems will have a much longer life.

Manufacturer (1)	Appliance (2)	Order No (3)	Quantity (4)	List Price (5) p
Bard Ltd	Urisac Portabag belt	7681	1	550
	*Urisac Portabag	7680	10	940
EMS Medical Ltd	Shepheard Sporran belt	T130	1	620
	*Drainage bag for use with above belt	T121	10	1180
Seton Products Ltd — see Bard Ltd				
H G Wallace Ltd (Medical-Assist Ltd)	Leg bag holster — Small 24"-30"	WH6176	1	758
	— Medium 30"-36"	WH7691	1	758
	— Large 36"-44"	WH91112	1	758
	*400ml Holster bag	400 H	10	1621
Warne-Franklin Medical	Portabelt for Portabag	800210	1	730
	*Portabag	800200	10	1325

*Plastics

PART IXB - INCONTINENCE APPLIANCES

TUBING AND ACCESSORIES

Manufacturer (1)	Appliance (2)	Order No (3)	Quantity (4)	List Price (5) p
Argyle	75cm Foam and Velcro leg strap (washable)	8887-600149	10	1540
	150cm Foam and Velcro abdomen strap (washable)	8887-600156	5	1445
	Suregrip general purpose tube 7mm 10 length 2.7m	8888-301226	50	3450
	Penrose tubing			
	6mm ID Length 44cm	8888-514604	50	2950
	8mm ID " "	8888-514802	50	2950
	10mm ID " "	8888-515007	50	2950
	13mm ID " "	8888-515205	50	2950
	16mm ID " "	8888-515403	50	2950
	19mm ID " "	8888-515601	50	2950
	25mm ID " "	8888-515809	50	2950
Bard Ltd				
	General purpose tubing 96"	1766-8	1	167
	Urinary drainage econ tube 48"	1399-4	1	106
	Adaptor for Uro sheath 8" (penile sheath to leg bag)	0538	1	84
	Uriplan leg bag straps (Washable)	15LS	5 pairs	975
	Leg bag straps, Latex	8440	10 pairs	200
	Leg bag straps, foam/velcro	8441	10 pairs	380
	Seton Products Ltd range			
	Urisac tapes	7667	10 pairs	420
Coloplast Ltd	Velcrobands (washable)	5050	10 pairs	2680
ConvaTec Ltd	Accuseal leg bag extension tube	S455	10	546
	Accuseal Catheter adaptor	S441	10	478
Downs Surgical Ltd - see Simcare				
EMS Medical Ltd	Velcro leg straps	T300	10	475
Eschmann Bros and Walsh Ltd - see Simcare				
Incare Medical Products	Leg Bag Straps 14" (Calf)	9804	1 pair	214
	Leg Bag Straps 23" (Thigh)	9802	1 pair	214

PART IXB – INCONTINENCE APPLIANCES

TUBING AND ACCESSORIES – cont

Manufacturer (1)	Appliance (2)	Order No (3)	Quantity (4)	List Price (5) p
GU Manufacturing Ltd – See SG & P Payne				
Kinpax & F T Mitchell Group Ltd	Velcro leg straps	VLS	1 Pair	140
	Leg bag connecting tube with mount	LBCTM	1	185
	Leg bag connecting tube	LBCT	1	110
Leyland Medical Ltd (Peoplecare) (See Aldington Laboratories Ltd)	Connecting tubes for Kipper bag	886104	1	212
	14" connecting tube for drip urinal	754136	1	211
	Connecting tube for all urinals with female connector	754135	1	322
S G & P Payne	6" Rubber extension tube		1	270
	Velcro leg strap		1	75
	Rubber leg strap		1	95
Portex Ltd	Stepped tapered adaptor	700/110/100	10	690
	Tapered adaptor (catheter to leg bag)	700/150/634	10	490
Redland Medical– see Bard Ltd				
Salt & Son Ltd	Heritage leg bag extension tube	ZL0021	2	163

TUBING AND ACCESSORIES - cont

Manufacturer (1)	Appliance (2)	Order No (3)	Quantity (4)	List Price (5) p
Seton Products Ltd - see Bard Ltd				
Simcare	Stopcock for use on chiron plastic urinal bags in place of screw cap	WS-155-20-E	1	360
	Rubber extension tube (with mounts)	WS-152-01-M	1	360
	Rubber tubing (1.5m long)	WS-152-20-R	1	841
	Plastic connector with tube	WS-152-25-C	1	241
	Female Connector for Mitcham bag	WH-566-01-G	1	166
	Leg Straps	WS-167-65-P	5 pairs	1050
	Night Bag Connector	WH-533-01-C	1	102
	Spare "O" rings for pp urinal	WR-045-01-R	5	95
	Uro-Flo Elastic Velcro Leg Straps	WS-167-35-H	5 pairs	342
	Paul (Penrose) tubing			
	6 mm	27-500-15	10	1032
	13 mm	27-500-23	10	1032
	19 mm	27-500-31	10	1032
	25 mm	27-500-58	10	1032
	32 mm	27-502-28	10	1032
	38 mm	27-502-36	10	1032
	44 mm	27-502-44	10	1032
	51 mm	27-502-52	10	1032

PART IXB — INCONTINENCE APPLIANCES

TUBING AND ACCESSORIES — cont

Manufacturer (1)	Appliance (2)	Order No (3)	Quantity (4)	List Price (5) p
Simpla Plastics Ltd	Foam leg bag straps	380810	20 pairs	1015
	Leg bag extension tube	380303	10	355
	Elasticated leg bag straps (washable)	380812	5 pairs	1000
Squibb Surgicare Ltd — See ConvaTec Ltd				
Thackraycare (C F Thackray Ltd)	Leg bag connecting tube	57-0559	10	655
	Aquadry Leg Straps	78-3579	5 pairs	875
H G Wallace Ltd (Medical—Assist Ltd)	Leg bag extension tube 30 cm	ET30	10	2346
	60 cm	ET60	10	2580
	Silgrip Elasticated Leg strap	EC1	5 pairs	1048
	Silgrip Side—Fix Leg strap (thigh fitting)	SF1	5 pairs	1048
	Silgrip Side—Fix Leg strap (calf fitting)	SF2	5 pairs	996

PART IXB – INCONTINENCE APPLIANCES

URINAL SYSTEMS

The devices listed below are specialist appliances which comprise several components and need to be correctly fitted by someone competent to do so. Generally patients should have 2 appliances, one to wear and one to wash.

In general the individual components can be prescribed separately for replacement purposes. With proper care and cleansing, each appliance should last for 6 months.

Manufacturer (1)	Appliance (2)	Order No (3)	Quantity (4)	List Price (5) p
Bard Ltd	Uriplan Mcguire urinal and adaptor waist sizes			
	66–81 cm	050802	1	4458
	81–96 cm	050803	1	4458
	96–112 cm	050804	1	4458
	Male day/night urinal 14 oz	0005	1	3496
	20 oz	0007	1	3095
	Mobile paraplegic day/night urinal	0019	1	3638
	Uriplan Mcguire Adaptor & Tubing	600532		602
C S Bullen Ltd	Child urinal with transverse bag	LU11	1	5925
	Child urinal with medium size long bag	LU18	1	5726
	Male urinal with large size long bag	LU412	1	6293
Downs Surgical Ltd – see Simcare				
Ellis, Son & Paramore Ltd	Hallam Modular Urinals	NS200	1	2687
	Spare bag	NS200(a)	1	143
	Spare belt	NS200(b)	1	319
GU Manufacturing Ltd – See S G & P Payne				

PART IXB – INCONTINENCE APPLIANCES

URINAL SYSTEMS – cont

Manufacturer (1)	Appliance (2)	Order No (3)	Quantity (4)	List Price (5) P
John Bell and Croyden	Fridjohn male urinal	U50	1	4061
	Male urinal – long bag day and night use	U51	1	3735
	Male urinal – short bag day and night use	U52	1	3735
Kinpax & F T Mitchell Group Ltd	MALE URINALS – All fitted with Taps			
	Day & night use, covered bag, with band & suspensory & leg strap with air vent	Fig 4A	1	4085
	Night use, covered bag, complete with band & suspensory	Fig 5	1	4970
	Day & night use, long tube, covered bag, complete with band and suspensory with air vent	Fig 6A	1	4830
	Day & night use, double bag, air vent, inflating rim, complete with band ' understraps	Fig 19	1	5115
	Day & night use, covered bag, diaphragm top, air vent	Fig 101	1	4420
	Day & night use, improved pattern, inflating rim, short air vent, complete with band and understrap	Fig 104	1	4850
	As above with extension tube	Fig 104ET	1	5120
	As above with long bag	Fig 104A	1	4920

PART IXB - INCONTINENCE APPLIANCES

URINAL SYSTEMS - cont

Manufacturer (1)	Appliance (2)	Order No (3)	Quantity (4)	List Price (5) p
Kinpax & F T Mitchell Group Ltd - cont	Day & night use, long bag, air vent, diaphragm top, with band and understrap	Fig 105	1	4705
	As above with short bag	Fig 106	1	4360
	As above with extension tube	Fig 106ET	1	4690
	Day & night use, long bag, air vent, complete with band and suspensory	Fig 107	1	4190
	Day use, to contain penis & scrotum, short bag, with band & understrap	Fig 111	1	3950
	Day & night use, to contain penis & scrotum, fitted with inner sheath & air vent	Fig 111A	1	4105
	Male jockey appliance	M200	1	4370
	Replacement belt for M200	JB/200	1	860
	Outer receiver	O/R	1	1000
	Inner sheath	I/S	5	1030
	Plastic bags	OLBWT	5	1130
	Rubber bag	RB/M200	1	1800
	Ring	SP/M200	1	75
	Stoke Mandeville male urinal (state size of sheath)	SM	1	4640
	Stoke Mandeville Replacement Sheath (state size of sheath)	SMS	1	460
	Stoke Mandeville male urinal with double bag (state size of sheath)	SMDB	1	5570
	Male PP urinal with rubber bag (state size of sheath)	PP1	1	4935
	Male PP urinal with 5 plastic bags (state size of sheath)	PP2	1	4640
	Spare Parts for PP Urinals:-			
	Flange with sheaths	PP3	1	2320
	Cone - small straight	PP4	1	920
	Cone - small curved	PP5	1	920
	Cone - medium straight	PP6	1	920
	Cone - medium curved	PP7	1	920
	Cone - large straight	PP8	1	920
	Cone - large curved	PP9	1	920
	Cone - ex-large straight	PP10	1	920

PART IXB - INCONTINENCE APPLIANCES

URINAL SYSTEMS - cont

Manufacturer (1)	Appliance (2)	Order No (3)	Quantity (4)	List Price (5) p
Kinpax &	Plastic bag small	OLBWT(S)	5	1130
F T Mitchell	Plastic bag large	OLBWT(L)	5	1130
Group Ltd — cont	Rubber bag	PP13	1	1800
	Rubber belt	RB	1	330
	Progress long life plastic inner sheath urinal	M700	1	1960
	Progress long life plastic scrotal urinal	M800	1	1960
	Fridjohn urinal	M600	1	5860
	YB wet urinal	M500	1	4755
	Essex appliance 1 Piece Belt	M400	1	3970
	Rubber Bag Coverlet	KM28	1	3980
	Plastic Bag Coverlet	KM29	1	3980
Leyland Medical Ltd (Peoplecare)	Thames urinal with standard bag and connecting tube	751100	1	5971
	Thames urinal with long bag and connecting tube	751102	1	5971
	Severn urinal with standard bag and connecting tube	752120	1	5971
	Severn urinal with long bag and connecting tube	752122	1	5971
	Severn urinal with 5 plastic bags and connecting tube	752124	1	5971
	Severn spare sheaths	758300	5	2340
	Mersey urinal with standard bag and connecting tube	753220	1	5971
	Mersey urinal with long bag and connecting tube	753222	1	5971
	Mersey urinal with 5 plastic bags and connecting tube	753224	1	5971
	Wye urinal with separate connecting tube & on/off valve	751300	1	1929
	Wye urinal with long night extension tube	751301	1	2249
	Wye urinal with short bag	751120	1	3214
	Wye urinal with long bag	751175	1	3214
	Arizona male urinal	751400	1	5971
	'55' male urinal	756200	1	5881
	Spare sheaths for '55' urinal	756212	6	2748

0308M/28

PART IXB — INCONTINENCE APPLIANCES

URINAL SYSTEMS — cont

Manufacturer (1)	Appliance (2)	Order No (3)	Quantity (4)	List Price (5) p
Leyland Medical Ltd (Peoplecare) — cont	Clyde with standard bag and connecting tube	852140	1	5971
	Clyde with long bag and connecting tube	852142	1	5971
	Clyde with five plastic bags and connecting tube	852144	1	5971
	Stoke Mandeville Pattern			
	Male Urinal 20mm sheath	754001	1	5971
	24mm "	754002	1	5971
	25mm "	754003	1	5971
	28mm "	754004	1	5971
	32mm "	754005	1	5971
	35mm "	754006	1	5971
	38mm "	754007	1	5971
	42mm "	754008	1	5971
	45mm "	754009	1	5971
	48mm "	754010	1	5971
	51mm "	754011	1	5971
	54mm "	754012	1	5971
	57mm "	754013	1	5971
	60mm "	754014	1	5971
	63mm "	754015	1	5971
	Spare sheaths on request		1	579
	Sahara one piece top PP urinal — with small rubber collection bag Paed	755109	1	5692
	— with five small plastic collection bags Paed	755110	1	5692
	— with standard collection bag and con tube Standard	755120	1	5692
	— with long collection bag and connection tube Standard	755130	1	5692
	— with five medium collection bags and connection tube Standard	755140	1	5692
	— with standard rubber bag and connection tube Large	755150	1	5692

PART IXB - INCONTINENCE APPLIANCES

URINAL SYSTEMS - cont

Manufacturer (1)	Appliance (2)	Order No (3)	Quantity (4)	List Price (5) p
Leyland Medical Ltd (Peoplecare) - cont	Sahara one piece top PP urinal - cont			
	- with long rubber bag and connection tube Large	755160	1	5692
	- with five medium plastic bags and connection tube Large	755170	1	5692
	Peoplecare PP Male urinal:			
	PP Flange 25mm Child			
	Sheath size 13mm	844113	1	1849
	16mm	844116	1	1849
	19mm	844119	1	1849
	22mm	844122	1	1849
	PP Flange 29mm Child			
	Sheath size 22mm	845122	1	1849
	25mm	845125	1	1849
	PP Flange 32mm Child			
	Sheath size 19mm	845219	1	1849
	22mm	845222	1	1849
	25mm	845225	1	1849
	PP Flange 38mm Adult			
	Sheath size 19mm	846319	1	1849
	22mm	846322	1	1849
	25mm	846325	1	1849
	29mm	846327	1	1849
	32mm	846332	1	1849
	PP Flange 44mm Adult			
	Sheath size 35mm	847435	1	1849
	38mm	847438	1	1849
	41mm	847441	1	1849
	PP standard bag Medium	881002	1	954
	Large	881003	1	1183
	PP curved top Small	874101	1	720
	Medium	874102	1	720
	Large	874103	1	720

PART IXB – INCONTINENCE APPLIANCES

		Order	Quantity	List
Manufacturer	Appliance	No		Price
(1)	(2)	(3)	(4)	(5)
				p

URINAL SYSTEMS – cont

Manufacturer (1)	Appliance (2)	Order No (3)	Quantity (4)	List Price (5) p
Leyland Medical Ltd (Peoplecare) – cont	Peoplecare PP Male urinal: – cont			
	PP straight top Small	875211	1	720
	Medium	875212	1	720
	Large	875213	1	720
	Ex Large	875214	1	720
	Transverse rubber bag with tap for above urinal	881001	1	1953
	Double based PP flanges for above urinal	846350	1	1849
	Rubber pubic flange, adult, for above urinal	854229	1	2132
	Kipper inco set	886100	1	3199
LRC Products Ltd	Dry Sheaths		144	1400
S G & P Payne	Male incontinence appliance – with rubber belt			
	– with combined rubber flange & understraps	MK1	1	4975
	– with rubber flange & – fabric face piece	MK2	1	5460
	– with combined rubber flange understraps & coned top	MK3	1	4415
	Lightweight male incontinence appliance			
	– with fabric face piece & separate long flanged plastic bag with foam pad	MK4	1	3154
	– with fabric facepiece separate flange & long flanged plastic bag with rubber belt	MK5	1	4430
	– with combined flange & understraps & long flanged plastic bag & Rubber belt	MK6	1	3885
	Replacements for above appliances			
	Rubber flange with feathered diaphragm	MK1, MK6 MK2,	1 1	2230 1440
	Rubber flange with diaprhragm	MK5	1	1440
	Rubber flange with feathered diaphragm and large reinforced top	MK3	1	2530

PART IXB - INCONTINENCE APPLIANCES

URINAL SYSTEMS - cont

Manufacturer (1)	Appliance (2)	Order No (3)	Quantity (4)	List Price (5) p
S G & P Payne - cont	Material face piece with belt and loop	MK2, MK4, MK5	1	1670
	Reinforced cone top	MK1	1	970
	Rubber reinforced cone top	MK2	1	970
	Plastic bag	MK1, MK2, MK3	1	245
	Rubber bag	MK1, MK2, MK3	1	1465
	Rubber belt	MK1, MK6, MK3	1	315
	Elastic belt	MK1, MK3	1	665
	Web belt	MK1, MK3	1	465
	Night connector	MK1	1	315
	Night drainage connector	MK2, MK3	1	315
	Long flange plastic bag	MK4	1	375
	Long flange plastic bag	MK5, MK6	1	330
	Material face piece with support belt, loop and scrotal		1	1895
	Payne's Urine Director		1	1780
	Stoke Mandeville condom Urinal Complete		1	4105
	Spare for above:-			
	Kipper Bags		1	2310
	Belt 38", 46", 60"		1	490
	Rubber tube & Connector		1	180
	Dry Incontinence Sheath		144	1195
	Tubing (rubber)		per metre	370
	Nylon Connectors		1	105
	PP Urinal Complete with Rubber Bag		1	4975
	PP Urinal Complete with Plastic Bag		1	4975
	Spares for above:			
	PP flange 1" with $\frac{1}{2}$" sheath		1	2230
	1" with $\frac{5}{8}$" sheath		1	2230
	1" with $\frac{3}{4}$" sheath		1	2230
	1" with $\frac{7}{8}$" sheath		1	2230
	$1\frac{1}{4}$" with $\frac{7}{8}$" sheath		1	2230
	$1\frac{1}{4}$" with 1" sheath		1	2230
	$1\frac{1}{2}$" with $1\frac{1}{8}$" sheath		1	2230
	$1\frac{1}{2}$" with $1\frac{1}{4}$" sheath		1	2230
	$1\frac{3}{4}$" with $1\frac{3}{8}$" sheath		1	2230
	$1\frac{3}{4}$" with $1\frac{1}{2}$" sheath		1	2230
	$1\frac{3}{4}$" with $1\frac{5}{8}$" sheath		1	2230
	Coned Top, Small Straight		1	970
	Small Curved		1	970
	Medium Straight		1	970
	Medium Curved		1	970
	Large Straight		1	970
	Large Curved		1	970
	Extra Large		1	970

PART IXB - INCONTINENCE APPLIANCES

URINAL SYSTEMS - cont

Manufacturer (1)	Appliance (2)	Order No (3)	Quantity (4)	List Price (5) p
S G & P Payne - cont	Replacements for above appliances:			
	Rubber bag with vent tube	MK1, MK3 MK6	1	1760
	Reinforced cone top with vent tube	MK1, MK2	1	1275
	Latex tubing (per metre)			
	8 mm bore		1	370
	10 mm bore		1	370
	Condom Set		1	4280
	Condom Set (40 oz bag)		1	5310
	Replacement parts for above urinals			
	Nylon studs		1	105
	Nylon stud with latex tube		1	180
	Waist belt for single	38"	GU 532/WB/38	1	490
	chambered bag	46"	GU 532/WB/46	1	490
		60"	GU 532/WB/60	1	490
Salt & Son Ltd	Male PP urinal			
	– rubber bag	ZL0001	1	3972
	– plastic bag (4)	ZL0001	1	3972
	Spare parts for above urinal			
	1" Flange 1/2" Sheath	ZL0051	1	1906
	1" Flange 5/8" Sheath	ZL0052	1	1906
	1" Flange 3/4" Sheath	ZL0053	1	1906
	1" Flange 7/8" Sheath	ZL0054	1	1906
	1 1/4" Flange 3/4" Sheath	ZL0057	1	1906
	1 1/4" Flange 7/8" Sheath	ZL0058	1	1906
	1 1/4" Flange 1" Sheath	ZL0059	1	1906
	1 1/2" Flange 3/4" Sheath	ZL0060	1	1906
	1 1/2" Flange 7/8" Sheath	ZL0061	1	1906
	1 1/2" Flange 1" Sheath	ZL0062	1	1906
	1 1/2" Flange 1.1/8" Sheath	ZL0063	1	1906
	1 1/2" Flange 1.1/4" Sheath	ZL0064	1	1906
	1 3/4" Flange 1.3/8" Sheath	ZL0065	1	1906
	1 3/4" Flange 1.1/2" Sheath	ZL0066	1	1906
	1 3/4" Flange 1.5/8" Sheath	ZL0067	1	1906

PART IXB — INCONTINENCE APPLIANCES

URINAL SYSTEMS — cont

Manufacturer (1)	Appliance (2)		Order No (3)	Quantity (4)	List Price (5) p
Salt & Son Ltd — cont	Cone — Small Straight		ZL0100	1	849
	Cone — Small Curved		ZL0101	1	849
	Cone — Medium Straight		ZL0102	1	849
	Cone — Medium Curved		ZL0103	1	849
	Cone — Large Straight		ZL0104	1	849
	Cone — Large Curved		ZL0105	1	849
	Cone — Ex Large Straight		ZL0106	1	849
	Pubic Pressure Flange Belt		ZL0034	1	1675
	— plastic bags — child		ZL0151	4	933
	— adult		ZL0152	4	933
	— rubber bag — adult		ZL0155	1	933
	— child		ZL0154	1	933
	— transverse		ZL0153	1	933
	— belt		ZL0010	1	284
Simcare	Male PP urinal, child, with integral flange Rubber Bag:				
	Straight Cone	Medium	WR-007-01-D	1	4760
	Plastic Bag:				
	Curved Cone	Small	WR-011-01-H	1	4653
		Medium	WR-013-01-R	1	4653
	Replacement PP flange with integral sheath for male pp urinals:				
		Sheath 13 mm	WS-025-13-K	1	2620
		Sheath 16 mm	WS-025-16-R	1	2620
		Sheath 19 mm	WS-025-19-X	1	2620
	Rubber PP Flange Child				
	Sheath 22 mm, Flange 25 mm		WS-025-22-L	1	2620
	Sheath 22 mm, Flange 29 mm		WS-029-22-D	1	2620
	Sheath 22 mm, Flange 32 mm		WS-032-22-D	1	2620
	Sheath 25 mm, Flange 29 mm		WS-029-25-K	1	2620
	Sheath 25 mm, Flange 32 mm		WS-032-25-K	1	2620

PART IXB - INCONTINENCE APPLIANCES

URINAL SYSTEMS - cont

Manufacturer (1)	Appliance (2)	Order No (3)	Quantity (4)	List Price (5) p
Simcare cont	Replacement curved rubber cone top for above urinals			
	Small	WS-130-01-S	1	1108
	Medium	WS-130-03-W	1	1108
	Large	WS-130-05-B	1	1108
	Replacement straight rubber cone top for above urinals			
	Small	WS-135-01-P	1	1108
	Medium	WS-135-03-T	1	1108
	Large	WS-135-05-X	1	1108
	Ex Large	WS-135-07-C	1	1108
	Replacement double-based PP flange			
	adult 32 mm opening	WS-160-32-V	1	2343
	38 mm opening	WS-160-38-J	1	2343
	44 mm opening	WS-160-44-D	1	2343
	Chailey male urinal, child with plastic bag	WR-105-01-B	1	4898
	Chailey male urinal, adolescent ' adult with			
	rubber bag	WP-100-01-P	1	4392
	plastic bag	WP-105-01-L	1	5563
	Spares for Chailey urinals 1 price curved top with integral sheath and under-straps			
	22 mm Sheath	WS-200-22-R	1	2931
	Adult 22 mm Sheath	WS-202-22-A	1	2931
	25 mm Sheath	WS-202-25-G	1	2931
	29 mm Sheath	WS-202-29-Q	1	2931
	32 mm Sheath	WS-202-32-D	1	2931
	35 mm Sheath	WS-202-35-K	1	2931
	38 mm Sheath	WS-202-38-R	1	2931
	44 mm Sheath	WS-202-44-L	1	2931

PART IXB – INCONTINENCE APPLIANCES

URINAL SYSTEMS – cont

Manufacturer (1)	Appliance (2)	Order No (3)	Quantity (4)	List Price (5) p
Simcare cont	– Rubber belt			
	61 cm	WS–101–61–A	1	432
	91 cm	WS–101–91–K	1	432
	– Rubber bags (suitable	WS–110–01–G	1	1393
	also for PP and Chiron	WS–110–05–Q	1	1911
	urinals)			
	– plastic bags (suitable also for PP urinals & Chiron urinals)			
	Wide Neck	WS–120–10–N	1	289
	Adult	WS–120–05–V	1	289
	Child	WS–120–01–M	1	289
	Male PP urinal, adult, with integral flange			
	rubber bag various sizes	WP–001–01–M	1	5515
		WP–003–01–V	1	5515
		WP–005–01–E	1	5515
	plastic bag various sizes	WP–011–01–S	1	5138
		WP–013–01–B	1	5138
		WP–015–01–K	1	5138
	Replacement PP flange for above	WS–038	1	2620
	Male PP urinal, adult, with double-based flange			
	– rubber bag various sizes	WP–025–01–Q	1	5515
		WP–028–01–D	1	5515
		WP–031–01–D	1	5515
	– plastic bag various sizes	WP–035–01–V	1	5138
		WP–038–01–J	1	5138
		WP–041–01–J	1	5138

PART IXB - INCONTINENCE APPLIANCES

URINAL SYSTEMS - cont

Manufacturer (1)	Appliance (2)	Order No (3)	Quantity (4)	List Price (5) p
Simcare cont	Replacement Sheath for above urinals	WS-160-01-J	10	101
	Rubber bag with vent tube for PP urinals Adult	WS-140-05-G	1	2286
	Rubber double bag, adult, for PP urinals	WS-140-08-N	1	2448
	Stoke Mandeville sheath type urinal	WP-110-01-U	1	2024
	Stoke Mandeville double rubber bag urinal	WP-113-01-H	1	6531
	Replacement Sheaths	WS-160-02-L	10	301
	Replacement bag for WP113	WS-140-07-L	1	2448
	" sheath for WP113	WS-162	1	685
	" net suspensory WP113	WS-107-05-Q	1	1449
	Chiron male rubber urinal with webbing belt	WP-124-01-S	1	4522
	Male one-piece urinal	WP-125-01-W	1	4306
	Surrey model L/weight urinal L - MK I	WP-130	1	4091
	- MK II	WP-133	1	4091
	Replacement bags for MK I & MK II Surrey urinal	WH-002	10	2560
	Replacement foam pads for Surrey urinal 76mm dia/32mm opening	WJ-275-32-W	5	504
	Chiron male plastic urinal (rubber sheaths)	WP-145-01-H	1	2340
	Chiron geriatric urinal (film type sheaths)	WP-148-01-V	1	3398
	Chiron urinal (rubber sheaths)	WP-151-01-V	1	3398

PART IXB - INCONTINENCE APPLIANCES

URINAL SYSTEMS - cont

Manufacturer (1)	Appliance (2)	Order No (3)	Quantity (4)	List Price (5) p
Simcare - cont	Replacement sheaths for WP145 & WP151	WS-168	1	432
	Replacement net suspensory for WP107, WP129 & WP145	WS-107-08-W	1	1016
	Male urinal for bed use	WP-136-01G	1	3817
	Pubic flange - large opening	WS-001-05H	1	1754
	Bag & top for Stoke-Mandeville urinal	WS-112-05Y	1	4637
	Transverse rubber bag & stopcock (child)	WS-145-01U	1	2584
	Non allergic film type sheath	WS-161-01N	10	80
Steeper (Orthopaedic) Ltd incorporating Donald Rose Ltd	Paraplegic male urinal for day or night use with porthole swan-neck top, adjustable elastic belt with linen front, 4 buttonholes and understraps suitable for sitting patients.	52	1	5436
	Male rubber urinal for day use, porthole top, straight neck and inner sheath, adjustable elastic belt with linen front, 4 buttonholes and understraps.	53	1	4015
	"Ditto" but with swan-neck	54	1	4341
	Male urinal, rabbit eared with inner sheath complete with waistband.	57	1	3850
	Adjustable waistbands for above.	59	1	377

PART IXB - INCONTINENCE APPLIANCES

URINAL SYSTEMS - cont

Manufacturer (1)	Appliance (2)	Order No (3)	Quantity (4)	List Price (5) p
Steeper (Orthopaedic) Ltd incorporating Donald Rose Ltd	Elastic waistband adjustable with linen front with 4 buttonholes and tape understraps for porthole type urinals.	60	1	682
	Male dribbling bag (rubber) curved with porthole diaphragm and adjustable webbing belt.	61	1	1961
	Pubic pressure urinal with double based flange, disposable film sheaths and 4 plastic bags.	64	1	3586
	Scrotal pouch for Rabbit eared urinals.	90	1	425
Thackraycare (Thackray C F Ltd)	Aquadry male urinal, scrotal support			
	Adult	78-5172	1	4455
	Adolescent	78-5148	1	4455
	Aquadry urinal, pubic pressure			
	Adult	47-0856	1	4455
	Adolescent	47-0864	1	4455
	Paediatric, rubber under strap	47-0848	1	4455
	Aquadry urinal, rubber understrap			
	Adult	78-5369	1	4455
	Adolescent	78-5164	1	4455
	Aquadry urinal, paediatric	78-5156	1	4455
	Aquadry urinal, long term	78-3625	1	4380

PART IXB - INCONTINENCE APPLIANCES

URINAL SYSTEMS - cont

Manufacturer (1)	Appliance (2)		Order No (3)	Quantity (4)	List Price (5) p
Thackraycare (Thackray C F Ltd) - cont	Drainage bag for use with Aquadry urinals (except drip type & long term)				
	250ml		78-5350	5	1085
	325ml		78-5377	5	1085
	Aquadry Pubic Pressure Flange				
	Child Flanges	1/2"	787000	1	2360
		5/8"	787019	1	2360
		3/4"	787027	1	2360
		7/8"	787035	1	2360
		1"	787043	1	2360
		1 1/8"	787051	1	2360
		1 1/4"	786470	1	2360
	Adult Flanges	1"	787078	1	2360
		1 1/8"	787086	1	2360
		1 1/4"	787094	1	2360
		1 3/8"	787108	1	2360
		1 1/2"	787116	1	2360
		1 5/8"	787124	1	2360
		1 3/4"	787132	1	2360
	Aquadry Pubic Pressure Cones Straight				
		Small	787140	1	935
		Medium	787159	1	935
		Large	787167	1	935
	Curved				
		Small	787175	1	935
		Medium	787183	1	935
		Large	787191	1	935
	Rubber Belt				
		Adult	787205	1	250
		Child	787213	1	250

PART IXB - INCONTINENCE APPLIANCES

URINAL SYSTEMS - cont

Manufacturer (1)	Appliance (2)	Order No (3)	Quantity (4)	List Price (5) p
Ward Surgical Appliance Co	Jockey Male Urinal	WM27	1	5530
	Varsity Male Urinal	WM14	1	4268
	Day use, covered bag complete with belt suspensory and thigh strap	Fig 4	1	353i
	Male Urinal Day and Night Use covered bag air vent, belt suspensory	FIG 4A	1	3655
	Male Urinal Day and Night Use with short bag and belt	FIG 104	1	3784
	As above with covered bag	Fig 104a	1	4100
	As above with double Chamber bag	Fig 104b	1	4262
	Male Urinal Day and Night Use with long bag and belt	FIG 105	1	3784
	Paraplegic Male Urinal	FIG 110	1	5170
	Stoke Mandeville Patter	WM18	1	4967
	Stoke Mandeville removeable rubber sheath, double chamber rubber bag, thigh strap and belt	WM18a	1	4461
	Male P P Urinal Rubber Bag	WM19	1	4628
	Stoke Mandeville spare Sheaths rubber	WM20	1	462
	Plastic Bags (4)	WM21	1	4101
	Replacement for Above P P Flange	WM22	1	2123
	P P Cone	WM23	1	839
	Rubber Bag	WM24	1	1150
	Plastic Bag	WM26	1	231

PART IXB – INCONTINENCE APPLIANCES

URINAL SYSTEMS – cont

Manufacturer (1)	Appliance (2)	Order No (3)	Quantity (4)	List Price (5) p
Ward Surgical Appliance Co – cont	Day use, covered bag complete with belt	Fig 2	1	3360
	Night use, covered Bag complete with belt suspensory and thigh strap	Fig 5	1	4440
	Day and Night use, covered bags, air vent complete with belt, suspensory and thigh strap	Fig 5a	1	4440
	Day and Night use, long tube rubber bag with air vent, complete with belt and thigh strap	Fig 6	1	4020
	Male Dribbling bag and tapes	Fig 9	1	1640
	Day and Night use, short covered bag	Fig 101	1	3784
	Day and Night use, short bag and belt	Fig 106	1	3784
	Male Urinal sheath and Disc Type with long rubber belt	WM53	1	4124
	Male Urinal Conical Top with short rubber bag	WM54	1	2354
	Male Urinal Conical Top with long rubber bag	WM55	1	2354
	Male Urinal Sheath and suspensory with short covered bag	WM56	1	4124
	Male Urinal Sheath and suspensory with Long covered bag	WM57	1	4124

PART IXB — INCONTINENCE APPLIANCES

URINAL SYSTEMS — cont

Manufacturer (1)	Appliance (2)	Order No (3)	Quantity (4)	List Price (5) p
Ward Surgical Appliance Co — cont	Night Urinal with long tube	WM59	1	1989
	Stoke Mandeville Sheath type urinal, with 30 rubber film sheaths, rubber bag and thigh strap and belt	WM49	1	3950
	St Peters Pattern SP Bag	WM76	1	2433
S R Willis & Sons Ltd	Male urinal for day and night use, air tube to bag, inner sheath and diaphragm to receiver, web belt and cotton suspensory bag	IU/9	1	4468
	Male urinal similar to IU/9 but bag covered with coutil and with elastic legstrap	IU/10	1	4650
	Male urinal with long narrow bag coutil covered, web belt and cotton suspensory bag	IU/365	1	4650
	Male urinal for day use the receiver to contain the penis and scrotum, web waist band and tape understraps	IU/11	1	4266
	Male urinal for night use, similar to IU/11 but the receiver designed for use in bed	IU/12	1	4266
	Male urinal to contain penis and scrotum (for the small built man) web belt and tape understraps	IU/11B/893C	1	4266
	Male urinal for day and night use, long rubber bag with two leg straps loops and straps, flanged received, air tube, diaphragm and short conical inner sheath, web band and cotton suspensory bag	IU/15/3977	1	4414
	Male urinal for day and night use, short rubber bag, detachable bag and night tube, web belt and cotton suspensory bag	IU/43	1	3557

PART IXB - INCONTINENCE APPLIANCES

URINAL SYSTEMS - cont

Manufacturer (1)	Appliance (2)	Order No (3)	Quantity (4)	List Price (5) p
S R Willis & Sons Ltd cont	Replacement 1 1/2" white web waist band for male urinals - sizes 29", 36", 44"-48"	IU/1465	1	400
	Replacement suspension bag - small, medium & large	IU/1458	1	449

CROSS REFERENCE INDEX
(INCONTINENCE APPLIANCES)

APPLIANCE RANGE	MANUFACTURER
"55"	Leyland Medical Ltd
A4	Franklin Medical
Accuseal	ConvaTec Ltd
Aldon	Aldington Laboratories Ltd
Alexa	Henleys Medical Supplies Ltd
Aqua	Thackraycare
Aquadry	Raymed (Thackray Chas F Ltd)
Argyle Florite	Sherwood Medical
Arizona	Leyland Medical Ltd
Bubble "U"	Simpla Plastics Ltd
Careline	Bradgate Unitech
Chailey	Simcare
Chiron	Simcare
Clyde	Leyland Medical Ltd
Contour	Coloplast Ltd
Conveen	Coloplast Ltd
Dribblet	C S Bullen Ltd
Dryaid	Aldington Laboratories Ltd
Essex	Kinpax & F T Mitchell Ltd
Freedom	Raymed (Thackray Chas F Ltd)
Fridjohn	John Bell & Croydon
"	Kinpax & F T Mitchell Ltd
Hallam	Ellis, Son & Paramore Ltd
Heritage	Salt & Son Ltd
Incontiaid	S G & P Payne
I.n.b.e.d.s.	Medical Assist Ltd
IU	S R Willis, & Sons Ltd
Jockey	Ward Surgical Applicances Co
Macpak	Hospital Management & Supplies Ltd
Macrodom	Hospital Management & Supplies Ltd
Medimates	Mediplus Ltd
Mersey	Leyland Medical Ltd
McGuire	Bard Ltd
Mitcham	Simcare
MK	S G & P Payne

PART IXB - INCONTINENCE APPLIANCES

CROSS REFERENCE INDEX - cont
(INCONTINENCE APPLIANCES)

APPLIANCE RANGE	MANUFACTURER
Paul (Penrose)	Simcare
Peniflow	Vygon (UK) Ltd
Penrose	Argyle
Peoplecare	Leyland Medical Ltd
Polymed	Aldington Laboratories Ltd
Portabag	Franklin Medical
Portabelt	Franklin Medical
Portasheath	Franklin Medical
Posey	Camp Ltd
Progress	Kinpax & F T Mitchell Ltd
Regard	Smith & Nephew Medical Ltd
Reliacath	Bard Ltd
S	Simpla Plastics Ltd
Sahara	Leyland Medical Ltd
Secure	Warne Franklin Medical Ltd
Severn	Leyland Medical Ltd
Shepheard	EMS Medical Ltd
Silgrip	H G Wallace Ltd
St Peters	Wards Surgical Appliances
Surrey	Simcare
Texas Catheter	Sherwood Medical
Thames	Leyland Medical Ltd
Tribag	LIC Ltd
Trident	Simpla Plastics Ltd
Tri-Form	H G Wallace Ltd
Unicorn	Universal Hospital Supplies
Urico	LIC Ltd
Uridom	Fry Surgical International Ltd
Uri-Drain	Sherwood Medical
Uridrop	North West Medical Supplies Ltd
Urifix Tape	Big Diagnostics
Urifix	EMS Medical
Urihesive	CovaTec Ltd
Uriplan	Bard Ltd
Urisac	Bard Ltd
Urisac Incontinence sheath	Seton Products Ltd
Uristrip	North West Medical Supplies Ltd
Uro-flo	Simcare
Uro-Sheath	Simpla Plastics Ltd
Varsity	Wards Surgical Appliances
Wye	Leyland Medical Ltd
YB	Kinpax & F T Mitchell Ltd

0308M/46

PART IXB - INCONTINENCE APPLIANCES

SUPPLIERS' ADDRESSES AND TELEPHONE NUMBERS
(INCONTINENCE APPLIANCES)

Aldington Laboratories Ltd, PO Box 6, Leyland, Preston, Lancs PR5 1XR (0772 431151)

Argyle - See Sherwood Medical Industry Ltd

Associated Hospital Supply: see Bio Diagnostic

Astra Meditec Ltd, PO Box 13, Stroud, Gloucestershire, GL5 3DL (045 383 3377)

Bard Ltd, Forest House, Brighton Road, Crawley, West Sussex RH11 9BP (0293-27888)

Bradgate Unitech Ltd, Ryhall Road Industrial Estate, Stamford, Lincs PE9 1UL (0780 64674)

John Bell and Croyden, 54 Wigmore Street, London W1H 0AU (071-935 5555)

Bio Diagnostics, Upton Industrial Estate, Rectory Road, Upton-upon-Severn Worcestershire WR8 0LX
(0386 554848)

C S Bullen Ltd, 3-7 Moss Street, Liverpool L6 1EY (051-207 6995/6/7/8)

Camp Ltd, Northgate House, Staple Gardens, Winchester, Hampshire, SO23 8ST (0962 55248)

Coloplast Ltd, Peterborough Business Park, Peterborough PE2 0FX (0733 239898)

ConvaTec Ltd, Reeds Lane, Moreton, Merseyside L46 1QW (051-677 2207)

Dow Corning Ltd, AVCO House, Castle Street, Reading, Berks RG1 1DZ (0734-596888)

Downs Surgical Ltd, see Simcare

Elan Surgical Ltd, 18 Ellingham Way, Ashford, Kent, TN23 2NF (0233-37785)

Ellis, Son & Paramore Ltd, Spring Street Works, Sheffield S3 8PD (0742-738921/21269)

EMS Medical Ltd, Unit 3, Stroud Industrial Estate, Oldends Lane, Stonehouse, Gloucester GL10 2DG
(045-382 5750)

Eschmann Bros & Walsh Ltd, see Simcare

Franklin Medical - see Warne-Franklin Medical Ltd

Fry Surgical International Ltd, Unit 17, Goldsworth Park Trading Estate, Woking, Surrey GU21 3BA
(0483 721404)

G U Manufacturing Co Ltd, - see S G & P Payne

Henleys Medical Supplies Ltd, Brownfields, Welwyn Garden City, Hertfordshire AL7 1NA (0707 333164)

Incare Medical Products a Division of Hollister Ltd, 43 Castle Street, Reading RG1 7SN (0734-597211)
(Retail Pharmacy Order Line 0800 521392)

Kinpax & F T Mitchell Group Ltd, 631 London Road, Westcliff-on-Sea, Essex SS0 9PE (0702-337339)

Leyland Medical Ltd (Peoplecare), PO Box 6, Leyland, Preston, Lancs PR5 1XR (0772 431151)

LIC Ltd, Unit B11, Armstrong Mall, Southwood Summit Centre, Farnborough, Hants GU14 0NR (0252 377778)

PART IXB — INCONTINENCE APPLIANCES

cont —

LRC Products Ltd, North Circular Road, London E4 8QA (081-527 2377)

Hospital Management & Supplies Ltd, Selinas Lane, Dagenham, Essex RM8 1QD (081 593 7511)

Medical-Assist Ltd (Wallace Products) Commerce Way, Colchester CO2 8HH (0206-572800)

Mediplus Ltd, 6 Eghams Court, Bostons Drive, Bourne End, Buckinghamshire SL8 5YS (06285-21672)

North West Medical Supplies Ltd, Green Arms Road, Bolton BL7 0ND (0204-852383)

S G & P, Payne Percy House, Brook street, Hyde, Cheshire SK14 2NS (061-3678561)

Peoplecare (see Leyland Medical)

Portex Limited, Hythe, Kent, CT21 6JL (0303-260551/60551)

Rand Rocket Ltd, ABCare House, Walsworth Road, Hitchin, Herts SG4 9SX (0462-58871)

Raymed — see Thackraycare (Thackray C F Ltd)

Redland Medical PLC — See Bard Ltd

Rehab Products — See Camp Ltd

Donald Rose Ltd see Steeper (Orthopaedic) Ltd

Salt & Son Ltd, Saltair House, Lord Street, Birmingham B7 4DS Tel. 021-359 5123

Seton Products Ltd, Tubiton House, Medlock Street, Oldham, Lancashire OL1 3HS (061-652 2222)

Sherwood Medical Industries Ltd, London Road, County Oak, Crawley, West Sussex RH10 2TL (0293 34501)

Simcare Peter Road, Lancing, West Sussex, BN15 8TJ (0903-761122)

Simpla Plastics Ltd, Phoenix Estate, Caerphilly Road, Cardiff CF4 4XG (0222-621000)

Smith & Nephew Medical Ltd, PO, Box 81, Hessle Road, Hull HU3 2BN (0482-25181)

Squibb Surgicare Ltd (see ConvaTec Ltd)

Steeper (Orthopaedic) Ltd, 59 North Worple Way, Mortlake, London SW14 8PS (081 878 6833)

Thackraycare (Thackray Chas F Ltd), 47 Great George Street, Leeds, LS1 3BB (0532-430028)

Universal Hospital Supplies, 313 Chase Road, London N14 6JA (081-882 6444)

Vygon (UK) Ltd, Bridge Road, Cirencester, Gloucestershire GL7 1PT (0285-67051)

Wallace H G Ltd, Whitehall Road, Colchester, Essex CO2 8JH (0206-45133)

Ward Surgical Appliance, Company 57A Brightwell Avenue, Southend-on-Sea, Essex SS1 1LU (6702-354064)

Warne-Franklin Medical, PO Box 138, Turnpike Road, Cressex Industrial Estate, High Wycombe, Bucks HP12 3NB (0494-32761)

Willis S R & Sons Ltd, 176 Albion Road, London N16 9JR (071-254-7373/3866)

STOMA APPLIANCES
(Colostomy, Ileostomy, Urostomy)

1. Prescribers and suppliers should note that products not included in the list are not prescribable (See Part 1 Clause 2).

2. Only basic information has been provided and prescribers may on occasions wish to seek further information about certain products eg when assessing a patient for the first time. If so this is always available from the manufacturers (addresses and telephone numbers are given at the end of the entry). Information may also be sought from stoma nurses and community pharmacists.

3. Where the prescriber has not specified the type of appliance or part thereof or accessory the pharmacy or appliance contractor must endorse the prescription form stating the type supplied and submit the invoice if requested by the Prescription Pricing Authority.

List of components and accessories:

Adhesive Discs/Rings/Pads/Plasters (page 158)

Adhesives (Pastes, sprays, solutions) (page 162)

Adhesive Removers (Sprays/liquid) (page 162)

Bag Closures (page 163)

Bag Covers (page 164)

Belts (page 167)

Colostomy Bags (page 178)

Colostomy Sets (page 198)

Deodorants (page 200)

Filters/Bridges (page 201)

Flanges (page 202)

Ileostomy Bags (page 208)

Ileostomy Sets (page 228)

Irrigation/Wash-Out Appliances (page 230)

Pressure Plates/Shield (page 231)

Skin Fillers and Protectives (Barrier creams, pastes, aerosols, lotions, gels) (page 235)

Skin Protectors (Wafers, blankets, foam pads, washers)(page 237)

PART IXC — STOMA APPLIANCES

PART IXC — STOMA APPLIANCES

ADHESIVE DISCS/RINGS/PADS/PLASTERS

Manufacturer (1)	Appliance (2)	Order No (3)	Quantity (4)	List Price (5) p

For a list of adhesive tapes prescribable under Drug Tariff see page 101

Manufacturer	Appliance	Order No	Quantity	List Price
C S Bullen Ltd	Double Sided Adhesive Plaster Zinc Oxide			
	3 1/2" x 3 1/2"	UF 33	10	342
	4" x 4"	UF 34	10	422
	5" x 5"	UF 35	10	712
	Double Sided Adhesive Plaster Acrylic base			
	3 1/2" x 3 1/2"	UF 62	10	317
	4" x 4"	UF 63	10	407
	5" x 5"	UF 64	10	685
	Flange Retention Strips			
	4" x 1"	UF 440	50	153
	4" x 2"	UF 441	50	206
Downs Surgical Ltd — see Simcare				
John Drew Ltd	Double Sided Plasters			
	Square	OST012A	10	230 Δ
	Round	OST012B	10	240 Δ
Eschmann Bros & Walsh Ltd — see Simcare				
Leyland Medical Ltd	Ostomy Double Sided			
	Plasters 25mm opening	LM 721031	25	1507
	No opening	LM 721035	25	1507
3M Health Care Ltd	Stomaseal Adhesive			
	Discs 10cm diam	1500	12	330

PART IXC — STOMA APPLIANCES

ADHESIVE DISCS/RINGS/PADS/PLASTERS — cont

Manufacturer (1)	Appliance (2)		Order No (3)	Quantity (4)	List Price (5) p
Salt & Son Ltd	Transacryl Double Sided				
	Plaster	25mm	833018	10	440
		32mm	833019	10	440
		38mm	833020	10	440
	Zopla D/S Plasters				
	Square	25mm	833078	10	331
		32mm	833079	10	331
		38mm	833080	10	331
	Circular	25mm	833081	10	384
		32mm	833082	10	384
		38mm	833083	10	384
	Kidney Seals		833087	10	342
	Reliaseal Double—sided hypo— allergic adhesive disc				
		13mm round	906009	10	1385
		13mm oval	906010	10	1385
		19mm round	906011	10	1385
		22mm round	906012	10	1385
		25mm round	906013	10	1385
		29mm round	906014	10	1385
		32mm round	906015	10	1385
		38mm round	906016	10	1385
T J Shannon Ltd	Easychange spare Plasters with Rings			5	500
	Rubber Retaining Ring		TJS 948h	5	506
	Plastic Locking Ring		TJS 962c	1	188
	Double Sided Plasters		TJS 948a	25	1265
A H Shaw & Partners Ltd	Double Sided Plasters 5" x 5" hole cut to size		NSI46	10	595
	With hole cut to size 4" x 4"		NSI49	10	575

PART IXC – STOMA APPLIANCES

ADHESIVE DISCS/RINGS/PADS/PLASTERS – cont

Manufacturer (1)	Appliance (2)		Order No (3)	Quantity (4)	List Price (5) p
Simcare	Chiron Clearseal				
	Plasters 100mm Square				
		19mm opening	WJ 050–19–K	10	548
		35mm opening	WJ 050–34–F	10	548
	Kidney Seals – Adhesive				
	Flange Retaining Strips				
		Small	WJ 250–51–T	10	383
		Large	WJ 250–75–J	10	383
	Double Sided				
	Adhesive Discs:				
	76mm diam				
		19mm opening	WJ 002–19–R	10	351
		25mm opening	WJ 002–25–L	10	351
	90mm diam				
		32mm opening	WJ 005–32–V	10	351
		38mm opening	WJ 005–38–J	10	351
	Chiron Double-Sided				
	Plasters:				
	90mm square				
		19mm opening	WJ–010–19N	10	478
		35mm opening	WJ–010–35L	10	478
	102mm square				
		19mm opening	WJ–011–19S	10	548
		35mm opening	WJ–011–35Q	10	548
	127mm square				
		19mm opening	WJ–012–19W	10	605
		35mm opening	WJ–012–35U	10	605
	150mm square				
		19mm opening	WJ–013–19B	10	675 ∇
	102mm × 76mm				
		19mm opening	WJ–014–19F	10	675 ∇
	102mm square				
		25mm opening	WJ–016–25J	10	675 ∇
	90mm square				
		25mm opening	WJ–017–25N	10	675 ∇
	125mm square				
		25mm opening	WJ–018–01C	10	740

PART IXC – STOMA APPLIANCES

ADHESIVE DISCS/RINGS/PADS/PLASTERS – cont

Manufacturer (1)	Appliance (2)	Order No (3)	Quantity (4)	List Price (5) p
Simcare cont				
	Elastic Rings for use with			
	Spout Bags	WD 600–12–E	3	174
	Carshalton Plasters			
	Acrylic 25mm	48–530–40	10	373
	32mm	48–530–59	10	373
	38mm	48–530–67	10	373
	Carshalton Plasters			
	Zinc Oxide 25mm	48–538–49	10	590
	32mm	48–538–57	10	590
	38mm	48–538–65	10	590
Ward Surgical Co	Double Sided Plasters with opening	WM 17	10	339

PART IXC - STOMA APPLIANCES

ADHESIVE (PASTES, SPRAYS, SOLUTIONS)

Manufacturer (1)	Appliance (2)	Order No (3)	Quantity (4)	List Price (5) p
Dow Corning Ltd	DC 355 Adhesive	DC 355	20 ml	272
	Medical Adhesive Spray B	895-6	150 ml/207 gm	897
Hollister Ltd	Medical Adhesive Aerosol	7730	170 g	1065
Salt and Son Ltd	Latex Adhesive Solution	833005	1 oz	151
Thackraycare (Thackray Chas F Ltd)	Aquadry Medical Adhesive	470651	20 ml	300

ADHESIVE REMOVERS (SPRAYS, LIQUIDS)

Dow Corning Ltd	Adhesive B Remover	896-6	150 ml/227 gm	706
Hollister Ltd	Adhesive Remover	7731	170 g	900
Salt and Son Ltd	Plaster Remover SPR (Rezolve)	812010	70 g	231

PART IXC – STOMA APPLIANCES

BAG CLOSURES

(Available separately from the bags)

Manufacturer (1)	Appliance (2)	Order No (3)	Quantity (4)	List Price (5) p
Clinimed Ltd	Biotrol Closure Clamps (Post-Op Bags)	3740	1	84
	Closure Clamps (Drainable Bags)	3750	1	84
ConvaTec Ltd	Clip	S 206	10	227
Downs Surgical Ltd – see Simcare				
John Drew Ltd	Clips	OST014	10	18 Δ
Eschmann Bros & Walsh Ltd – see Simcare				
Hollister Ltd	Drainable Bag Clamp	7765	1	79
			20	1297
	Premium Bag clamp	7770	1	82
Salt & Son Ltd	Closure Clips	833044	5	147
T J Shannon Ltd	Closing Tape		reel	136
A H Shaw & Partners Ltd	Drainable Bag Clips	NSI 58	1	60
	Rubber Bag fastening Ring	NSI 54	1	90
Simcare	Carshalton Clamp	48-540-12	5	784
	Closure Clips for Odourproof Bags	WN 110-01-E	10	506
	Bag Clamp	32-285-17	10	662
Simpla Plastics Ltd	Ileo Bag Clamps	130406	20	440
Squibb Surgicare Ltd – See ConvaTec Ltd				
Thackraycare (Chas F Thackray Ltd)	Stomastar Drainage Clips	784451	10	585

0309M/8

PART IXC — STOMA APPLIANCES

BAG COVERS

Manufacturer (1)	Appliance (2)	Order No (3)	Quantity (4)	List Price (5) p
C S Bullen Ltd	Night Bag Cover	UF 57	1	688
	Day " "	UF 58	1	688
Clinimed Ltd	Biotrol Stoma Bag Covers	32–100	5	665
Coloplast Ltd	Closed MC2000/MC2002			
	White	9011	5	1660
	Flesh	9021	5	1660
	Open MC2000/MC2002			
	White	9012	5	1660
	Flesh	9022	5	1660
	Mini Decorated Open			
	MC2000 White	9013	5	1660
	Flesh	9023	5	1660
	URO 2002 4260 White	9014	5	1660
	" " 4240	9015	5	1660
	" " 4241	9016	5	1660
	Comfort 2	9002	5	1660
	ILEO B (Standard)	9003	5	1660
ConvaTec Ltd	Surgicare System 2 Pouch Covers			
	Mini 32/38mm pouches	S 198	3	527
	45/57mm pouches	S 199	3	527
	Large Urostomy pouches	S 200	3	557
	Standard Drainable pouches & urostomy pouches	S 201	3	557
	Small 38/45mm closed pouches, small drainable pouches, combihesive closed pouches	S 203	3	557
	Medium 57 & 70mm closed pouches	S 204	3	557
Downs Surgical Ltd — see Simcare				
John Drew Ltd	Bag Covers	OST011	1	123 Δ
Eschmann Bros & Walsh Ltd — see Simcare				

PART IXC – STOMA APPLIANCES

BAG COVERS – cont

Manufacturer (1)	Appliance (2)	Order No (3)		Quantity (4)	List Price (5) p
Hollister Ltd	Closed Bag	7036	†	30	2400
				5	325
	Drainable Bag	7038	†	30	2400
				5	325
Kinpax & F T Mitchell Group Ltd	Bag Cover	KM 51		1	345
North West Ostomy Supplies (Wholesale) Ltd	Ostocovers (white or coloured)			3	600
Salt & Son Ltd	Salts Cotton Bag Cover (appliance to be stated)	833029		1	289
	Eakin Bag Covers Size of opening				
	Small 32mm	839030		1	336
	45mm	839031		1	336
	64mm	839032		1	336
	Large 32mm	839033		1	336
	45mm	839034		1	336
	64mm	839035		1	336
A H Shaw & Partners Ltd	Night Bag Cover Cotton	NSI 47		1	410
	Day Bag Cover Cotton	NSI 48		1	390
	Lycra	NSI 44		1	410
	Night Bag Cover Lycra	NSI 45		1	445
Simcare	Bag Cover, Day Size	WN 124–01–C		1	882
	Night Size	WN 125–04–N		1	882
	Cover to Fit Redifit Bags				
	25mm & 32mm opening	WN 103–01–M		1	607
	38mm, 44mm & 51mm opening	WN 103–04–T		1	607
	64mm & 75mm opening	WN 103–07–A		1	607
	Stomabag Covers White	32–238–84		5	1950
	Coloured	32–239–81		5	1950
	"Symphony" Bag Cover	32–286–06		5	347

† to be deleted 1 November 1990

0309M/10

PART IXC – STOMA APPLIANCES

BAG COVERS – cont

Manufacturer (1)	Appliance (2)	Order No (3)	Quantity (4)	List Price (5) p
Simpla Plastics	Colo Bag Covers Normal	130207	5	797
Ltd	Casual	130206	5	792
	Ileo Bag Covers	130209	5	822
Squibb Surgicare Ltd – see ConvaTec Ltd				
Steeper (Orthopaedic) Ltd incorporating Donald Rose Ltd	White Linen Cover	82	1	598
Warne–Franklin Medical Ltd	Ostopore Pouch covers			
	Small	749040	5	1530
	Large	749050	5	1530
Welland Medical Ltd	Bag Shields			
	Small (25–44mm)	FSA–200	10	257
	Large (10,51,60 mm)	FSA–301	10	257

PART IXC - STOMA APPLIANCES

BELTS

Manufacturer (1)	Appliance (2)	Order No (3)	Quantity (4)	List Price (5) p
C S Bullen Ltd	Elastic Belt, 4" deep with wire ring retainer			
	Small	UF 70	1	1217
	Medium	UF 71	1	1217
	Large	UF 72	1	1217
	1 1/2" Belt with aluminium retaining shield			
	Small	UF 51	1	814
	Medium	UF 52	1	814
	Large	UF 53	1	814
	1 1/2" Elastic Belt with wire ring retainer			
	Small	UF 44	1	831
	Medium	UF 45	1	831
	Large	UF 46	1	831
	1" Elastic Belt with plastic retainer ring shield	UF 47	1	879
	Waterproof Canvas retaining shield			
	Small	UF 48	1	1314
	Medium	UF 49	1	1314
	Large	UF 50	1	1314
	St Marks Belt	UF 551	1	3410
	Fitting windows in Stoma belt for use with Ileostomy bags or colostomy cups	UF 561	1	402
Cambmac Instruments Ltd	Dansac			
	Belt plus plates (5) 19-44mm	09063-0000	5	2635
	Belt plus plates (5) 50-63mm	09075-0000	5	2635
Clinimed Ltd	Biotrol Waist Belt	3780	1	310
Coloplast Ltd	Ileo Belt	0402	1	548
	K-Flex Belt	0420	1	417
ConvaTec Ltd	Belt	S 210	1	227

Downs Surgical Ltd - see Simcare

PART IXC — STOMA APPLIANCES

BELTS — cont

Manufacturer (1)	Appliance (2)	Order No (3)	Quantity (4)	List Price (5) p
John Drew Ltd	Waistband, Metal Ends	OST009A	1	240 Δ
	Plastic Ends	OST009B	1	749 Δ
	Day Belts	OST018	1	1754 Δ
	Night Belts	OST019	1	1193 Δ
	Belt 4" Deep Stoma Hole	OST020A	1	572 Δ
	Stoma/Bones	OST020B	1	626 Δ
Ellis, Son & Paramore Ltd	St Mark's Colostomy Belt	NS207	1	2682
	Shield for the above	NS207a	1	876
	Clifton Night Colostomy Belt	NS208	1	1067
Eschmann Bros & Walsh Ltd —	see Simcare			
Hollister Ltd	Adjustable Ostomy Belt Small	7098	1	500
			10	4163
	Medium	7100	1	500
			10	4163
	Large	7099	1	500
			10	4163
	Premium Belt Adaptor	420	10	686

PART IXC — STOMA APPLIANCES

BELTS — cont

Manufacturer (1)	Appliance (2)	Order No (3)	Quantity (4)	List Price (5) p
Kinpax & F T Mitchell Group Ltd				
	3" Belt	KM 22	1	1150
	3" Belt One Piece	KM 23	1	1495
	4" Belt One Piece	KM 24	1	1515
	St Mark's Pattern Col. Belt			
	Male	KM 30	1	4430
	Female	KM 31	1	4430
	St Mark's Coutil Ostomy belt	KM 32	1	3001
	Ostomy Web and Elastic Belt with Button and Buckle			
	Fastening 1"	KM 25	1	640
	2"	KM 26	1	755
	3"	KM 27	1	870
	Ostomy Girdle and Panti Brief Hole over Stoma made with Suspenders or understrap	KM 21	1	3715
Leyland Medical Ltd	Birkbeck Elastic Waistband			
	and Shield 19mm	LM 725219	5	3596
	38mm	LM 725238	5	3596
	54mm	LM 725254	5	3596
	Birkbeck Retaining ring — for use with above			
	19mm	LM 725319	5	683
	38mm	LM 725338	5	683
	54mm	LM 725354	5	683

PART IXC - STOMA APPLIANCES

BELTS - cont

Manufacturer (1)	Appliance (2)	Order No (3)	Quantity (4)	List Price (5) p
Leyland Medical Ltd cont	Birkbeck Elastic Waist Band	LM 725100	5	2733
	White Rubber Belting 28mm wide	LM 810063	per metre	299
	72mm wide	LM 811001	per metre	617
	White Sausage Belt	LM 810004	per metre	615
	Waist and Support Strap	LM 886103	1	510
J C Peacock & Son Ltd	St Marks Pattern Belt	Peak 1	1	3815
E Sallis Ltd	Colostomy Belt for Night Use	14a	1	508 Δ
		14b	1	807 Δ
		14c	1	421 Δ
	Day Use	15a	1	2223 Δ
		15b	1	621 Δ
	St Mark's Hospital Pattern Colostomy Belt	16	1	2038 Δ
	Colostomy shield	17	1	737 Δ
	Zipped Pocket (fitted to 15a, 15b and 16)	21	1	378 Δ
Salt & Son Ltd	Salger Adjustable Elastic Belt	600600	1	266
	With Velcro Fastening	600601	1	266
	Rubber front Belt with Straps and Buckles	877001	1	446
	25mm Single Elastic Belt with 2 loops: Standard 35" long	877002	1	266
	Ex-large 42" long	877024	1	266

PART IXC – STOMA APPLIANCES

BELTS – cont

Manufacturer (1)	Appliance (2)	Order No (3)	Quantity (4)	List Price (5) p
Salt & Son Ltd – cont	25mm Double Elastic Belt with 4 loops	877003	1	370
	25mm Rubber Belt with 2 fastening studs	877004	1	306
	25mm Single Elastic Belt with suspender ends	877007	1	266
	102mm Elastic Belt with waterproof panel	877008	1	1075
	With 4 loops & retaining ring	877009	1	1433
	Saltair Ileostomy Girdle	877010	1	3565
	25mm Button Belt	877011	1	266
	Button and Loop Belt	877012	1	266
	Baby Lycra Belt	877013	1	1058
	With Velcro Fastening Standard 35" long	877022	1	266
	Ex–large 42" long	877023	1	266
	150mm Elastic Belt with Waterproof Panel	877017	1	1312
	Colostomy Belt	877018	1	5581
	Saltair Ileostomy Elastic Night Belt	877019	1	1063
	Eakin Elasticated Belt Small	839029	1	263
	Large	839036	1	263
T J Shannon Ltd	Elastic Belt and Shield (with Velcro Fastening)	TJS 948c	1	627
	Elastic Belt (with button and Buckle Fastening)	TJS 962d	1	378

PART IXC — STOMA APPLIANCES

BELTS — cont

Manufacturer (1)	Appliance (2)	Order No (3)	Quantity (4)	List Price (5) P
Shaw A H & Partners	Col Belt 4" wide elastic web made to measure	NSI 10	1	1075
	4" Ostomy belt with groin strap	NSI 10A	1	1235
	With lace fastenings	NSI 11	1	1310
	With Wire Spring	NSI 12	1	1205
	Double Zip Panel	NSI 36	1	625
	Col Belt with Under-strap or Suspenders 6" wide made to measure	NSI 13	1	1445
	With lace fastenings	NSI 14	1	1965
	Col Belt with Under-strap or Suspenders 8" wide made to measure	NSI 15	1	2080
	With lace fastenings	NSI 16	1	2470
	10" Belt made to measure	NSI 17	1	2350
	With Zip Panel	NSI 18	1	2970
	12" Belt made to measure	NSI 19	1	2585
	With Zip Panel	NSI 20	1	3145
	14" Belt made to measure	NSI 21	1	2635
	With Zip Panel	NSI 22	1	3295
	Col/Ileo Adjustable Belt 1" wide	NSI 23	1	625
	4" wide 3 sections	NSI 24	1	1580
	6" wide 3 sections	NSI 25	1	1990

PART IXC — STOMA APPLIANCES

BELTS — cont

Manufacturer (1)	Appliance (2)	Order No (3)	Quantity (4)	List Price (5) p
A H Shaw & Partners — cont	Col Belt, Elastic with Nylon fronts made to measure			
	10" wide	NSI 33	1	2760
	12" wide	NSI 34	1	2855
	14" wide	NSI 35	1	3085
	Colostomy Night Belt in net or rayon, no hole, for use with dressing pad	NSI 32	1	1161
Simcare	Web and Elastic Belt			
	25mm wide	WL–002–25–B	1	803
	51mm wide	WL–002–51–C	1	936
	75mm wide	WL–002–75–S	1	1069
	Short Web End and Buckle	WL–005–25–P	1	542
	Web and Elastic Belt			
	25mm wide	WL–008–25–C	1	878
	Narrow Belt			
	Flange diam 32mm	WL–111–32–F	1	1669
	38mm	WL–111–38–T	1	1669
	51mm	WL–111–51–K	1	1669
	White Leno Belts with Velcro Fasten Flange diam			
	38mm	WL–120–38–U	1	1669

BELTS - cont

Manufacturer (1)	Appliance (2)		Order No (3)	Quantity (4)	List Price (5) P
Simcare cont	Redifit Adjustable				
	Belt	Small	WL-123-01-H	1	675
		Medium	WL-123-04-P	1	675
		Large	WL-123-07-V	1	675
	Web and Elastic Belt				
	Child	25mm wide	WL-129-25-Y	1	675
		38mm wide	WL-129-38-J	1	941
	Elastic non-slip belt		WL-132-25-Y	1	941
	Non Slip Belt		WL-133-01-N	1	1376
	Rubber 'Sausage' Belt		WL-135-12-C	1	1752
		Tubular Belt	WL-138-01-K	1	1752
		Narrow Belt	WL-144-01-X	1	509
	Night Belt Two Way				
	Stretch	Small	WL-236-01-H	1	1880
		Medium	WL-236-04-P	1	1880
		Large	WL-236-07-V	1	1880
		Ex Large	WL-236-09-A	1	1880
	Carshalton Belt Small		48-522-14	1	712
		Medium	48-522-22	1	712
		Large	48-524-19	1	712
	Stoma belt	Small 17"-26"	32-247-83	1	446
		Medium 26"-43"	32-248-80	1	446

BELTS — cont

Manufacturer (1)	Appliance (2)	Order No (3)	Quantity (4)	List Price (5) p
Simpla Plastics Ltd	Belt/Collar	130105	1	306
Squibb Surgicare Ltd — see ConvaTec Ltd				
Steeper (Orthopaedic) Ltd incorporating Donald Rose Ltd	Day Colostomy Belt, made to measure. All sizes	1	1	3776
	Night colostomy belt, made to measure, in white cellular material. All sizes	2	1	2780
	Nylon Elastic Colostomy belt hook & eye fastening, complete with 2 pairs suspenders or understraps. All sizes	3	1	3900
	Gabriel type colostomy belt with 2 prs suspenders or understraps. All sizes	4	1	4408
	Two-way stretch elastic pull-on colostomy belt. All sizes	6	1	1061
	Adjustable rubber belts with window	70	1	1072
	Adjustable elastic belt with buckle fastening and celluloid hook ends	77	1	804
	Double elastic waistband with cellulosed hook ends.	81	1	804

BELTS — cont

Manufacturer (1)	Appliance (2)	Order No (3)	Quantity (4)	List Price (5) P
Steeper (Orthopaedic) Ltd incorportating Donald Rose Ltd — cont	Wide second stage rubberised ileostomy belt with 2 straps, and buttonholed ends for use with ileostomy boxes, or with celluloid hook ends for use with ileostomy bags	86	1	2215
	AS ABOVE — with under-straps or suspenders	87	1	2491
	Fitting "windows" in belt for use with Ileostomy bags or colostomy cups, or 4 stiched holes for studs of colostomy cups or shields	15	1	415
Thackraycare (Chas F Thackray Ltd)	Schacht Belt 36"	780251	1	465
	Slimline Belt and Belt Plate	784141	1	1160
	Stomastar Belt	783870	1	395
	Stomalite Mk 2 Belt and Belt Plate	786217	1	310
	Ostomy Panty girdle White/ Skin colour ostomy adaption and waterproofing as required	784192	1	2675
	Ostomy Girdle — White/Skin colour ostomy adaption and waterproof backing as required	784206	1	2675
	4" Nightbelt, waterproof backing	784265	1	1075

PART IXC — STOMA APPLIANCES

BELTS — cont

Manufacturer (1)	Appliance (2)	Order No (3)	Quantity (4)	List Price (5) p
Ward Surgical Co	Web and Elastic Belt with button and buckle fastening			
	1" wide	WM 25	1	591
	2" wide	WM 51	1	760
	3" wide	WM 75	1	865
	Colostomy/Ileostomy Bath Belt	WM 50	1	1355
	Hookend (Plastic) Elastic Belt	WM 86	1	823
Warne–Franklin Medical Ltd	Ostopore Belt			
	Normal Width			
	Waist 17"–34"	749000	5	2440
	28"–56"	749010	5	2440
	Narrow Width			
	Waist 17"–34"	749020	5	2440
	28"–56"	749030	5	2440

PART IXC — STOMA APPLIANCES

COLOSTOMY BAGS

Manufacturer (1)	Appliance (2)		Order No (3)	Quantity (4)	List Price (5) P
Cambmac	Dansac Combi Colo F				
Instruments Ltd	Opaque	25mm	01525-1000	100	12240
		30mm	01530-1000	100	12240
		38mm	01538-1000	100	12240
		44mm	01544-1000	100	12240
		50mm	01550-1000	100	12240
		63mm	01563-1000	100	12240
	Clear	25mm	01525-2000	100	12240
		30mm	01530-2000	100	12240
		38mm	01538-2000	100	12240
		44mm	01544-2000	100	12240
		50mm	01550-2000	100	12240
		63mm	01563-2000	100	12240
	Small –				
	Opaque or Clear	25mm		100	12240
		30mm		100	12240
		38mm		100	12240
	Dansac Mini				
	(Opaque)	30mm	11109-1000	100	8555
	Dansac Standard				
	Colo 1	22mm	11122-4000	100	10995
	2	30mm	11230-4000	100	10995
	3	32mm	11332-4000	100	10995
	4	38mm	11438-4000	100	10995
	Dansac Combi-Micro C & S,				
	Opaque	25mm	22025-1300	30	5258
		32mm	22032-1300	30	5258
		38mm	22038-1300	30	5258
		44mm	22044-1300	30	5258
		50mm	22050-1300	30	5258
		63mm	22063-1300	30	5258
	Dansac Combi-Micro C & S				
	Clear	25mm	22025-2300	30	5258
		32mm	22032-2300	30	5258
		38mm	22038-2300	30	5258
		44mm	22044-2300	30	5258
		50mm	22050-2300	30	5258
		63mm	22063-2300	30	5258
	Dansac Combi-Micro C & S Cut to Fit – Clear				
	Starter hole	10mm – 38mm	22110-2300	30	5258
		38mm – 63mm	22138-2300	30	5258

PART IXC - STOMA APPLIANCES

COLOSTOMY BAGS - cont				
Manufacturer (1)	Appliance (2)	Order No (3)	Quantity (4)	List Price (5) p
Cambmac Inst Ltd Cont.	Dansac Combi-Micro C & S Cut to Fit - Opaque			
	Starter hole 10mm - 38mm	22110-1300	30	5258
	38mm - 63mm	22138-1300	30	5258
	Dansac Combi-Micro Mini			
	Petit C (closed)	24610-3303	30	4530
Clinimed Ltd	Biotrol colos closed stoma bag, with skin protector			
	25mm	32-525	30	5020
	30mm	32-530	30	5020
	35mm	32-535	30	5020
	40mm	32-540	30	5020
	45mm	32-545	30	5020
	50mm	32-550	30	5020
	60mm	32-560	30	5020
	Biotrol Integrale closed stoma bag, with skin protector & flatus filter			
	starter hole	32-415	30	5310
	25mm	32-425	30	5310
	30mm	32-430	30	5310
	35mm	32-435	30	5310
	40mm	32-440	30	5310
	45mm	32-445	30	5310
	50mm	32-450	30	5310
	60mm	32-460	30	5310
	70mm	32-470	30	5310
	Biotrol Biopore closed stoma bag, with filter & microporous adhesive			
	25mm	32-325	50	5440
	30mm	32-330	50	5440
	35mm	32-335	50	5440
	40mm	32-340	50	5440
	45mm	32-345	50	5440
	50mm	32-350	50	5440
	Biotrol preference closed stoma bag, with filter, skin protector, soft backing material			
	(white) starter hole	32-610	30	4915
	25mm	32-625	30	4915
	30mm	32-630	30	4915
	35mm	32-635	30	4915
	40mm	32-640	30	4915
	45mm	32-645	30	4915
	50mm	32-650	30	4915
	60mm	32-660	30	4915

0309M/24

COLOSTOMY BAGS - cont

Manufacturer (1)	Appliance (2)		Order No (3)	Quantity (4)	List Price (5) p
Clinimed Ltd Cont.	Biotrol preference closed stomabag, with filter, skin protector, adhesive, soft backing material				
	(skin colour)	15mm	36-615	30	4915
		25mm	36-625	30	4915
		30mm	36-630	30	4915
		35mm	36-635	30	4915
		40mm	36-640	30	4915
		45mm	36-645	30	4915
		50mm	36-650	30	4915
		60mm	36-660	30	4915
	Biotrol Integrale Elite closed stomabag, with filter, skin protector & soft cover				
	starter hole	15mm	32-815	30	5310
		25mm	32-825	30	5310
		30mm	32-830	30	5310
		35mm	32-835	30	5310
		40mm	32-840	30	5310
		45mm	32-845	30	5310
		50mm	32-850	30	5310
		60mm	32-860	30	5310
		70mm	32-870	30	5310
	Elite closed skin tone	starter hole	36-810	30	5310
		25mm	36-825	30	5310
		30mm	36-830	30	5310
		35mm	36-835	30	5310
		40mm	36-840	30	5310
		45mm	36-845	30	5310
		50mm	36-850	30	5310
		60mm	36-860	30	5310
		70mm	36-870	30	5310
Coloplast Ltd	MC 2000				
		25mm	5625	30	5370
		30mm	5630	30	5370
		35mm	5635	30	5370
		40mm	5640	30	5370
		45mm	5645	30	5370
		50mm	5650	30	5370
		55mm	5655	30	5370
		60mm	5660	30	5370
	MC 2000 Opaque				
		25mm	5725	30	5370
		30mm	5730	30	5370
		35mm	5735	30	5370
		40mm	5740	30	5370
		45mm	5745	30	5370
		50mm	5750	30	5370
		55mm	5755	30	5370
		60mm	5760	30	5370

PART IXC — STOMA APPLIANCES

COLOSTOMY BAGS - cont

Manufacturer (1)	Appliance (2)		Order No (3)	Quantity (4)	List Price (5) p
Coloplast Ltd Cont.	PC 3000 Clear				
		25mm	8725	30	4940
		30mm	8730	30	4940
		35mm	8735	30	4940
		40mm	8740	30	4940
		45mm	8745	30	4940
		50mm	8750	30	4940
		55mm	8755	30	4940
	PC 3000 Opaque				
		25mm	8825	30	4940
		30mm	8830	30	4940
		35mm	8835	30	4940
		40mm	8840	30	4940
		45mm	8845	30	4940
		50mm	8850	30	4940
		55mm	8855	30	4940
	Perfect Transparent				
	stoma sizes	30mm	8030	30	4860
		40mm	8040	30	4860
	Perfect Opaque				
	stoma sizes	30mm	8130	30	4860
		40mm	8140	30	4860
	K-Flex Transparent (F)				
	stoma sizes	10mm	2910	30	5010
		30mm	2913	30	5010
		40mm	2914	30	5010
	K-Flex Opaque				
	stoma sizes	30mm	2923	30	5010
		40mm	2924	30	5010
	Comfort Size 2				
	Extra No 1	24mm	0101	100	6600
	No 2	30mm	0102	100	8000
		40mm	0114	100	8000

PART IXC – STOMA APPLIANCES

COLOSTOMY BAGS – cont

Manufacturer (1)	Appliance (2)			Order No (3)	Quantity (4)	List Price (5) p
Coloplast Ltd	Extra	No 3	30mm	0103	100	9600
Cont.			50mm	0115	100	9700
	Regular	No 1	24mm	0001	100	5500
		No 2	30mm	0002	100	6600
		No 3	30mm	0003	100	7900
		No 5	24mm	0005	100	7300
ConvaTec Ltd	Colodress One Piece					
	Closed Pouches (Opaque)					
	19mm starter hole			S801	30	5093
	32mm precut			S803	30	5093
	38mm "			S805	30	5093
	45mm "			S806	30	5093
	50mm "			S807	30	5093
	Colodress Plus					
	Closed Pouches (Opaque)					
	19mm starter hole			S861	30	5093
	25mm Precut			S862	30	5093
	32mm "			S863	30	5093
	38mm "			S864	30	5093
	45mm "			S865	30	5093
	50mm "			S866	30	5093
	(Clear)					
	19mm starter hole			S871	30	5093
	25mm precut			S872	30	5093
	32mm "			S873	30	5093
	38mm "			S874	30	5093
	45mm "			S875	30	5093
	50mm "			S876	30	5093
Downs Surgical Ltd – see Simcare						
John Drew Ltd	Colostomy Spare Bags DC/2			OST008	50	2105

PART IXC — STOMA APPLIANCES

COLOSTOMY BAGS — cont

Manufacturer (1)	Appliance (2)		Order No (3)	Quantity (4)	List Price (5) p
Eschmann Bros & Walsh Ltd — see Simcare					
Hollister Ltd	Karaya seal only, without flatus filter (Transparent)				
	Gasket size:	1.0"	7162	30	4328
		1.25"	7168	30	4328
		1.5"	7163	30	4328
		1.75"	7169	30	4328
		2.0"	7164	30	4328
		2.5"	7165	30	4328
		3.0"	7166	30	4328
	With flatus filter (Opaque)				
	Gasket size:	1.0"	2112	30	4328
		1.25"	2118	30	4328
		1.5"	2113	30	4328
		1.75"	2119	30	4328
		2.0"	2114	30	4328
		2.5"	2115	30	4328
		3.0"	2116	30	4328
	Regular seal only, with flatus filter (Transparent)				
	Gasket size:	1.0"	2172	50	5088
		1.25"	2178	50	5088
		1.5"	2173	50	5088
		1.75"	2179	50	5088
		2.0"	2174	50	5088
		2.5"	2175	50	5088
		3.0"	2176	50	5088
	Karaya seal with micro-porous adhesive, flatus filter (Opaque)				
	Gasket size:	1.0"	3312	30	5247
		1.25"	3318	30	5247
		1.5"	3313	30	5247
		1.75"	3319	30	5247
		2.0"	3314	30	5247
		2.5"	3315	30	5247
		3.0"	3316	30	5247

PART IXC - STOMA APPLIANCES

COLOSTOMY BAGS - cont

Manufacturer (1)	Appliance (2)	Order No (3)	Quantity (4)	List Price (5) p
Hollister Ltd - cont	Karaya seal with micro-porous adhesive, flatus filter (Transparent)			
	Gasket size: 1.0"	3322	30	5247
	1.25"	3328	30	5247
	1.5"	3323	30	5247
	1.75"	3329	30	5247
	2.0"	3324	30	5247
	2.5"	3325	30	5247
	3.0"	3326	30	5247
	Holligard seal only with flatus filter (Transparent)			
	Gasket size: 1.0"	4162	30	4996
	1.25"	4168	30	4996
	1.5"	4163	30	4996
	1.75"	4169	30	4996
	2.0"	4164	30	4996
	2.5"	4165	30	4996
	3.0"	4166	30	4996
	Holligard seal with micro-porous adhesive, flatus filter (Opaque)			
	Gasket size: 1.0"	4112	30	5510
	1.25"	4118	30	5510
	1.5"	4113	30	5510
	1.75"	4119	30	5510
	2.0"	4114	30	5510
	2.5"	4115	30	5510
	3.0"	4116	30	5510
	Microporous II only, with flatus filter (Transparent)			
	Gasket size: 1.0"	3142	50	5506
	1.25"	3148	50	5506
	1.5"	3143	50	5506
	1.75"	3149	50	5506
	2.0"	3144	50	5506
	2.5"	3145	50	5506
	3.0"	3146	50	5506

COLOSTOMY BAGS — cont

Manufacturer (1)	Appliance (2)	Order No (3)	Quantity (4)	List Price (5) p
Hollister Ltd — cont	Loop Ostomy Equipment			
	Karaya Seal			
	Gasket size: 3.5"	7344	10	5302
	4.5"	7345	10	5302
	Drainable Bags,			
	size: 3.5"	7346	20	5302
	4.5"	7347	20	5302
	Closed stoma bag with karaya 5 seal microporous II adhesive deodorising flatus filter and quiet film Opaque			
	Gasket size: 1.0"	3532	15	2652
	1.25"	3538	15	2652
	1.5"	3533	15	2652
	1.75"	3539	15	2652
	2.0"	3534	15	2652
	2.5"	3535	15	2652
	3.0"	3536	15	2652
	Closed stoma bag with synthetic seal microporous II adhesive deodorising flatus filter and quiet film Transparent			
	Gasket size: 1.0"	3542	15	2766
	1.25"	3548	15	2766
	1.5"	3543	15	2766
	1.75"	3549	15	2766
	2.0"	3544	15	2766
	2.5"	3545	15	2766
	3.0"	3546	15	2766

PART IXC – STOMA APPLIANCES

COLOSTOMY BAGS – cont

Manufacturer (1)	Appliance (2)	Order No (3)	Quantity (4)	List Price (5) p
Hollister Ltd – contd	Closed stoma bag with karaya 5 seal microporous II adhesive deodorising flatus filter and quiet film Transparent			
	Gasket size: 1.0"	3552	15	2652
	1.25"	3558	15	2652
	1.5"	3553	15	2652
	1.75"	3559	15	2652
	2.0"	3554	15	2652
	2.5"	3555	15	2652
	3.0"	3556	15	2652
	Closed stoma bag with synethetic seal microporous II adhesive deodorising flatus filter and quiet film Opaque			
	Gasket size: 1.0"	3562	15	2766
	1.25"	3568	15	2766
	1.5"	3563	15	2766
	1.75"	3569	15	2766
	2.0"	3564	15	2766
	2.5"	3565	15	2766
	3.0"	3566	15	2766
Kinpax & F T Mitchell Group Ltd	White Rubber Colostomy Bags			
	Night Bag Screw–cap outlet	KM 46	1	1405
	Day " " "	KM 44	1	1220
	Night Bag Spout outlet	KM 49	1	1160
	Day " " "	KM 48	1	1100
	Night Bag Tap outlet	KM 47	1	1405
	Day " " "	KM 45	1	1220
	Black Butyl Bags odourless			
	Night Bag Screw–cap outlet	KM 40	1	2560
	Day " " "	KM 38	1	2195
	Night Bag Spout outlet	KM 43	1	2320
	Day " " "	KM 42	1	2320
	Night Bag Tap outlet	KM 41	1	2560
	Day " " "	KM 39	1	2440

COLOSTOMY BAGS - cont

Manufacturer (1)	Appliance (2)			Order No (3)	Quantity (4)	List Price (5) p
Leyland Medical Ltd	White rubber day bag					
	Spout outlet	19mm		LM 885101	1	929
		25mm		LM 885102	1	929
		28mm		LM 885103	1	929
	White rubber night bag					
	Spout outlet	19mm		LM 885111	1	1003
		25mm		LM 885112	1	1003
		28mm		LM 885113	1	1003
Palex (Cambridge Selfcare Diagnostics Limited)	Closed stoma bag with C L resin seal microporous adhesive and deodorising					
	flatus filter	19mm	startar hole	BCLF19	30	5100 |
		25mm	precut	BCLF25	30	5100 |
		32mm	"	BCLF32	30	5100 |
		38mm	"	BCLF38	30	5100 |
		44mm	"	BCLF44	30	5100 |
		51mm	"	BCLF51	30	5100 |
		64mm	"	BCLF64	30	5100 |
Salt & Son Ltd	Kombo Closed Bag with					
	Karaya Medium	30mm		531630	30	4741
		40mm		531640	30	4741
		50mm		531650	30	4741
		60mm		531660	30	4741
	With Karaya & Filter					
	Medium	30mm		531631	30	5766
		40mm		531641	30	5766
		50mm		531651	30	5766
		60mm		531661	30	5766
	Kombo Drainable Bag with					
	Karaya Medium	30mm		531730	30	4541
		40mm		531740	30	4541
		50mm		531750	30	4541
		60mm		531760	30	4541
		80mm		531780	30	4541
	With Karaya & Filter					
	Medium	30mm		531731	30	6244
		40mm		531741	30	6244
		50mm		531751	30	6244
		60mm		531761	30	6244
		80mm		531781	30	6244

PART IXC - STOMA APPLIANCES

COLOSTOMY BAGS - cont

Manufacturer (1)	Appliance (2)		Order No (3)	Quantity (4)	List Price (5) p
Salt & Son Ltd	Simplicity 1 Closed				
- cont		30mm	511330	30	5346
		40mm	511340	30	5346
		50mm	511350	30	5346
		60mm	511360	30	5346
	Simplicity 1 Paediatric				
		13mm Starter	621212	30	3481
	Solo Closed Bag				
	Medium	30mm	531830	30	1561
		40mm	531840	30	1561
		50mm	531850	30	1561
		60mm	531860	30	1561
	With Filter				
	Medium	30mm	531831	30	2357
		40mm	531841	30	2357
		50mm	531851	30	2357
		60mm	531861	30	2357
	Solo Drainable Bag				
	Medium	30mm	531930	30	1854
		40mm	531940	30	1854
		50mm	531950	30	1854
		60mm	531960	30	1854
		80mm	531980	30	1854
	With Filter				
	Medium	30mm	531931	30	2338
		40mm	531941	30	2338
		50mm	531951	30	2338
		60mm	531961	30	2338
		80mm	531981	30	2338
	Supasac Closed Bag				
	Medium	Starter	713644	30	1890
	Coloset Closed Bag				
	Medium	Starter	713655	30	1212
	Small	Starter	713656	30	798
	Large	Starter	713658	30	1005
	Medium	Starter	713659	30	918
	Medium	Starter	713685	30	1614
	Medium	Starter	713688	30	1350

PART IXC - STOMA APPLIANCES

COLOSTOMY BAGS - cont

Manufacturer (1)	Appliance (2)		Order No (3)	Quantity (4)	List Price (5) p
Salt & Son Ltd	Eakin Closed Bag				
− cont	White	32mm	839018	20	3234
		45mm	839019	20	3234
		64mm	839020	20	3234
		90mm	839021	20	4070
	Clear	32mm	839022	20	3234
		45mm	839023	20	3234
		64mm	839024	20	3234
		90mm	839025	20	4070
T J Shannon Ltd	Night Bags		TJS 948e	1	2147
	Day Bags		TJS 948f	1	1877
	Disposable Bags		TJS 948g	100	930
	Day Bags		TJS 948j	1	2147
	Night Bags		TJS 948k	1	2342
	Easychange Spare Bags			100	3750
	Bags with Elastic Necks			50	1875
	Disposable Bags and Plasters sealed both ends			12	514
A H Shaw & Partners Ltd	Hainsworth Bags with Body Mould Adhesive hole size 1", 1 1/4", 1 1/2", 2"		NSI 63	20	3225
	Hainsworth Bags with Healwell Adhesive hole size 1", 1 1/4", 1 1/2", 2"		NSI 39	20	1690
	Stick on Bags with Plasters		NSI 62	10	645
	Shaw double seal 11" x 6"		NSI 64	100	770
	Colostomy Bags 12" x 8"		NSI 65	100	845

PART IXC – STOMA APPLIANCES

COLOSTOMY BAGS – cont

Manufacturer (1)	Appliance (2)	Order No (3)	Quantity (4)	List Price (5) p
Simcare	Redifit Continuation bags with Karaya			
	32mm	WA 009-32-N	20	5604
	38mm	WA 009-38-V	20	5604
	44mm	WA 009-44-V	20	5604
	51mm	WA 009-51-S	20	5604
	64mm	WA 009-64-C	20	5604
	75mm	WA 009-75-H	20	5604
	Non-Adhesive bags with Karaya			
	44mm	WA 010-44-M	20	5604
	51mm	WA 010-51-J	20	5604
	bags without Karaya			
	38mm	WA 012-38-B	20	4252
	Redifit Hospital bags (closed) with Karaya			
	44mm	WA 033-44-L	20	5604
	51mm	WA 033-51-H	20	5604
	64mm	WA 033-64-S	20	5604
	Opaque Fronted			
	38mm	WB 005-38-R	10	1094
	44mm	WB 005-44-L	10	1094
	51mm	WB 005-51-H	10	1094
	Chiron Disposable Bags for 19mm stoma			
	305mm x 102mm	WD 119-01-L	10	773
	305mm x 127mm	WD 119-02-N	10	773
	Chironseal Disposable Bags For 22mm stoma			
	305mm x 102mm	WD 022-01-E	10	869
	305mm x 127mm	WD 022-02-G	10	869
	230mm x 127mm	WD 022-03-J	10	869
	305mm x 150mm	WD 022-04-L	10	869
	305mm x 205mm	WD 022-05-N	10	999
	305mm x 255mm	WD 022-06-Q	10	999

COLOSTOMY BAGS – cont

Manufacturer (1)	Appliance (2)		Order No (3)	Quantity (4)	List Price (5) p
Simcare cont	Chironseal Disposable Bags				
	For 38mm stoma				
	305mm x 102mm		WD 038-01-L	10	869
	305mm x 150mm		WD 038-02-N	10	869
	230mm x 127mm		WD 038-03-Q	10	869
	305mm x 150mm		WD 038-04-S	10	869
	305mm x 205mm		WD 038-05-U	10	999
	305mm x 255mm		WD 038-06-W	10	999
	Chiron Clearseal Disposable Bags				
	Sealed Both Ends for				
	22mm Stoma	Small	WD 222-02-U	10	1160
	38mm Stoma	Small	WD 238-02-B	10	1160
		Medium	WD 238-03-D	10	1160
	Chiron Reinforced Disposable Bags Open at Top		WD 438-01-M	10	1160
	Sealed at Both Ends		WD 525-01-A	10	1160
			WD 538-01-T	10	1160
			WD 538-02-V	10	1160
	Spout Outlet Bag PVC		WD 600-10-A	10	2383
	Adhesive Stoma Bag				
		25mm	32-232-80	90	9841
		32mm	32-233-88	90	9841
		38mm	32-234-85	90	9841
		44mm	32-240-07	90	9841
		51mm	32-235-82	90	9841
		64mm	32-237-87	90	9841
	With Filter	25mm	32-242-87	90	11061
		32mm	32-243-84	90	11061
		38mm	32-244-81	90	11061
		44mm	32-241-04	90	11061
		51mm	32-245-89	90	11061
		64mm	32-246-86	90	11061

PART IXC — STOMA APPLIANCES

COLOSTOMY BAGS — cont

Manufacturer (1)	Appliance (2)		Order No (3)	Quantity (4)	List Price (5) p
Simcare cont	Omni — 1-piece Closed				
	Bag	25mm	32-311-00	30	5550
		32mm	32-311-19	30	5550
		38mm	32-311-27	30	5550
		44mm	32-311-35	30	5550
		51mm	32-311-43	30	5550
	EC1 Range (Beige)	10-44mm	32-330-06	30	5470
		25mm	32-330-14	30	5470
		32mm	32-330-22	30	5470
		38mm	32-330-30	30	5470
		44mm	32-330-49	30	5470
		51mm	32-330-57	30	5470
		64mm	32-330-65	30	5470
	(Clear)	10-44mm	32-334-05	30	5470
		25mm	32-334-13	30	5470
		32mm	32-334-21	30	5470
		38mm	32-334-48	30	5470
		44mm	32-334-56	30	5470
		51mm	32-334-80	30	5470
		64mm	32-334-99	30	5470
	Symphony 'WC Disposable'				
	Closed bag	25mm	32-335-10	30	5809
		32mm	32-335-29	30	5809
		38mm	32-335-37	30	5809
		44mm	32-335-45	30	5809
		51mm	32-335-53	30	5809

PART IXC — STOMA APPLIANCES

COLOSTOMY BAGS — cont

Manufacturer (1)	Appliance (2)		Order No (3)	Quantity (4)	List Price (5) p
Simpla Plastics Ltd	Sassco Closed				
	Normal Size	32mm	100806	100	11513
		40mm	100807	100	11513
		45mm	100808	100	11513
	Phoenix Closed				
	Normal Size	32mm	101425	100	11857
		40mm	101426	100	11857
		45mm	101427	100	11857
	Casual Size	32mm	101420	100	11030
		40mm	101421	100	11030
		45mm	101422	100	11030
	Simplaseel Closed				
	Normal Size	Adjust	100500	30	5429
		26mm	100524	30	5429
		32mm	100525	30	5429
		40mm	100526	30	5429
		45mm	100527	30	5429
		50mm	100528	30	5429
	Casual Size	32mm	100520	30	5050
		40mm	100521	30	5050
		45mm	100522	30	5050

PART IXC – STOMA APPLIANCES

COLOSTOMY BAGS – cont

Manufacturer (1)	Appliance (2)	Order No (3)	Quantity (4)	List Price (5) p
Squibb Surgicare Ltd – See ConvaTec Ltd				
Thackraycare (Chas F Thackray Ltd)	Schacht			
	Colostomy Pouches	78 5474	100	3230
	Stomastar Non–Drain			
	Self Adhesive 1"	78 4338	10	1165
	1 1/4"	78 4346	10	1165
	1 1/2"	78 4354	10	1165
	2"	78 4389	10	1165
	Stomastar Non–Drain			
	Self Adhesive with			
	belt plate 1"	78 4443	10	1380
	1 1/4"	78 4478	10	1380
	1 1/2"	78 4486	10	1380
	2"	78 4494	10	1380
	2 1/2"	78 5067	10	1380
	3"	78 5075	10	1380

PART IXC – STOMA APPLIANCES

COLOSTOMY BAGS – cont

Manufacturer (1)	Appliance (2)		Order No (3)	Quantity (4)	List Price (5) p
Thackraycare (Chas F Thackray Ltd) – cont					
	Stomastar Non–Drain				
	with belt plate	1"	78 3765	10	1165
		1 1/4"	78 3773	10	1165
		1 1/2"	78 3781	10	1165
		2"	78 3803	10	1165
		2 1/2"	78 4974	10	1165
		3"	78 4982	10	1165
Ward Surgical Co	Colostomy Disposable Bags, sealed both ends				
	12" x 4" with 4" x 3" Plasters		WM15	10	667
	12" x 5" with 4" x 4" Plasters		WM16	10	667
	Celluloid Colostomy Cup with Sponge or Solid Rim, Small, Medium or Large		WM10	1	2768
	With Sponge Rubber or Solid Rim, Belt Fitting		WM11	1	3158
	Rubber Colostomy Bag for above with Mount Outlet		WM12	1	1150
	St Marks Shields (celluloid) 4 studs		WM13	1	602
Warne–Franklin Medical Ltd	Ostopore Colo KAV Transparent	32mm	740032	30	6330
		38mm	740038	30	6330
		45mm	740045	30	6330
		51mm	740051	30	6330
		64mm	740064	30	6330
	Ostopore Colo AV Opaque	25mm	742025	30	3660
		32mm	742032	30	3660
		38mm	742038	30	3660
		45mm	742045	30	3660
		51mm	742051	30	3660

PART IXC - STOMA APPLIANCES

		COLOSTOMY BAGS - cont		

Manufacturer (1)	Appliance (2)		Order No (3)	Quantity (4)	List Price (5) p
Warne—Franklin Medical Ltd — cont	Ostopore Colo KV Opaque	32mm	743032	30	4620
		38mm	743038	30	4620
		45mm	743045	30	4620
		51mm	743051	30	4620
		64mm	743064	30	4620
		76mm	743076	30	4620
	Ostopore Colo KAV Opaque	25mm	744025	30	4980
		32mm	744032	30	4980
		38mm	744038	30	4980
		45mm	744045	30	4980
		51mm	744051	30	4980
		64mm	744064	30	4980
Welland Medical Ltd	Welland Colostomy Bag with filter (Skin colour)	10mm (Starter hole)	FSC 110	30	4530
		25mm	FSC 125	30	4530
		32mm	FSC 132	30	4530
		38mm	FSC 138	30	4530
		44mm	FSC 144	30	4530
		51mm	FSC 151	30	4530
		60mm	FSC 160	30	4530
	(Clear)	10mm	FSC 410	30	4530
		25mm	FSC 425	30	4530
		32mm	FSC 432	30	4530
		38mm	FSC 438	30	4530
		44mm	FSC 444	30	4530
		51mm	FSC 451	30	4530
		60mm	FSC 460	30	4530
	Colostomy Bag with Soft Backing (Skin Colour)	10mm	FSC 910	30	4650
		25mm	FSC 925	30	4650
		32mm	FSC 932	30	4650
		38mm	FSC 938	30	4650
		44mm	FSC 944	30	4650
		51mm	FSC 951	30	4650
		60mm	FSC 960	30	4650
	(Clear)	10mm	FSC 710	30	4650
		25mm	FSC 725	30	4650
		32mm	FSC 732	30	4650
		38mm	FSC 738	30	4650
		44mm	FSC 744	30	4650
		51mm	FSC 751	30	4650
		60mm	FSC 760	30	4650

PART IXC — STOMA APPLIANCES

COLOSTOMY BAGS — cont

Manufacturer (1)	Appliance (2)	Order No (3)	Quantity (4)	List Price (5) p

PART IXC - STOMA APPLIANCES

COLOSTOMY SETS

Manufacturer (1)	Appliance (2)	Order No (3)	Quantity (4)	List Price (5) p
Downs Surgical Ltd - see Simcare				
John Drew	Colostomy Appliance DC/2	OST007	1	1310
Francol Surgical Ltd	† Francol Colostomy Set Regular 29mm, 40mm, 57mm		10	1855
	† Odour Barrier 29mm, 40mm, 57mm		10	3185
T J Shannon Ltd	Colostomy Appliance	TJS 962	1	1425
	Easychange Colostomy Appliance		1	376
	Colostomy Outfit	TJS 948A	1	6336
		TJS 948NA	1	6136
		TJS 948T	1	3360
	Adhesive Appliance	TJS 948B	1	4092
A H Shaw & Partners	Complete Colostomy outfit comprising of a 4" wide elastic web belt with groinstrap 26", 28" etc to 42" 1 Colostomy Facepiece (Flange) 100 Colostomy bags 11" x 6"	NSI 6	1	2985
	Complete Colostomy outfit comprising of a 4" wide elastic web belt with groinstrap 26", 28" etc to 42" 1 3" inner diameter Facepiece 100 Colostomy bags 12" x 8"	NSI 7	1	3045
	Complete Colostomy Outfit comprising of an adjustable 4" wide elastic web belt with groinstrap 26", 28" etc to 42" 1 Colostomy Facepiece 100 Colostomy bags 11" x 6"	NSI 8	1	3265

† to be deleted 1 October 1990

PART IXC – STOMA APPLIANCES

COLOSTOMY SETS – cont

Manufacturer (1)	Appliance (2)	Order No (3)	Quantity (4)	List Price (5) p
Simcare	Chiron Appliances Adhesive model with Spout Bag			
	Mk I	WE 001-38-W	1	5502
	Mk III	WE 007-38-X	1	5502
Thackraycare (Chas F Thackray Ltd)	Schacht Odourproof Colostomy Appliance	785466	1	2785
	Slimline Odourproof Colostomy Appliance	470503	1	3025

PART IXC – STOMA APPLIANCES

DEODORANTS

Manufacturer (1)	Appliance (2)	Order No (3)	Quantity (4)	List Price (5) p
Clinimed Ltd	Limone Ostomy Deodorant Spray	3905	50ml	340
Coloplast Ltd	Ostobon Deodorising Powder tube	4750	22 g	296
Downs Surgical Ltd – see Simcare				
Francol Surgical Ltd	Sween Deodorant	1523	1 1/4 oz	355 Δ
Loxley Medical	Nilodor		7.5 ml	146
			15.0 ml	266
Salt and Son Ltd	Noroma	833021	1 oz	185
		833056	8 oz	601
T J Shannon Ltd	Colostomy Plus		1	228
A H Shaw & Partners Ltd	Forest Breeze	NSI 61	1	255
Simcare	Chironair Odour Control Liquid	WN–003–01–F	4 oz	448
Simpla Plastics Ltd	Dor	130103	7 ml	137
Thackraycare (Chas F Thackray Ltd)	Atmocol Pocket Spray	785911	25 ml	180
	Stomogel Deodorising Gel	785830	50 g	260
Warne–Franklin Medical Ltd	Translet Plus One Male	703001	7 ml	243
	Plus Two Female	703002	7 ml	243

73

PART IXC – STOMA APPLIANCES

FILTERS/BRIDGES

Manufacturer (1)	Appliance (2)	Order No (3)	Quantity (4)	List Price (5) p
Clinimed Ltd	Biotrol Flatus Filters	35–500	50	890
Coloplast Ltd	Filtrodor Filters	0509	50	1400
	Maclet Filter Washers	0502	20	2200
ConvaTec Ltd	System 2 Closed Pouch Filters	S. 208	30	656
Cuxson Gerrard	Flatus Patches 3.8cm x 3.8cm	FLA 830 (T33)	50	210
Downs Surgical Ltd – see Simcare				
Eschmann Bros & Walsh Ltd – see Simcare				
Hollister Ltd				
	Replacement Filter elements for series 366 Drainable bags	7766	20 100	236 1177
Salt & Son Ltd	Metal Bridges – ready-fixed to Light Weight & LWU disposable bags	† 833050 833052	10 20	352 704 |
	– for use with other disposable bags	† 833051 833053	5 30	176 1056 |
Simcare	Doublesure Flatus Filter (pack)	WJ 130–11–N	10	270
	Stoma Bridge	32–298–07	20	241
	Spare filters for Beta and mini range	32–297–34	20	568
Squibb Surgicare Ltd – See ConvaTec Ltd				

† to be deleted 1 December 1990

PART IXC — STOMA APPLIANCES

FLANGES

Manufacturer (1)	Appliance (2)	Order No (3)	Quantity (4)	List Price (5) p
C S Bullen Ltd	Lenbul			
	1" diameter 2" base	UF 24	1	773
	1 1/2" diameter 3" base	UF 25	1	1140
	2" diameter 4" base	UF 26	1	1331
	Lightweight Plastic Flanges			
	Small	UF 73	1	314
	Medium	UF 74	1	314
	Large	UF 75	1	314
Downs Surgical Ltd — see Simcare				
John Drew Ltd	Kapok Flanges 1" — 1 1/2"	OST021	1	1284 Δ
Eschmann Bros & Walsh Ltd — see Simcare				
Kinpax & F T Mitchell Group Ltd	St Mark 's Pattern Soft Rubber Flanges	KM54	1	1040
Leyland Medical Ltd	St Mark 's Flanges made in two Rubbers with Hard Centre			
	25mm int diam,16mm deep, 76mm base	LM 841101	2	2609
	32mm int diam, 16mm deep, 76mm base	LM 841103	2	2609
	32mm int diam, 10mm deep, 76 base	LM 841104	2	2609
	38mm int diam, 16mm deep, 76mm base	LM 841105	2	2609
	38mm int diam, 10mm deep, 76mm base	LM 841106	2	2609
	44mm int diam, 16mm deep, 102mm base	LM 841107	2	2609

PART IXC — STOMA APPLIANCES

FLANGES — cont

Manufacturer (1)	Appliance (2)	Order No (3)	Quantity (4)	List Price (5) p
Leyland Medical Ltd — cont	St Mark 's Flanges made in two Rubbers with Hard Centre — cont			
	51mm int diam, 16mm deep, 102mm base	LM 841109	2	2609
	25mm int diam13mm deep, 76mm base	LM 841110	2	2609
	St Mark 's Flanges made in Soft Honey Coloured Rubber			
	25mm int diam, 13mm deep, 51mm base	LM 842101	2	1521
	32mm int diam, 16mm deep, 76mm base	LM 842103	2	1521
	32mm int diam, 10mm deep, 76mm base	LM 842104	2	1521
	38mm int diam, 16mm deep, 76mm base	LM 842105	2	1521
	38mm int diam, 10mm deep, 76mm base	LM 842106	2	1521
	44mm int diam, 16mm deep, 102mm base	LM 842107	2	1521
	51mm int diam, 16mm deep, 102mm base	LM 842109	2	1521
	25mm int diam, 13mm deep, 76mm base	LM 842111	2	1521
	Any of the above Flanges are available with a Diaphragm, or Cowl, or Dressing Retainer at the extra cost of:			264
	St Mark 's Flanges. Black Firm Rubber			
	25mm int diam, 13mm deep, 51mm base	LM 843101	2	1740
	32mm int diam, 16mm deep, 76mm base	LM 843103	2	1740
	32mm int diam, 10mm deep, 76mm base	LM 843104	2	1740
	38mm int diam, 16mm deep, 76mm base	LM 843105	2	1740

PART IXC - STOMA APPLIANCES

FLANGES - cont

Manufacturer (1)	Appliance (2)	Order No (3)	Quantity (4)	List Price (5) p
Leyland Medical Ltd - cont	St Mark's Flanges, Black Firm Rubber - cont 38mm int diam, 10mm deep, 76mm base	LM 843106	2	1740
	44mm int diam, 16mm deep, 102mm base	LM 843107	2	1740
	51mm int diam, 16mm deep, 102mm base	LM 843109	2	1740
	Birbeck Flanges, White Rubber 20mm int diam, 16mm deep, 75mm base	LM 722019	2	1740
	38mm int diam, 16mm deep, 90mm base	LM 722038	2	1740
	58mm int diam, 16mm deep, 110mm base	LM 722054	2	1740
Salt & Son Ltd	Latex Foam Diaphragm with Rigid Face Piece Flanges 38mm	811002	1	3000
	Latex Sheath for use with 811002 Flanges	811003	1	500
	SF1 Soft Rubber Flanges 25mm	822001	1	536
	SF2 Semi-Rigid Flange 25mm	822002	1	848
	SF3 Hard Rubber Flange 25mm	822003	1	612
	SF4 Soft Rubber Flange 38mm	822004	1	536
	SF5 Semi-Rigid Flange 38mm	822005	1	917
	SF6 Semi-Rigid Hard Rubber Flange 38mm	822006	1	612
	SF7 Soft Rubber Flange 51mm	822007	1	674
	SF8R Flexible (recessed) Flange 32mm	822008	1	848
	Baby Flange with Diaphragm 19mm	822009	1	713
	Salger Polythene Flange 40mm	600340	1	151
	Salger Polythene Flange 57mm	600357	1	151

PART IXC – STOMA APPLIANCES

FLANGES – cont

Manufacturer (1)	Appliance (2)	Order No (3)	Quantity (4)	List Price (5) p
T J Shannon Ltd	Flange Ring	TJS 962 e	1	189
A H Shaw & Partners Ltd	Rubber Adhesive Flange	NSI 1	1	450
	Rubber Non–Stick Flange	NSI 2	1	555
	Adhesive Flange & Diaphragm	NSI 3	1	710
	Non–Stick Inner Diaphragm	NSI 4	1	215

	Colostomy facepiece
	  rubber–foam face hole
	  diameter 1 3/4", 2", 2 1/2", 3"
		NSI 9	1	830

Simcare	Chiron Flanges, 38mm int diam			
	10mm deep	WK–102–38–K	1	1273
	25mm 13mm deep	WK–103–25–E	1	1273
	32mm 16mm deep	WK–104–32–F	1	1273
	38mm 16mm deep	WK–104–38–T	1	1273
	Rubber Flange 38mm int diam 16mm deep	WK–108–38–L	1	1273
	St Mark 's Pattern Flanges 25mm diam 13mm deep			
	51mm base	WK–111–25–B	1	1084
	76mm base	WK–113–25–K	1	1084
	32mm diam 10mm deep 76mm base	WK–115–32–Q	1	1084
	32mm diam, 16mm deep 76mm base	WK–117–32–Y	1	1084
	38mm diam, 10mm deep 76mm base	WK–119–38–V	1	1084
	38mm diam, 16mm deep 76mm base	WK–121–38–R	1	1084
	44mm diam, 16mm deep 102mm base	WK–123–44–U	1	1084
	51mm diam, 16mm deep 102mm base	WK–125–51–A	1	1084

	St Mark 's pattern flanges
	  38mm with dressing
	  retainer
		WK–126–01–N	1	1356

	38mm with 16mm canopy	WK–126–02–Q	1	1357

PART IXC – STOMA APPLIANCES

FLANGES – cont

Manufacturer (1)	Appliance (2)	Order No (3)	Quantity (4)	List Price (5) p
Simcare – cont	Flanges all Blue Rubber 25mm int diam,			
	13mm deep, 51mm base	WK-132-25-R	1	1150
	38mm int diam, 10mm deep, 76mm base	WK-135-38-P	1	1150
	38mm int diam, 16mm deep, 76mm base	WK-138-38-C	1	1150
	Flanges Blue and Brown 25mm int diam, 13mm			
	deep, 76mm base	WK-141-25-S	1	1672
	38mm int diam 10mm deep, 76mm base	WK-144-38-Q	1	1672
	38mm int diam 16mm deep, 76mm base	WK-147-38-D	1	1672
	Chiron Plastic Flanges, flexible without diaphragm			
	32mm int diam 13mm deep	WK-155-32-M	1	636
	38mm int diam 13mm deep	WK-155-38-A	1	636
	Rubber Flanges, double base hole			
	25mm int diam	WK-160-25-Y	1	1460
	38mm int diam	WK-160-38-J	1	1687
	Belt Flanges 19mm	32-269-80	1	21
	25mm	32-270-81	1	21
	32mm	32-271-89	1	21
	38mm	32-272-86	1	21
	44mm	32-275-88	1	21
	51mm	32-273-83	1	21
	64mm	32-274-80	1	21
	Redifit belt flange	WL-124-01-M	1	50

PART IXC — STOMA APPLIANCES

FLANGES — cont

Manufacturer (1)	Appliance (2)	Order No (3)	Quantity (4)	List Price (5) p
Thackraycare (Chas F Thackray Ltd)	Slimline Padded Flanges	78 4125	1	400
	Schacht Colo Flanges and Locking Rings	78 4583	1	470
	Schacht Ileo Flanges and Locking Rings	78 4575	1	470
	Standard Rubber Ileo Flanges 0.75"	78 5555	1	750
	1"	78 5601	1	750
	1 1/4"	78 5571	1	750
	1 3/8"	78 5547	1	750
	1 1/2"	78 5539	1	750
Ward Surgical Co	Plastic/rubber airfilled flange	WM 88	1	1344
	St Mark 's standard flange	WM 100	1	833
	St Mark's flange with diaphragm	WM 101	1	1077

PART IXC – STOMA APPLIANCES

		Order	Quantity	List
Manufacturer (1)	Appliance (2)	No (3)	(4)	Price (5) p

ILEOSTOMY BAGS

Manufacturer (1)	Appliance (2)	Order No (3)	Quantity (4)	List Price (5) p
C S Bullen Ltd	Lenbul			
	Day Bag with screw outlet	F 5	1	1061
	Night Bag " " "	F 6	1	1168
	Day Bag with large outlet	F 7	1	1101
	Night Bag " " "	F 8	1	1212
	Day Bag with metal strip	F 9	1	1273
	Night Bag " " "	F 10	1	1273
	One Piece Flange and Bag			
	1"	F 91	1	2433
	2"	F 92	1	2433
	Lightweight 1"	F 93	1	141
	2"	F 94	1	141
Cambmac Instruments Ltd	Dansac Combi D + A			
	Opaque 19mm	03819-1110	30	6330
	22mm	03822-1110	30	6330
	25mm	03825-1110	30	6330
	32mm	03832-1110	30	6330
	38mm	03838-1110	30	6330
	50mm	03850-1110	30	6330
	63mm	03863-1110	30	6330
	Dansac Combi Ileo F			
	Opaque 22mm	03522-1010	100	13610
	30mm	03530-1010	100	13610
	Small Size Opaque 19mm	03619-1010	100	13610
	25mm	03625-1010	100	13610
	Gigant Bag	03908-4020	10	2485
	Dansac Sterile postop			
	30mm	83430-4020	25	3585
	50mm	83450-4020	25	3585
	Dansac Combi – Micro D & S precut opaque			
	Starter hole 25 mm diam	32125-1310	30	5600
	32 mm diam	32132-1310	30	5600
	38 mm diam	32138-1310	30	5600
	44 mm diam	32144-1310	30	5600
	50 mm diam	32150-1310	30	5600
	63 mm diam	32163-1310	30	5600
	Dansac Combi – Micro D & S Precut clear			
	Starter hole 25 mm diam	34525	30	5600
	32 mm diam	34532	30	5600
	38 mm diam	34538	30	5600
	44 mm diam	34544	30	5600
	50 mm diam	34550	30	5600
	63 mm diam	34563	30	5600

PART IXC – STOMA APPLIANCES

ILEOSTOMY BAGS – cont

Manufacturer (1)	Appliance (2)	Order No (3)	Quantity (4)	List Price (5) p
Cambmac Instruments Ltd – contd	Dansac Combi – Micro Mini Petit D (drainable)	34610–4323	30	4710
	Dansac Combi – Micro Infant Drainable Stoma Bag			
	cut to fit 10–25 mm	31010–2320	30	4470
	Starter hole – Opaque			
	Stoma hole, range 10–38 mm	32010–1310	30	5600
	38–63 mm	32038–1310	30	5600
	Starter hole – clear			
	Stoma hole, range 10–38 mm	32010–2310	30	5600
	38–63 mm	32038–2310	30	5600
Clinimed Ltd	Biotrol Ileo S Drainable Stoma			
	Bags with skin starter hole	32–715	30	5450
	protector (white) 20mm	32–720	30	5450
	25mm	32–725	30	5450
	30mm	32–730	30	5450
	35mm	32–735	30	5450
	40mm	32–740	30	5450
	45mm	32–745	30	5450
	50mm	32–750	30	5450
	60mm	32–760	30	5450
	70mm	32–770	30	5450
	Biotrol Preference Drainable			
	Stoma Bags starter hole	34–615	30	5450
	20mm	34–620	30	5450
	25mm	34–625	30	5450
	30mm	34–630	30	5450
	35mm	34–635	30	5450
	40mm	34–640	30	5450
	45mm	34–645	30	5450
	50mm	34–650	30	5450
	60mm	34–660	30	5450
	Biotrol Elite Drainable Bags:			
	starter hole	34–815	30	5450
	20mm	34–820	30	5450
	25mm	34–825	30	5450
	30mm	34–830	30	5450
	35mm	34–835	30	5450
	40mm	34–840	30	5450
	45mm	34–845	30	5450
	50mm	34–850	30	5450
	60mm	34–860	30	5450
	70mm	34–870	30	5450

PART IXC – STOMA APPLIANCES

		ILEOSTOMY BAGS – cont		

Manufacturer (1)	Appliance (2)	Order No (3)	Quantity (4)	List Price (5) p
Clinimed Ltd – contd	Biotrol Post-op Drainable Stoma Bags (clear)			
	Small	32–210	30	5500
	Large	32–215	30	7770
	Elite drainable			
	skin tone starter hole	38–810	30	5450
	20mm	38–820	30	5450
	25mm	38–825	30	5450
	30mm	38–830	30	5450
	35mm	38–835	30	5450
	40mm	38–840	30	5450
	45mm	38–845	30	5450
	50mm	38–850	30	5450
	60mm	38–860	30	5450
	70mm	38–870	30	5450
Coloplast Ltd	Ileo B – Clear 20mm	0401	100	11900
	Decorated White 20mm	0405	100	11900
	Mini Decorated White 20mm	0404	100	11800
	MC 2000 – Clear 20mm	5920	30	5700
	25mm	5925	30	5700
	30mm	5930	30	5700
	35mm	5935	30	5700
	40mm	5940	30	5700
	45mm	5945	30	5700
	50mm	5950	30	5700
	55mm	5955	30	5700
	60mm	5960	30	5700
	MC 2000 – Opaque 20mm	6320	30	5700
	25mm	6325	30	5700
	30mm	6330	30	5700
	35mm	6335	30	5700
	40mm	6340	30	5700
	45mm	6345	30	5700
	50mm	6350	30	5700
	55mm	6355	30	5700
	60mm	6360	30	5700
	MC 2000 – Mini Opaque 20mm	5820	30	5370
	25mm	5825	30	5370
	30mm	5830	30	5370
	35mm	5835	30	5370
	40mm	5840	30	5370
	Sterile Post-Op Bag with Emptying Device	2200	100	18100
	Sterile Post-Op Bag	2202	100	11800
	Large Open Adjust 10mm–70mm	6100	30	5640
	K Flex Transparent 10mm	2900	30	5550
	40mm	2904	30	5550

PART IXC - STOMA APPLIANCES

	ILEOSTOMY BAGS - cont			

Manufacturer (1)	Appliance (2)	Order No (3)	Quantity (4)	List Price (5) p
ConvaTec Ltd	Ileodress Drainable Pouches Opaque			
	19mm starter hole	S 831	10	1864
	25mm precut	S 832	10	1864
	32mm precut	S 833	10	1864
	38mm precut	S 835	10	1864
	45mm precut	S 836	10	1864
	50mm precut	S 837	10	1864
	64mm precut	S 840	10	1864
	Ileodress Drainable Pouches Clear			
	19mm starter hole	S 841	10	1864
	38mm precut	S 845	10	1864
	45mm precut	S 846	10	1864
	50mm precut	S 847	10	1864
	64mm precut	S 850	10	1864
	Stomadress drainable pouch for paediatric use			
	8mm starter hole	S 880	15	2397
	Ileodress One Piece Drainable Pouch, Small			
	19 mm starter hole	S 851	10	1825
	25 mm starter hole	S 852	10	1825
	32 mm starter hole	S 853	10	1825
	38 mm starter hole	S 855	10	1825
	45 mm starter hole	S 856	10	1825
	50 mm starter hole	S 857	10	1825
	64 mm starter hole	S 860	10	1825
Downs Surgical Ltd - see Simcare				
John Drew Ltd	Ileostomy Bags D1/1	OST002	50	5665 Δ
	D1/6	OST004	50	4044 Δ
Eschmann Bros & Walsh Ltd - see Simcare				
Hollister Ltd	Karaya seal only, (Transparent) 12" length			
	Gasket size: 1.0"	7212	30	5290
	1.25"	7218	30	5290
	1.5"	7213	30	5290
	1.75"	7219	30	5290
	2.0"	7214	30	5290
	2.5"	7215	30	5290
	3.0"	7216	30	5290

ILEOSTOMY BAGS – cont

Manufacturer (1)	Appliance (2)	Order No (3)	Quantity (4)	List Price (5) p
Hollister Ltd – contd	Karaya seal with regular adhesive (transparent) 12" length			
	Gasket size: 1.0"	7222	30	6071
	1.25"	7228	30	6071
	1.5"	7223	30	6071
	1.75"	7229	30	6071
	2.0"	7224	30	6071
	2.5"	7225	30	6071
	3.0"	7226	30	6071
	Karaya seal with micro-porous adhesive (trans parent) 12" length			
	Gasket size: 1.0"	3222	30	6071
	1.25"	3228	30	6071
	1.5"	3223	30	6071
	1.75"	3229	30	6071
	2.0"	3224	30	6071
	2.5"	3225	30	6071
	3.0"	3226	30	6071
	16" Length			
	Gasket size 1.0"	3272	30	6071
	1.25"	3278	30	6071
	1.5"	3273	30	6071
	1.75"	3279	30	6071
	2.0"	3274	30	6071
	2.5"	3275	30	6071
	3.0"	3276	30	6071
	Karaya seal with micro-porous adhesive (trans parent) 12" length			
	Gasket size: 1.0"	3112	30	5846
	1.25"	3118	30	5846
	1.5"	3113	30	5846
	1.75"	3119	30	5846
	2.0"	3114	30	5846
	2.5"	3115	30	5846
	3.0"	3116	30	5846
	(Opaque) 9" length			
	Gasket size: 1.0"	3132	30	6071
	1.25"	3138	30	6071
	1.5"	3133	30	6071
	1.75"	3139	30	6071
	2.0"	3134	30	6071

0309M/57

PART IXC – STOMA APPLIANCES

ILEOSTOMY BAGS – cont

Manufacturer (1)	Appliance (2)	Order No (3)	Quantity (4)	List Price (5) p
Hollister Ltd – contd	Drainable stoma bag with karaya 5 seal microporous II adhesive and quiet film			
	Gasket size: 1.0"	3602	15	2979
	1.25"	3608	15	2979
	1.5"	3603	15	2979
	1.75"	3609	15	2979
	2.0"	3604	15	2979
	2.5"	3605	15	2979
	3.0"	3606	15	2979
	Premium Drainable bag with synthetic seal			
	25mm	3642	15	2979
	32mm	3648	15	2979
	38mm	3643	15	2979
	44mm	3649	15	2979
	51mm	3644	15	2979
	64mm	3645	15	2979
	Premium Drainble bag with integral flatus filter and twenty replacement filters			
	25mm	3662	15	3314
	32mm	3668	15	3314
	38mm	3663	15	3314
	44mm	3669	15	3314
	51mm	3664	15	3314
	64mm	3665	15	3314
Kinpax & F T Mitchell Group Ltd	White Rubber Ileostomy Bags			
	Night Bag Screw-cap outlet	KM 46	1	1307
	Day " " "	KM 44	1	1134
	Night Bag Spout outlet	KM 49	1	1080
	Day " " "	KM 48	1	1021
	Night Bag Tap outlet	KM 47	1	1307
	Day " " "	KM 45	1	1134

PART IXC – STOMA APPLIANCES

ILEOSTOMY BAGS – cont

Manufacturer (1)	Appliance (2)	Order No (3)	Quantity (4)	List Price (5) p
Kinpax & F T Mitchell Group Ltd – contd	Black Butyl Bags odourless			
	Night Bag Screw–cap outlet	KM 40	1	2381
	Day " " "	KM 38	1	2041
	Night Bag Spout outlet	KM 43	1	2155
	Day " " "	KM 42	1	2155
	Night Bag Stopcock outlet	KM 41	1	2381
	Day " " "	KM 39	1	2268
Leyland Medical Ltd	Black Rubber Day Bag			
	(Birkbeck) 19mm	LM 723225	1	2076
	38mm	LM 723230	1	2076
	54mm	LM 723235	1	2076
	Black Rubber Night Bag			
	(Birkbeck) 19mm	LM 723275	1	2374
	38mm	LM 723280	1	2374
	54mm	LM 723295	1	2374
	Pink Rubber Day Bag			
	(Birkbeck) 19mm	LM 724225	1	2076
	38mm	LM 724230	1	2076
	54mm	LM 724235	1	2076
	Night Bag			
	19mm	LM 724275	1	2374
	38mm	LM 724280	1	2374
	54mm	LM 724295	1	2374
	White Rubber Day Bag			
	38mm	LM 882111	1	929
	44mm	LM 882112	1	929
	51mm	LM 882113	1	929
	Screw–cap 38mm	LM 882115	1	1003
	With air vent 38mm	LM 882114	1	1111
	White Rubber Child's Bag			
	19mm	LM 882101	1	895
	25mm	LM 882102	1	895
	28mm	LM 882103	1	895
	White Rubber Child's Bag Night Bag			
	19mm	LM 882121	1	1096
	25mm	LM 882122	1	1096
	28mm	LM 882123	1	1096

0309M/59

PART IXC — STOMA APPLIANCES

ILEOSTOMY BAGS — cont

Manufacturer (1)	Appliance (2)		Order No (3)	Quantity (4)	List Price (5) p
Leyland Medical Ltd — contd	Latex Rubber Day Bag				
		38mm	LM 882140	1	1009
		44mm	LM 882147	1	1009
		51mm	LM 882144	1	1009
	Night Bag				
		19mm	LM 882150	1	1115
		25mm	LM 882152	1	1115
		28mm	LM 882154	1	1115
	Birkbeck Disposable Plastic Bag		LM 724000	100	1256
Salt & Son Ltd	KR AR Black Rubber				
	Screw Bag	Special	161099	1	2387
	Large	25mm	161125	1	2387
		29mm	161129	1	2387
		32mm	161132	1	2387
		35mm	161135	1	2387
		38mm	161138	1	2387
		44mm	161144	1	2387
		51mm	161151	1	2387

PART IXC — STOMA APPLIANCES

ILEOSTOMY BAGS — cont

Manufacturer (1)	Appliance (2)		Order No (3)	Quantity (4)	List Price (5) p
Salt & Son Ltd — cont	KR AR Black Rubber Screw Bag				
	Small	25mm	161225	1	2387
		32mm	161232	1	2387
		38mm	161238	1	2387
		44mm	161244	1	2387
		51mm	161251	1	2387
	KR WP Black Rubber				
	Screw Bag	Special	163099	1	3077
	Large	25mm	163125	1	3077
		32mm	163132	1	3077
		38mm	163138	1	3077
	Small	25mm	163225	1	3077
		32mm	163232	1	3077
		38mm	163238	1	3077
	KR AR MB Black Rubber				
	Screw Bag Special		165099	1	3077
	Large	25mm	165125	1	3077
		32mm	165132	1	3077
		38mm	165138	1	3077
		44mm	165144	1	3077
		51mm	165151	1	3077
	Small	25mm	165225	1	3077
		32mm	165232	1	3077
		38mm	165238	1	3077
	KR WP MB Black Rubber				
	Screw Bag	Special	168099	1	3586
	Large	25mm	168125	1	3586
		32mm	168132	1	3586
		38mm	168138	1	3586
		44mm	168144	1	3586
		51mm	168151	1	3586
	Small	25mm	168225	1	3586
		32mm	168232	1	3586
		38mm	168238	1	3586

PART IXC – STOMA APPLIANCES

ILEOSTOMY BAGS – cont

Manufacturer (1)	Appliance (2)		Order No (3)	Quantity (4)	List Price (5) p
Salt & Son Ltd – cont	KR AR Black Rubber				
	Spout Bag	Special	171099	1	1732
	Large	25mm	171125	1	1732
		29mm	171129	1	1732
		32mm	171132	1	1732
		38mm	171138	1	1732
		44mm	171144	1	1732
		51mm	171151	1	1732
	Small	25mm	171225	1	1732
		32mm	171232	1	1732
		38mm	171238	1	1732
		44mm	171244	1	1732
		51mm	171251	1	1732
	KR WP Black Rubber				
	Spout Bag	Special	173099	1	2328
	Large	25mm	173125	1	2328
		32mm	173132	1	2328
		38mm	173138	1	2328
	Small	25mm	173225	1	2328
		32mm	173232	1	2328
		38mm	173238	1	2328
	KR AR MB Black Rubber				
	Spout Bag	Special	175099	1	2245
	Large	25mm	175125	1	2245
		32mm	175132	1	2245
		38mm	175138	1	2245
		44mm	175144	1	2245
		51mm	175151	1	2245
	Small	25mm	175225	1	2245
		32mm	175232	1	2245
		38mm	175238	1	2245

PART IXC - STOMA APPLIANCES

ILEOSTOMY BAGS - cont

Manufacturer (1)	Appliance (2)	Order No (3)	Quantity (4)	List Price (5) p
Salt & Son Ltd	KR WP MB Black Rubber			
- cont	Spout Bag Special	178099	1	2867
	Large 25mm	178125	1	2867
	32mm	178132	1	2867
	38mm	178138	1	2867
	44mm	178144	1	2867
	51mm	178151	1	2867
	Small 25mm	178225	1	2867
	32mm	178232	1	2867
	38mm	178238	1	2867
	Light White Drainable Bag			
	Large 25mm	273125	30	3898
	32mm	273132	30	3898
	38mm	273138	30	3898
	Small 25mm	273225	30	3898
	32mm	273232	30	3898
	38mm	273238	30	3898
	Medium 25mm	273325	30	3898
	32mm	273332	30	3898
	38mm	273338	30	3898
	Coloset Drainable Bag			
	Medium Starter	713689	30	1752

PART IXC – STOMA APPLIANCES

ILEOSTOMY BAGS – cont

Manufacturer (1)	Appliance (2)		Order No (3)	Quantity (4)	List Price (5) p
Salt & Son Ltd – cont	Light White Drainable Adhesive Bag				
	Large	25mm	274125	30	4422
		32mm	274132	30	4422
		38mm	274138	30	4422
		44mm	274144	30	4422
	Small	25mm	274225	30	4422
		32mm	274232	30	4422
		38mm	274238	30	4422
	Medium	25mm	274325	30	4422
		32mm	274332	30	4422
		38mm	274338	30	4422
	Black Rubber Screw Bag (for use with flange)				
		Special	362099	1	2269
		Large	362129	1	2269
		Small	362229	1	2269

PART IXC — STOMA APPLIANCES

ILEOSTOMY BAGS — cont

Manufacturer (1)	Appliance (2)			Order No (3)	Quantity (4)	List Price (5) P
Salt & Son Ltd — cont	Black Rubber Spout Bag (for use with flange)					
			Special	372099	1	1637
			Large	372129	1	1637
			Small	372229	1	1637
	White Rubber Screw Bag (for use with flange)					
			Large	461129	1	757
			Small	461229	1	757
	White Rubber Spout Bag (for use with flange)					
			Large	472129	1	622
			small	472229	1	622
	Salger Clear Drainable Bag					
		Medium	40mm	600240	10	873
			57mm	600257	10	873
	Eakin Drainable					
	Clear Bag	Wide	90mm	839005	20	7933
	White Bag					
		Large	32mm	839006	20	3738
			45mm	839007	20	3738
			64mm	839008	20	3738
	Clear Bag					
		Large	32mm	839009	20	3738
			45mm	839010	20	3738
			64mm	839011	20	3738
	White Bag					
		Small	32mm	839012	20	3738
			45mm	839013	20	3738
			64mm	839014	20	3738
	Clear Bag					
		Small	32mm	839015	20	3738
			45mm	839016	20	3738
			64mm	839017	20	3738
	Cohflex Paediatric Drainable Bag		10mm starter	632310	30	4460	

PART IXC - STOMA APPLIANCES

ILEOSTOMY BAGS - cont

Manufacturer (1)	Appliance (2)	Order No (3)	Quantity (4)	List Price (5) p
Salt & Son Ltd	Eakin Fistula Bag			
- cont	Large	839026	10	9015
	Small Starter	839027	20	7773
	Medium Starter	839028	20	10114
	Simplicity 1 Drainable			
	30mm	510330	30	5576
	40mm	510340	30	5576
	50mm	510350	30	5576
	60mm	510360	30	5576
	Simplicity 1 Paediatric			
	13mm Starter	622212	30	3481
A H Shaw & Partner Ltd	Hainsworth Drainable Bag with Body Mould Adhesive hole sizes: 7/8", 1", 1 1/4", 1 1/2"	NSI 57	20	3225
	Black Rubber Day Bag			
	(with screw cap) 19mm	NSI 66	1	1815
	38mm		1	1815
	54mm		1	1815
	Black Rubber Night Bag			
	(with screw cap) 19mm	NSI 67	1	1930
	38mm		1	1930
	54mm		1	1930
Simcare	Redifit Continuation			
	with Karaya and 25mm	WA018-25S	20	5605
	medium bags 32mm	WA018-32P	20	5605
	38mm	WA018-38C	20	5605
	44mm	WA018-44W	20	5605
	51mm	WA018-51T	20	5605
	64mm	WA018-64D	20	5605
	With Karaya and			
	small bags 25mm	WA020-25N	20	5605
	32mm	WA020-32K	20	5605
	38mm	WA020-38X	20	5605
	Redifit bags with			
	Karaya 25mm	WA027-25T	20	5605
	32mm	WA027-32Q	20	5605
	44mm	WA027-44X	20	5605
	51mm	WA027-51U	20	5605
	64mm	WA027-64E	20	5605

0311M/5

PART IXC — STOMA APPLIANCES

ILEOSTOMY BAGS — cont

Manufacturer (1)	Appliance (2)		Order No (3)	Quantity (4)	List Price (5) p
Simcare cont	Cavendish Odourproof				
	Plastic Bag	25mm	WC 010-25-X	10	2496
		32mm	WC 010-32-U	10	2496
		38mm	WC 010-38-H	10	2496
	Cavendish Plastic Bag with				
	adhesive flange	25mm	WC 013-25-L	10	3007
		32mm	WC 013-32-H	10	3007
		38mm	WC 013-38-V	10	3007
	Cavendish Clear PVC Bag				
		25mm	WD 650-25-R	10	2512
		32mm	WD 650-32-N	10	2512
		38mm	WD 650-38-B	10	2512
	Chiron Rubber Night Bag		WF 031-01-V	1	1408
	Day Bag				
	Spout outlet	38mm	WF 051-38-G	1	1266
	Chiron White Rubber				
	Night Bag Spout				
	outlet	38mm	WF 061-38-M	1	1376
	Day Bags Screw cap				
	outlet	38mm	WF 001-38-E	1	1473
		44mm	WF 001-44-Y	1	1473
		51mm	WF 001-51-V	1	1473
	Day Bags Screw cap				
	outlet, body side				
		38mm	WF 002-38-J	1	1473

PART IXC — STOMA APPLIANCES

ILEOSTOMY BAGS — cont

Manufacturer (1)	Appliance (2)	Order No (3)	Quantity (4)	List Price (5) p
Simcare cont	Chiron Day Bag, Latex Rubber Screw cap			
	outlet 38mm	WF 003-38-N	1	1280
	Chiron Black Butyl Bags, Odourless, Day Use			
	38mm	WF 005-38-W	1	2559
	44mm	WF 005-44-R	1	2559
	51mm	WF 005-51-N	1	2559
	Chiron White Rubber Bag (Children) 38mm	WF 011-38-K	1	1165
	Chiron Rubber Bag (Children) 38mm	WF 012-38-P	1	1280
	Chiron White Rubber Night Bag Screw cap			
	outlet 38mm	WF 021-38-Q	1	1695
	51mm	WF 021-51-G	1	1695
	Chiron Latex Rubber Night Bag Screw cap			
	outlet 38mm	WF 023-38-Y	1	1695

PART IXC - STOMA APPLIANCES

ILEOSTOMY BAGS - cont

Manufacturer (1)	Appliance (2)		Order No (3)	Quantity (4)	List Price (5) p
Simcare cont	Chiron Black Butyl				
	Night Bag	38mm	WF 025-38-H	1	3071
		44mm	WF 025-44-C	1	3071
	Drainable Adhesive Stoma				
	Bag	19mm	32-250-89	60	7195
		25mm	32-251-86	60	7195
		32mm	32-252-83	60	7195
		38mm	32-253-80	60	7195
		51mm	32-254-88	60	7195
	Omni-1-Piece Drainable				
	Patterned Bag	19mm	32-299-04	20	3818
		25mm	32-299-12	20	3818
		32mm	32-299-20	20	3818
		38mm	32-299-39	20	3818
		44mm	32-299-47	20	3818
	Clear Bag	19mm	32-318-01	20	3818
		25mm	32-318-28	20	3818
		32mm	32-318-36	20	3818
		38mm	32-318-44	20	3818
		44mm	32-318-52	20	3818
		56mm	32-318-60	20	3818
	EC1 Range	10-44mm	32-331-62	30	5730
		19mm	32-331-03	30	5730
		25mm	32-331-11	30	5730
		32mm	32-331-38	30	5730
		38mm	32-331-46	30	5730
		44mm	32-331-54	30	5730
	EC1 Range				
†	Post Op	32mm	32-332-00	20	3940
		38mm	32-332-19	20	3940
		44mm	32-332-27	20	3940
		51mm	32-332-35	20	3940
		64mm	32-332-43	20	3940
	EC1 Range Post Op				
	Small outline 10-64mm		32-332-78	20	3940
	Large outline 10-90mm		32-332-51	10	2788
	EC1 Mini		32-333-08	30	5730
	(Beige)		32-333-16	30	5730

† to be deleted 1 November 1990

0311M/8

ILEOSTOMY BAGS - cont

Manufacturer (1)	Appliance (2)	Order No (3)	Quantity (4)	List Price (5) p
Simpla Plastics Ltd	Sassco Ileostomy Bags			
	Size 26mm	110801	100	13218
	32mm	110802	100	13218
	Simplaseel Drainable Bags			
	Opaque Size 26mm	110524	30	5513
	32mm	110525	30	5513
	40mm	110526	30	5513
	45mm	110527	30	5513
	50mm	110528	30	5513
	Simplaseel Post-op Drainable Bag	140501	10	2989
	Simplaseel Paediatric Drainable Bag	120705	30	4795
Suibb Surgicare Ltd - see ConvaTec Ltd				
Steeper (Orthopaedic Ltd incorporating Donald Rose Ltd	Celluloid cup with chute	69	1	1952
	Rubber bag, spring-in-neck with vulcanite screw outlets Small	71	1	1199
	Medium	72	1	1662
	Large	73	1	1702
	Donald Rose registered design rubber bags with celluloid collars, solid, flat or fluid rims.	76	1	1814
	New improved rubber bag only, complete with collar.	79	1	1969
	New improved rubber bag but with tap outlet and with skirt. Extra. Also extra to RD Bags	80	1	239
	Shaped rubber night bag with long vertical spring vulcanite screw outlet	85	1	1863

PART IXC — STOMA APPLIANCES

ILEOSTOMY BAGS — cont

Manufacturer (1)	Appliance (2)		Order No (3)	Quantity (4)	List Price (5) p
Thackraycare (Chas F Thackray Ltd)	Schacht Ileostomy Pouches		47 0511	50	1840
	Stomalite Mk 2 Ileo Day Bag	1"	78 5989	5	1620
		1¼	78 5997	5	1620
		1½"	78 6004	5	1620
	Stomalite Mk 2 Ileo Night Bag	1"	78 6012	5	1620
		1¼"	78 6047	5	1620
		1½"	78 6055	5	1620
	Stomastar Drain with belt plate	1"	78 3838	10	1380
		1¼"	78 3846	10	1380
		1½"	78 3854	10	1380
		2"	78 3862	10	1380
		2½"	78 4990	10	1380
		3"	78 5008	10	1380
	Stomastar Drain Self Adhesive with Belt Plate	1"	78 4397	10	1595
		1¼"	78 4419	10	1595
		1½"	78 4427	10	1595
		2"	78 4435	10	1595
		2½"	78 5105	10	1595
		3"	78 5113	10	1595

PART IXC - STOMA APPLIANCES

ILEOSTOMY BAGS - cont

Manufacturer (1)	Appliance (2)	Order No (3)	Quantity (4)	List Price (5) p
Thackraycare (Chas F Thackray Ltd) cont	Stomastar Drain Self			
	Adhesive 1"	78 4249	10	1380
	1¼"	78 4257	10	1380
	1½"	78 4281	10	1380
	2"	78 4303	10	1380
	2½"	78 4311	10	1380
	3"	78 4850	10	1380
	Raymed Butyl Day Bag			
	Screw outlet	78 5679	1	2090
	Tap outlet	78 5822	1	2190
Ward Surgical Co	White rubber ileostomy bag with St Mark's flange attached	WM 99	1	2107
	With screw outlet			
	Day Size	WM 01	1	949
	Night Size	WM 02	1	1069
	Ureterostomy bag with tap outlet Night Size	WM 47	1	1518
	19mm, 35mm or 54mm opening Day Size	WM 48	1	1421
	White rubber ileostomy bag with spout outlet			
	Day Size	WM 03	1	949
	Night Size	WM 04	1	1069
	With tap outlet			
	Day Size	WM 05	1	1391
	Night Size	WM 06	1	1548
	White rubber Transverse ileostomy bag with tap outlet	WM 07	1	2226
	Black rubber bag with screw outlet			
	19mm, 35mm or 54mm			
	Day Size	WM 08	1	1390
	Night Size	WM 09	1	1451

PART IXC — STOMA APPLIANCES

ILEOSTOMY BAGS — cont

Manufacturer (1)	Appliance (2)		Order No (3)	Quantity (4)	List Price (5) p
Warne—Franklin Medical Ltd	Ostopore Ileo KAV				
	Transparent	32mm	741032	30	5940
		38mm	741038	30	5940
		45mm	741045	30	5940
		51mm	741051	30	5940
		64mm	741064	30	5940
		76mm	741076	30	5940
	Ostopore Ileo AV				
	Opaque	19mm	745019	30	3840
		25mm	745025	30	3840
		32mm	745032	30	3840
		38mm	745038	30	3840
		45mm	745045	30	3840
	Ostopore Ileo KAV				
	Opaque	19mm	746019	30	5550
		25mm	746025	30	5550
		32mm	746032	30	5550
		38mm	746038	30	5550
		45mm	746045	30	5550
		51mm	746051	30	5550
	Mini Pouch	25mm	751025	30	3240
		32mm	751032	30	3240
		38mm	751038	30	3240
		45mm	751045	30	3240
		51mm	751051	30	3240

PART IXC — STOMA APPLIANCES

ILEOSTOMY SETS

Manufacturer (1)	Appliance (2)		Order No (3)	Quantity (4)	List Price (5) p
C S Bullen Ltd	The SR-F Set		SR-F	1	4906
	The OPR-F Appliance		OPR-F	1	7119
	The LOP-F7 Appliance		LOP-F7	1	3413
Downs Surgical Ltd — see Simcare					
John Drew Ltd	Ileostomy Appliance	D1/1	OSTOO 1	1	2979 Δ
		D1/6	OSTOO 3	1	2552 Δ
Leyland Medical Ltd	Birkbeck Ileostomy	19mm	LM 720119	1	7248
	Appliance "A"	38mm	LM 720138	1	7248
		54mm	LM 720154	1	7248
	Appliance "B"	19mm	LM 720519	1	4676
		38mm	LM 720538	1	4676
		54mm	LM 720554	1	4676
A H Shaw & Partners Ltd	Shaw Ileostomy Outfit 5" wide elastic web belt Sizes: 26", 28" etc, to 42"		NSI 5	1	4595

Steeper (Orthopaedic) Ltd
  incorporating
  Donald Rose Ltd
	Donald Rose Ileostomy
	Appliance First stage
			68	1	4439

	Second stage		75	1	4390
	New improved		78	1	4660
Thackraycare (Chas F Thackray Ltd)	Schacht Odourproof Ileostomy Appliance		470538	1	2925

PART IXC — STOMA APPLIANCES

ILEOSTOMY SETS — cont

Manufacturer (1)	Appliance (2)	Order No (3)	Quantity (4)	List Price (5) p

PART IXC — STOMA APPLIANCES

IRRIGATION/WASH — OUT APPLIANCES — (Replacements Parts)
(SLEEVES/DRAINS/BAGS/CONES/LUBRICANTS)
NB. Complete Appliances are not prescribable

Manufacturer (1)	Appliance (2)	Order No (3)	Quantity (4)	List Price (5) p
Astra Meditec	Medena Ileostomy Catheter	M8730	5	360
Cambmac Instru-ments Ltd	Irri Drain with Ring holder for	95047 — 2620	20	1630
	Silicone Ring	09547 — 0000	1	325
	Irridrain (adhesive)	95038 — 2520	20	1630
	Water Container	95200 — 0000	1	1275
	Clamp	95210 — 0000	1	550
	Cone	95205 — 0000	1	820
	Brush	95220 — 0000	1	140
	Tube	95215 — 0000	1	98
	Belt	09000 — 0000	5	2635
Clinimed Ltd	Biotrol Irrigation Sleeves	3061	50	2800
	Cone	3062	1	200
Coloplast Ltd	Disposable Sleeve	1540	30	2400
	Disposable Sleeve	1560	30	2400
	Colotip	1110	1	450
	Irrigator Bag	1511	1	852
	Supporting Plate	1120	1	428
	Irrigation Belt	0420	1	417
Hollister Ltd	Stoma Cone/Irrigator Kit	7718	1	1462
	Irrigator Drain	7724	20	2045
	Replacement Cones	7723	10	5186
			1	633
	Stoma Lubricant	7740	1	359
Ward Surgical Co	Wash—out Cup	WM 77	1	2177
	Cap	WM 78	1	116
	Belt	WM 79	1	630
	Tube	WM 80	1	410

PART IXC — STOMA APPLIANCES

PRESSURE PLATES/SHIELDS

Manufacturer (1)	Appliance (2)		Order No (3)	Quantity (4)	List Price (5) p
Coloplast Ltd	Supporting Plate		1120	1	428
Downs Surgical Ltd — see Simcare					
John Drew Ltd	Pressure Plates	Oval	OSTO 10A	1	246 Δ
		Round	OSTO 10B	1	246 Δ
		4 Slot	OSTO 10C	1	369 Δ
Eschmann Bros & Walsh Ltd — see Simcare					
Kinpax &	St Mark's Shield	4"	KM52	1	620
F T Mitchell		5"	KM52	1	620
Group Ltd		6"	KM52	1	620
	St Mark's Shield	4"	KM52	1	770
	with rubber	5"	KM52	1	770
	rim	6"	KM52	1	770

PART IXC - STOMA APPLIANCES

PRESSURE PLATES/SHIELDS - cont

Manufacturer (1)	Appliance (2)		Order No (3)	Quantity (4)	List Price (5) p
Salt & Son Ltd	Plastic Retaining Shield				
		Single	833008	1	249
		Double	833009	1	384
	SS Wire Retaining Ring				
		Large	833010	1	249
		Medium	833011	1	237
		Small	833012	1	231
	Plastic Retaining Shield				
		Large	833030	1	305
	Light White Anti-Sag ring for Belt use		833038	1	118
	For Velcro Belt Fastening		833086	1	126
	Ring		833039	1	98
	Convex Plate for Light White Bag	25mm	833046	5	1069
		32mm	833047	5	1069
		38mm	833048	5	1069
	Pressure Plate for Simplicity, Kombo & Solo	30mm	833057	1	155
		40mm	833058	1	155
		50mm	833059	1	155
		60mm	833060	1	155
	Pressure Plate Kombo	30mm	833088	1	155
		40mm	833089	1	155
		50mm	833090	1	155
		60mm	833091	1	155
	Eakin Support Frame	32mm	839037	1	97
		45mm	839038	1	97
		64mm	839039	1	97
		90mm	839040	1	97

PART IXC – STOMA APPLIANCES

PRESSURE PLATES/SHIELDS – cont

Manufacturer (1)	Appliance (2)	Order No (3)	Quantity (4)	List Price (5) p
T J Shannon Ltd	Facepiece	TJS 948b	1	754
Simcare				
	Surrey Model Plastic Pressure Plate			
	25 mm	WK 001–25–P	1	573
	32 mm	WK 001–32–L	1	573
	Standard Plastic Pressure Plates to use with Lightweight Bag			
	Attached Flange			
	25 mm int diameter	WK 004–25–C	1	573
	32 mm " "	WK 004–32–Y	1	573
	38 mm " "	WK 004–38–M	1	573
	Stainless Wire Pressure Frames, Hook and Lug			
	To fit 25 mm Flange	WK 012–25–Y	1	699
	32 mm "	WK 012–32–V	1	699
	38 mm "	WK 012–38–J	1	699
	44 mm "	WK 012–44–D	1	699
	51 mm "	WK 012–51–A	1	699

PART IXC – STOMA APPLIANCES

PRESSURE PLATES/SHIELDS – cont

Manufacturer (1)	Appliance (2)		Order No (3)	Quantity (4)	List Price (5) p
Simcare cont					
	Cotton Facepiece		WS 300-01-P	1	1738
	Body Plates	25mm	48-526-48	1	396
		32mm	48-526-56	1	396
		38mm	48-526-64	1	396
Thackraycare (Chas F Thackray Ltd)	Slimline Rubber Retaining Ring		784133	5	275

PART IXC – STOMA APPLIANCES

SKIN FILLERS AND PROTECTIVES
(Barrier Creams, Pastes, Aerosols, Lotions, Powders and Gels)

Manufacturer (1)	Appliance (2)	Order No (3)	Quantity (4)	List Price (5) p
C S Bullen Ltd	Balspray Aerosol	UF 95	1	589
	Karaya Gum Powder	UF 65	70 g	380
Clinimed Ltd	Clinimed Barrier Wipes	3800	50	890
Coloplast Ltd	Comfeel Barrier Cream	4720	60 g	288
	Comfeel Protective Film			
	Sachets	4735	30	690
	Applicator	4731	1	318
ConvaTec Ltd	Orabase Paste	S103	30 g	140
		S104	100 g	310
	Orahesive Powder	S106	25 g	161
	Stomahesive Paste	S105	60 g	541
Downs Surgical Ltd – see Simcare				
Eschman Bros & Walsh Ltd – see Simcare				
Hollister Ltd	Karaya Paste	7910	128 g	533
	Karaya Powder	7905	1	633
	Skin Gel	7916	28 g	463
Salt & Son Ltd	Karaya Powder 402 Puffer Pack	833004	1	347
	Ostomy Cleaning Soap (Spirit of Soap)	833007	110 ml	209
†	Saltair 'Protect' Balsam Spray	833026	150 g	550
	Skin Prep Wipes	840001	50	1129
	United Skin Barrier Paste	840033	70 g	508
Simcare	Chiron Barrier Cream	WM102-01-A	52 g	385
	Karaya Gel	WM086-01-E	35 g	462
	Karaya Powder	WM083-01-R	100 g	543
	Derma-gard Skin Wipes	32-291-06	50	1128
Simpla Plastics Ltd	Simpla Gel	130101	1	484

† To be deleted 1 October 1990

PART IXC — STOMA APPLIANCES

SKIN FILLERS AND PROTECTIVES
(Barrier Creams, Pastes, Aerosols, Lotions, Powders and Gels) — cont

Manufacturer (1)	Appliance (2)	Order No (3)	Quantity (4)	List Price (5) p
Squibb Surgicare Ltd — See ConvaTec Ltd				
Thackraycare (Thackray Chas F Ltd)	Stomobar Barrier Cream	785857	20 g	180
	Stomosal Deodorizing and Antiseptic Solution	785849	200 ml	412
	Skin Sheild	781630	50	700
Warne–Franklin Medical Ltd	Translet Barrier Cream	703003	51 g	211
	Wipes	732730	30	458

PART IXC — STOMA APPLIANCES

SKIN PROTECTORS (Wafers, Blankets, Foam Pads, Washers)

Manufacturer (1)	Appliance (2)		Order No (3)	Quantity (4)	List Price (5) p
C S Bullen Ltd	Karaya Gum Washers in tins				
	2" diameter				
	Regular 2" x 7/8" opening		UF 601	10	1032
2" x 1 1/8" "			UF 602	10	1032
	Extra Hard 2" x 7/8" "		UF 6601	10	1032
	2" x 1 1/8" "		UF 6602	10	1032
	2.5" diameter				
	Regular 2 1/2" x 1 1/4"				
	opening		UF 603	10	1196
	Extra Hard 2 1/2" x 1 1/2"				
	opening		UF 6603	10	1196
	3" diameter				
	Regular 3" x 7/8" opening		UF 604	10	1371
	3" x 1 1/8" "		UF 605	10	1371
	3" x 1 1/2" "		UF 606	10	1371
	3" x 2" "		UF 607	10	1371
	Extra Hard				
	3" x 7/8" opening		UF 6604	10	1371
	3" x 1 1/8" "		UF 6605	10	1371
	3" x 1 1/2" "		UF 6606	10	1371
	3" x 2" "		UF 6607	10	1371
Cambmac Instruments Ltd	Karaya Rings	19mm	06019-0000	25	3035
		22mm	06022-0000	25	3035
		25mm	06025-0000	25	3035
		32mm	06032-0000	25	3035
		38mm	06038-0000	25	3035
		50mm	06050-0000	25	3035
		63mm	06063-0000	25	3035
Clinimed Ltd	Biotrol Skin Protectors				
		20cm x 20 cm	32-072	5	3000
		10cm x 10cm	32-075	10	1250
		10cm Dia.	32-076	10	1250

0311M/22

SKIN PROTECTORS (Wafers, Blankets, Foam Pads, Washers) — cont

Manufacturer (1)	Appliance (2)	Order No (3)	Quantity (4)	List Price (5) p
Coloplast Ltd	Coloplast Protective Sheets			
	Non Sterile 10cm x 10cm	3210	10	1540
	15cm x 15cm	3215	5	1785
	20cm x 20cm	3220	5	3245
	formerly comfeel protective sheets			
	Coloplast Protective Rings			
	10mm	2310	30	2550
	15mm	2315	30	2550
	20mm	2320	30	2550
	25mm	2325	30	2550
	30mm	2330	30	2550
	40mm	2340	30	2550
	50mm	2350	30	2550
ConvaTec Ltd	Stomahesive Wafers			
	100mm x 100mm	S 100	5	799
	200mm x 200mm	S 101	3	1950
	Varihesive Wafers			
	100mm x 100mm	S 108	5	740
Downs Surgical Ltd — see Simcare				
John Drew Ltd	K Seal Karaya Gum Washers			
	Small	OSTO 13B	20	813 Δ
	Large	OSTO 13A	20	925 Δ
Eschman Bros & Walsh Ltd — see Simcare				
Francol Surgical Ltd	Spare Plaster Face Plate			
	29mm		20	1685
	40mm		20	1685
	57mm		20	1685
Hollister Ltd	Hollihesive Skin Barrier			
	4" x 4"	7700	5	808
	8" x 8"	7701	4	2459

SKIN PROTECTORS (Wafers, Blankets, Foam Pads, Washers) — cont

Manufacturer (1)	Appliance (2)			Order No (3)	Quantity (4)	List Price (5) p
Salt & Son Ltd	Salger Karaya Washers					
	with Foam	40mm		600440	5	991
		57mm		600457	5	991
	Salts Saltair Twin Pack					
		Small		833001	1	737
		Large		833002	1	1021
	Salts Small Karaya					
	Washers			833003	10	601
	Foam Cushions	25mm		833014	5	197
		32mm		833015	5	197
		38mm		833016	5	197
		51mm		833017	5	197
	Salts Dri Pads	40mm		833024	5	200
	Foam Seals as in small					
	twin pack			833031	10	149
	Salts Large Karaya					
	Washers			833084	10	971
	Foam Seals as in large					
	twin pack			833085	10	149
	Cohesive Washers	Small	50mm	839002	20	2454
		Large	95mm	839001	10	1623
	Realistic Washers					
		13mm		833070	10	1214
		19mm		833071	10	1214
		22mm		833072	10	1214
		25mm		833073	10	1214
		29mm		833074	10	1214
		32mm		833075	10	1214
		38mm		833076	10	1214
	United Skin Barrier Wafer					
	4" x 4" (10cm x 10cm)			840040	5	769
	8" x 8" (20cm x 20cm)			840041	3	1810

PART IXC – STOMA APPLIANCES

SKIN PROTECTORS (Wafers, Blankets, Foam Pads, Washers) – cont

Manufacturer (1)	Appliance (2)	Order No (3)	Quantity (4)	List Price (5) p
T J Shannon Ltd	Foam Sponge Rings	TJS 962b	1	62
	Kaygee Washers 2 1/2" base			
	(1 1/8" or 7/8" hole)		10	560
	2 3/4" base			
	(1 3/8" or 7/8" hole)		10	560
A H Shaw & Partners Ltd	Shaw Healwell Squares			
	hole sizes 1", 1 1/4", 1 1/2"	NSI 53	12	785
	Body Mould Squares			
	hole sizes 1", 1 1/4", 1 1/2"	NSI 56	5	835
	Washers			
	hole sizes 1", 1 1/4"	NSI 59	10	765
	Rings			
	hole sizes 1", 1 1/4", 1 1/2"	NSI 55	5	765
	Shaw Healwell Rings			
	hole sizes 1", 1 1/4", 1 1/2"	NSI 52	12	680
	5" x 5" Healwell Rings			
	hole sizes 1", 1 1/4", 1 1/2"	NSI 60	12	945
Simcare	White Foam Pads			
	76mm diam			
	25mm opening	WJ 275–25–A	5	368
	29mm opening	WJ 275–29–J	5	504
	32mm opening	WJ 275–32–W	5	504
	38mm opening	WJ 275–38–K	5	504
	90mm diam 32mm opening	WJ 290–32–L	5	504
	38mm opening	WJ 290–38–Y	5	504

PART IXC - STOMA APPLIANCES

SKIN PROTECTORS (Wafers, Blankets, Foam Pads, Washers) - cont

Manufacturer (1)	Appliance (2)	Order No (3)	Quantity (4)	List Price (5) p
Simcare cont	Black Foam Pads 76mm diam			
	25mm opening	WJ-475-25N	5	472
	Karaya Washers to fit			
	(Redifit) Bag 25mm	WM 080-25-T	10	1088
	32mm	WM 080-32-Q	10	1088
	38mm	WM 080-38-D	10	1088
	44mm	WM 080-44-X	10	1088
	51mm	WM 080-51-U	10	1088
	Downs Adhesive Karaya Gum Washers 22mm centre opening			
	51mm base	WM 051-23-C	10	882
	29mm centre opening			
	51mm base	WM 051-28-N	10	882
	22mm centre opening			
	70mm base	WM 070-23-J	10	1088
	29 mm centre opening			
	70mm base	WM 070-28-U	10	1088
	Karaya Gum Sheets 300mm x 100mm	WM 089-01-S	1	544
	Karaya Rings 19mm	32-263-87	20	1981
	25mm	32-264-84	20	1981
	32mm	32-265-81	20	1981
	38mm	32-266-89	20	1981
	51mm	32-267-86	20	1981
	Seel-a-Peel Squares			
	100mm sq	32-292-03	20	3100
	150mm sq	32-292-11	5	1909

PART IXC - STOMA APPLIANCES

SKIN PROTECTORS (Wafers, Blankets, Foam Pads, Washers) - cont

Manufacturer (1)	Appliance (2)	Order No (3)	Quantity (4)	List Price (5) p
Simcare cont	Rings			
	19mm	32-293-00	20	1812
	25mm	32-293-19	20	1812
	32mm	32-293-27	20	1812
	38mm	32-293-35	20	1812
	44mm	32-293-43	20	1812
Simpla Plastics Ltd	Simplaseel Wafer			
	100mm × 100mm	130320	10	1387
Squibb Surgicare - See ConvaTec Ltd				
Thackraycare (Thackray Chas F Ltd)	Schacht Foam Rings			
	Colostomy	78 4885	10	710
	Ileostomy	78 4893	10	710

PART IXC - STOMA APPLIANCES

STOMA CAPS/DRESSINGS

Manufacturer (1)	Appliance (2)		Order No (3)	Quantity (4)	List Price (5) p
C S Bullen Ltd	Rubber Cap to protect flange whilst bathing		UF 61	1	369
Cambmac Instrument Ltd	Dansac Minicap (Opaque)	30mm 44mm	01930-1000 01944-1000	50 50	4075 4075
Coloplast Ltd	Colocap		1014	100	8100
ConvaTec Ltd	Colodress Stoma Cap		S 821	30	2600
Downs Surgical Ltd - see Simcare					
Eschmann Bros & Walsh Ltd - see Simcare					
Hollister Ltd	Hollister Stoma Cap	51mm 76mm	7184 7186	50 50	4341 4341
Palex (Cambridge Selfcare Diagnostics Limited)	Mini Stoma Cap		MINI 1	30	2450 |
Salt & Son Ltd	Simplicity 1. Stoma caps		510250	30	2593
Simcare	Leisure Pouch		32-287-11	20	1836
Squibb Surgicare - See ConvaTec Ltd					

PART IXC – STOMA APPLIANCES

STOMA CAPS/DRESSINGS – cont

Manufacturer (1)	Appliance (2)	Order No (3)	Quantity (4)	List Price (5) p
Steeper (Orthopaedic) Ltd incorporating Donald Rose Ltd	Celluloid colostomy shield 10cm (4") diameter with 4 studs	7	1	435
	Waterproof material squares 16.5cm x 16.5cm (6 1/2" x 6 1/2") for use with colostomy dressings.	9	12	293
	All solid rim celluloid colostomy cup with 4 studs	12	1	1854
	All Celluloid colostomy cup with 4 studs and chute	13	1	2231
	Two zip fasteners fitted to colostomy belt	16	1	729
	Waterproof front, fitted to colostomy belt	17	1	601
	Donald Rose rubber ileo/colostomy bath belt with internal chamber for dressings, with stud fastenings for adjustment	31	1	1807
	Woven understraps with buttonhold ends	47	1 pair	279
	1 sq yd Waterproof material	91	1	284

PART IXC — STOMA APPLIANCES

TUBING

Manufacturer (1)	Appliance (2)	Order No (3)	Quantity (4)	List Price (5) P
Eschmann Bros & Walsh Ltd — see Simcare				
Hollister Ltd	Urostomy Drain Tube	7328	10	1813
	Urostomy Drain Tube for fitting to LO-Profile Urostomy Bags	7330	8	1686
	Premium Urostomy drain tube adaptor	7331	10	1485
Salt & Son Ltd	Salts Night Tube Adaptor	833043	2	75
Simcare	Carshalton Connector	11-110-19	10	318
Steeper (Orthopaedic) Ltd incorporating Donald Rose Ltd	Metal Spring Tubing Clip	28	1	203

PART IXC – STOMA APPLIANCES

TWO PIECE OSTOMY SYSTEMS

Manufacturer (1)	Appliance (2)	Order No (3)	Quantity (4)	List Price (5) p
Cambmac Instruments Ltd	Dansac Supersquare System – 2 Piece:			
	Max Stoma Size 50 mm: Base Plate			
	100mm x 100mm	06510-0000	10	2325
	Closed Bag:			
	Opaque Standard	02550-1000	100	10630
	Clear Standard	02550-2000	100	10630
	Opaque Small	02650-1000	100	10630
	Clear Small	02650-2000	100	10630
	Drainable Bag:			
	Opaque Standard	04550-1010	30	3080
	Clear Standard	04550-2010	30	3080
	Opaque Small	04650-1010	30	3080
	Clear Small	04650-2010	30	3080
	Max Stoma Size 80 mm: Base Plate			
	125mm x 125mm	06512-0000	10	4290
	Closed Bag:			
	Opaque Standard	02480-1000	100	13480
	Clear Standard	02480-2000	100	13480
	Drainable Bag:			
	Opaque Standard	04480-1010	30	4450
	Clear Standard	04480-2010	30	4450
Coloplast Ltd	MC2002			
	Base Plates			
	40mm flange 15mm stoma	6742	5	1090
	40mm flange 25mm stoma	6743	5	1090
	60mm flange 35mm stoma	6764	5	1090
	60mm flange 45mm stoma	6765	5	1090
	Pouches 40mm closed clear	6641	30	2970
	40mm closed opaque	6642	30	2970
	40mm open clear	6541	30	3270
	40mm open opaque	6542	30	3270
	60mm closed clear	6661	30	2970
	60mm closed opaque	6662	30	2970
	60mm open clear	6561	30	3270
	60mm open opaque	6562	30	3270

0311M/31

PART IXC — STOMA APPLIANCES

TWO PIECE OSTOMY SYSTEMS — cont				
Manufacturer (1)	Appliance (2)		Order No (3)	Quantity (4)	List Price (5) p

Manufacturer	Appliance		Order No	Quantity	List Price p
Coloplast Ltd— cont	MC2002 — cont				
	Belt Plates	40mm	4270	10	440
		60mm	4271	10	440
	UR02002				
	Base Plates	40mm flange	4245	5	1120
		60mm "	4265	5	1120
	Bags	40mm Large	4240	20	4240
		40mm Small	4241	20	4240
		60mm Large	4260	20	4240
	Night Drainage Bag		4210	10	1090
	Conseal				
	Base Plate	40mm	1200	5	1030
		50mm	1250	5	1030
	Colostomy Plug	40 x 35 mm	1235	10	930
		40 x 45 mm	1245	10	930
		50 x 35 mm	1285	10	930
		50 x 45 mm	1295	10	930
	Closed Bag	40 mm	1210	30	2790
		50 mm	1260	30	2790
	Discharge Bag	40 mm	1220	50	250
		50 mm	1270	50	250
ConvaTec Ltd	System 1:				
	Stomahesive Flanges				
		32mm	S1	4	670
		38mm	S2	4	670
		45mm	S3	4	670
		57mm	S5	4	670
	Ostomy Pouches		S40	100	3474
	System 2:				
	Stomahesive Flanges Wafer size 100mm x 100mm				
		32mm flange	S239	10	1888
		38mm "	S240	10	1888
		45mm "	S241	10	1888
		57mm "	S242	10	1888
		70mm "	S243	10	1888
	Stomahesive Flexible Flanges Wafer size 100mm x 100mm				
		32mm flange	S244	5	944
		38mm "	S245	5	944
		45mm "	S246	5	944
		57mm "	S247	5	944
		70mm "	S248	5	944

PART IXC - STOMA APPLIANCES

		Order	Quantity	List
Manufacturer	Appliance	No		Price
(1)	(2)	(3)	(4)	(5)
				p

TWO PIECE OSTOMY SYSTEMS - cont

Manufacturer (1)	Appliance (2)	Order No (3)	Quantity (4)	List Price (5) p
ConvaTec Ltd - Cont	System 2			
	Wafer size 127mm x			
	127mm (70mm flange)	S250	10	3824
	Wafer size 152mm x			
	152mm (100mm flange)	S251	10	4590
	Drainable Pouches			
	Standard, white			
	32mm	S274	10	866
	38mm	S275	10	866
	45mm	S276	10	866
	57mm	S277	10	866
	70mm	S278	10	866
	Combihesive Closed Pouches			
	with integral filter (Beige)			
	38mm flange	S295	30	2639
	45mm "	S296	30	2639
	57mm "	S297	30	2639
	70mm "	S298	30	2639
	Combihesive Flexible			
	Flanges			
	Wafer size			
	100mm x 100mm			
	32mm flange	S351	5	1070
	38mm "	S352	5	1070
	45mm "	S353	5	1070
	Wafer size			
	127mm x 127mm			
	57mm flange	S354	5	1165
	70mm "	S355	5	1165
	Accordion Flanges			
	Wafer size 100mm x			
	100mm (70mm flange)	S235	10	3135
	Wafer size 127mm x			
	127mm (100mm flange)	S236	10	5532
	Closed Pouches for			
	38mm flange	S260	30	2555
	45mm "	S261	30	2555
	57mm "	S262	30	2555
	70mm "	S263	30	2555

PART IXC — STOMA APPLIANCES

TWO PIECE OSTOMY SYSTEMS — cont

Manufacturer (1)	Appliance (2)	Order No (3)	Quantity (4)	List Price (5) p
ConvaTec Ltd — Cont	**Closed Pouches**			
	with S3			
	Pouch Film for:			
	38mm flange	S264	30	2555
	45mm "	S265	30	2555
	57mm "	S266	30	2555
	70mm "	S267	30	2555
	Combihesive Mini Pouches			
	with S3			
	Pouch Film for:			
	32mm flanges	S290	20	1447
	38mm "	S291	20	1447
	45mm "	S292	20	1447
	57mm "	S293	20	1447
	Combihesive Drainable Pouches			
	Standard Clear			
	with S3			
	Pouch Film for:			
	45mm flanges	S230	10	874
	57mm "	S231	10	874
	70mm "	S232	10	874
	100mm "	S233	10	1545
	Standard Beige			
	with S3			
	Film Pouch for:			
	32mm flanges	S269	10	874
	38mm "	S270	10	874
	45mm "	S271	10	874
	57mm "	S272	10	874
	70mm "	S273	10	874
	Small Beige			
	with S3			
	Pouch Film for:			
	32mm flanges	S279	10	874
	38mm "	S280	10	874
	45mm "	S281	10	874
	57mm "	S282	10	874
	70mm "	S283	10	874
	Urostomy Pouches			
	Standard for:			
	32mm flanges	S300	10	1868
	38mm "	S301	10	1868
	45mm "	S302	10	1868
	57mm "	S303	10	1868
	70mm "	S316	10	2023
	100mm "	S317	10	3047

0311M/34

PART IXC – STOMA APPLIANCES

TWO PIECE OSTOMY SYSTEMS – cont

Manufacturer (1)	Appliance (2)		Order No (3)	Quantity (4)	List Price (5) p
ConvaTec Ltd – Cont	Small for:				
	32mm flanges		S310	10	1868
	38mm "		S311	10	1868
	45mm "		S312	10	1868
	57mm "		S313	10	1868
	Urostomy Pouches with Accuseal Tap, clear				
	Standard for:				
	32mm flanges		S360	10	1915
	38mm "		S361	10	1915
	45mm "		S362	10	1915
	57mm "		S363	10	1915
Eschmann Bros & Walsh Ltd see Simcare					
Hollister Ltd	Premium				
	2 Piece Drainable Bag – Clear		460	10	834
	2 Piece Drainable Bag – 102mm		4606	10	1794
	2 Piece Drainable Bag – Opaque		461	10	834
	2 Piece Urostomy Bag	1"	4702	10	1840
	" " " "	1.5"	4703	10	1840
	" " " "	2"	4704	10	1840
	2 Piece Closed Bag – Clear	1"	4503	15	1217
	" " " "	2"	4504	15	1217
	" " " "	2.5"	4505	15	1217
	2 Piece Closed Bag – Opaque	1"	4513	15	1217
	" " " "	2"	4514	15	1217
	" " " "	2.5"	4515	15	1217
	Skin Barrier Floating Flange	25mm	4402	5	983
		38mm	4403	5	983
		51mm	4404	5	983
		64mm	4405	5	983
		102mm	4406	5	1074
Salt & Son Ltd	Simplicity Flanges				
	Standard	30mm	500130	5	226
		40mm	500140	5	226
		50mm	500150	5	226
		60mm	500160	5	226

PART IXC - STOMA APPLIANCES

TWO PIECE OSTOMY SYSTEMS - cont

Manufacturer (1)	Appliance (2)		Order No (3)	Quantity (4)	List Price (5) p
Salt & Son Ltd	Simplicity 2 Flange				
- cont		30mm	520130	5	1118
		40mm	520140	5	1118
		50mm	520150	5	1118
		60mm	520160	5	1118
	Simplicity 2 Drainable				
		30mm	521330	15	1486
		40mm	521340	15	1486
		50mm	521350	15	1486
		60mm	521360	15	1486
		70mm	521370	15	1486
	Simplicity 2 Closed				
		30mm	520330	30	2676
		40mm	520340	30	2676
		50mm	520350	30	2676
		60mm	520360	30	2676
		70mm	520370	30	2676
	Simplicity 2 Post Op				
		30mm	520230	30	2933
		40mm	520240	30	2933
		50mm	520250	30	2933
		60mm	520260	30	2933
		70mm	520270	30	2933
	Simplicity 2 Transverse Flange		520530	5	1631
	Simplicity 2 Transverse Bag Starter		520630	10	3334
	Flange with Cohesive				
	Washer	30mm	502130	5	1144
		40mm	502140	5	1144
		50mm	502150	5	1144
	Clear Closed Bag				
	Medium	40mm	530940	30	1247
		50mm	530950	30	1247
		60mm	530960	30	1247
		70mm	530970	30	1247

0311M/36

PART IXC - STOMA APPLIANCES

TWO PIECE OSTOMY SYSTEMS - cont

Manufacturer (1)	Appliance (2)			Order No (3)	Quantity (4)	List Price (5) p
Salt & Son Ltd - cont	Clear Drainable Bag					
	Medium	40mm		531340	30	1422
		50mm		531350	30	1422
		60mm		531360	30	1422
	Post-Operative Closed					
	Bag	Large	40mm	530240	30	1235
		50mm		530250	30	1235
		60mm		530260	30	1235
	Pink Closed Bag					
	Medium	40mm		530340	30	1235
		50mm		530350	30	1235
		60mm		530360	30	1235
Simcare	Beta 2 Piece kit			32-294-08	1	4127
	Beta 2 Piece spare Bags			32-294-16	90	11362
Squibb Surgicare Ltd - See ConvaTec Ltd						

PART IXC – STOMA APPLIANCES

TWO PIECE OSTOMY SYSTEMS – cont

Manufacturer (1)	Appliance (2)	Order No (3)	Quantity (4)	List Price (5) p
Warne–Franklin Medical Ltd	Translet Range			
	Premier Colostomy Set (1 adhesive ring and 6 bags)			
	27mm opening	731127	15	5175
	40mm opening	731140	15	5175
	57mm opening	731157	15	5175
	Premier Spare Bags			
	28cm length	732100	10	397
	18cm length	732150	10	397
	Royal Colostomy Set (1 adhesive ring and 6 odour proof bags)			
	27mm opening	731027	15	7215
	40mm opening	731040	15	7215
	57mm opening	731057	15	7215
	Royal Spare Bags			
	28cm length	732000	10	630
	18cm length	732050	10	630

PART IXC — STOMA APPLIANCES

TWO PIECE OSTOMY SYSTEMS — cont

Manufacturer (1)	Appliance (2)		Order No (3)	Quantity (4)	List Price (5) p
Warne—Franklin	Translet Adhesive				
Medical Ltd — cont	Rings	27mm	732327	5	531
		40mm	732340	5	531
		57mm	732357	5	531
	Translet Microporous Spare				
	Adhesive Rings	27mm	732427	5	531
		40mm	732440	5	531
		57mm	732457	5	531

PART IXC — STOMA APPLIANCES

UROSTOMY BAGS

Manufacturer (1)	Appliance (2)		Order No (3)	Quantity (4)	List Price (5) p
C S Bullen Ltd	Lenbul				
	Day Bag with tap		U 5	1	1232
	Night Bag with tap		U 6	1	1408
	Day Bag with large opening		U 7	1	1278
	Night Bag with large opening		U 8	1	1461
	Day Bag with metal strip		U 9	1	1378
	One Piece Flange and Bag				
		1"	U 91	1	2587
		2"	U 92	1	2587
	Babies' Bag and Flange				
	With night–tube	1¼"	U 78	1	3596
		2"	U 79	1	3596
	Without night–tube	1¼"	U 80	1	3596
		2"	U 81	1	3596
	Child's Rubber Cap and Bag				
		Small	U 82	1	2437
		Large	U 83	1	2437
	With metal strip				
		Small	U 84	1	2437
		Large	U 85	1	2621
Coloplast Ltd	Stoma Urine Bags	Maxi	1005	30	5820
		Midi	1006	30	5820

PART IXC - STOMA APPLIANCES

UROSTOMY BAGS - cont

Manufacturer (1)	Appliance (2)	Order No (3)	Quantity (4)	List Price (5) p
Downs Surgical Ltd - see Simcare				
John Drew Ltd	Urostomy Bags D½	OSTO 06	50	6992 Δ
	Rubber Bags	OSTO 16	1	1198 Δ
		OSTO 17	1	1257 Δ
Eschmann Bros and Walsh Ltd - see Simcare				
Hollister Ltd	Karaya Seal with Regular Adhesive (Transparent) 12" Length			
	Gasket Size: 1.0"	7482	20	5403
	1.25"	7488	20	5403
	1.5"	7483	20	5403
	1.75"	7489	20	5403
	2.0"	7484	20	5403
	9" length			
	Gasket Size: 0.75"	7417	20	5403
	1.0"	7412	20	5403
	1.25"	7418	20	5403
	1.5"	7413	20	5403
	1.75"	7419	20	5403
	2.0"	7414	20	5403
	Lo-Profile Urostomy Bag with Microporous II Adhesive and Karaya 5 Seal			
	Gasket Size: 0.75"	1437	10	4793
	1.0"	1432	10	4793
	1.25"	1438	10	4793
	1.5"	1433	10	4793
	1.75"	1439	10	4793
	2.0"	1434	10	4793

PART IXC — STOMA APPLIANCES

UROSTOMY BAGS — cont

Manufacturer (1)	Appliance (2)		Order No (3)	Quantity (4)	List Price (5) p
Hollister Ltd cont					
	Adhesive only				
	Gasket Size:	0.75"	1427	10	3640
		1.0"	1422	10	3640
		1.25"	1428	10	3640
		1.5"	1423	10	3640
		1.75"	1429	10	3640
		2.0"	1424	10	3640
	Regular Adhesive only, (Beltless) (Transparent)				
	9" length				
	Gasket Size:	0.75"	7447	20	4110
		1.0"	7442	20	4110
		1.25"	7448	20	4110
		1.5"	7443	20	4110
		1.75"	7449	20	4110
		2.0"	7444	20	4110
	Regular Adhesive only, with Belt Lugs (Transparent)				
	12" length				
	Gasket Size:	1.0"	7472	20	4110
		1.25"	7478	20	4110
		1.5"	7473	20	4110
		1.75"	7479	20	4110
		2.0"	7474	20	4110
	16" length				
	Gasket Size:	1.0"	7452	20	4110
		1.25"	7458	20	4110
		1.5"	7453	20	4110
		1.75"	7459	20	4110
		2.0"	7454	20	4110

PART IXC — STOMA APPLIANCES

UROSTOMY BAGS — cont

Manufacturer (1)	Appliance (2)		Order No (3)	Quantity (4)	List Price (5) p
Hollister Ltd cont					
	9" length				
	Gasket Size:	0.75"	7407	20	4110
		1.0"	7402	20	4110
		1.25"	7408	20	4110
		1.5"	7403	20	4110
		1.75"	7409	20	4110
		2.0"	7404	20	4110
	Karaya Seal with Regular Adhesive)Transparent)				
	16" length				
	Gasket size:	1.0"	7462	20	5403
		1.25"	7468	20	5403
		1.5"	7463	20	5403
		1.75"	7469	20	5403
		2.0"	7464	20	5403
Kinpax & F T Mitchell Group Ltd	White rubber urostomy bags				
	Night bag screw cap outlet		KM 46	1	1405
	Day " " " "		KM 44	1	1220
	Night bag spout "		KM 49	1	1160
	Day " " "		KM 48	1	1100
	Black Butyl bag odourless				
	Night bag screw cap outlet		KM 40	1	2560
	Day " " " "		KM 38	1	2195
	Night bag spout outlet		KM 43	1	2320
	Day " " "		KM 42	1	2320
	Night bag tap outlet		KM 41	1	2560
	Day " " "		KM 39	1	2440
Leyland Medical Ltd	Birkbeck Black Rubber				
	Day Bag 19mm		LM 723125	1	2374
	Night Bag 19mm		LM 723175	1	2590

9/90

PART IXC – STOMA APPLIANCES

UROSTOMY BAGS – cont

Manufacturer (1)	Appliance (2)		Order No (3)	Quantity (4)	List Price (5) p
Leyland Medical Ltd cont	Pink Rubber				
	Day Bag	19mm	LM 724125	1	2374
	Night Bag	19mm	LM 724175	1	2590
	White Rubber Day Bag				
		19mm	LM 883111	1	1290
		25mm	LM 883112	1	1290
		28mm	LM 883113	1	1290
	Night Bag	19mm	LM 883121	1	1325
		25mm	LM 883122	1	1325
		28mm	LM 883123	1	1325
	White Rubber Glasgow Bag				
		Small tap	LM 884230	1	1575
		Large tap	LM 884232	1	1575
	White Rubber Transverse Bag Right	Small	LM 884104	1	1575
		Medium	LM 884105	1	1575
		Large	LM 884106	1	1575
	White Rubber Transverse Bag Left	Small	LM 884114	1	1575
		Medium	LM 884115	1	1575
		Large	LM 884116	1	1575
	Latex Rubber Day Bag	19mm	LM 883140	1	1305
		25mm	LM 883142	1	1305
		28mm	LM 883144	1	1305
	Night Bag	19mm	LM 883150	1	1448
		25mm	LM 883152	1	1448
		28mm	LM 883154	1	1448
Salt & Son Ltd	KR AR Black Rubber Tap Bag	Special	181099	1	3053

PART IXC - STOMA APPLIANCES

UROSTOMY BAGS - cont

Manufacturer (1)	Appliance (2)		Order No (3)	Quantity (4)	List Price (5) p
Salt & Son Ltd cont	Large	19mm	181119	1	3053
		25mm	181125	1	3053
		32mm	181132	1	3053
		38mm	181138	1	3053
	Medium	19mm	181319	1	3053
		25mm	181325	1	3053
		32mm	181332	1	3053
		38mm	181338	1	3053
	KR WP Black Rubber Tap Bag				
		Special	183099	1	3629
	Large	19mm	183119	1	3629
		25mm	183125	1	3629
		32mm	183132	1	3629
		38mm	183138	1	3629
	Medium	19mm	183319	1	3629
		25mm	183325	1	3629
		32mm	183332	1	3629
		38mm	183338	1	3629
	KR AR MB Black Rubber Tap Bag				
		Special	185099	1	3463
	Large	19mm	185119	1	3463
		25mm	185125	1	3463
		32mm	185132	1	3463
		38mm	185138	1	3463
	Medium	19mm	185319	1	3463
		25mm	185325	1	3463
		32mm	185332	1	3463
		38mm	185338	1	3463
	KR WP MB Black Rubber Tap Bag				
		Special	188099	1	4158
	Large	19mm	188119	1	4158
		25mm	188125	1	4158
		32mm	188132	1	4158
		38mm	188138	1	4158

PART IXC - STOMA APPLIANCES

UROSTOMY BAGS - cont

Manufacturer (1)	Appliance (2)	Order No (3)	Quantity (4)	List Price (5) p
Salt & Son Ltd – cont	KR WP MB Black Rubber Tap Bag			
	Medium 19mm	188319	1	4158
	25mm	188325	1	4158
	32mm	188332	1	4158
	38mm	188338	1	4158
	Light White Urostomy Bag with Realistic			
	Large 25mm	292125	20	8706
	32mm	292132	20	8706
	38mm	292138	20	8706
	Light White Clear Urostomy Bag with Realistic			
	Large 25mm	293125	20	8706
	32mm	293132	20	8706
	38mm	293138	20	8706
	Light White Clear Urostomy Bag with Realistic			
	Small 25mm	293225	20	8706
	32mm	293232	20	8706
	38mm	293238	20	8706
	Light White Urostomy Bag			
	Large 25mm	294125	20	6542
	32mm	294132	20	6542
	38mm	294138	20	6542

0311M/46

PART IXC — STOMA APPLIANCES

UROSTOMY BAGS — cont

Manufacturer (1)	Appliance (2)			Order No (3)	Quantity (4)	List Price (5) p
Salt & Son Ltd – cont	Light White Clear Urostomy Bag					
		Large	25mm	296125	20	6542
			32mm	296132	20	6542
			38mm	296138	20	6542
	Light White Clear Urostomy Bag					
		Small	25mm	296225	20	6542
			32mm	296232	20	6542
			38mm	296238	20	6542
	Light White Urostomy Adhesive Bag					
		Large	25mm	298125	20	6909
			32mm	298132	20	6909
			38mm	298138	20	6909
	Light White Clear Urostomy Adhesive Bag					
		Large	25mm	299125	20	6909
			32mm	299132	20	6909
			38mm	299138	20	6909

0311M/47

PART IXC — STOMA APPLIANCES

UROSTOMY BAGS — cont

Manufacturer (1)	Appliance (2)	Order No (3)	Quantity (4)	List Price (5) p
Salt & Son Ltd — cont	Light White Clear Urostomy Adhesive Bag			
	Small 25mm	299225	20	6909
	32mm	299232	20	6909
	38mm	299238	20	6909
	AR White Rubber Tap Bag			
	Large 25mm	281125	1	1245
	32mm	281132	1	1245
	38mm	281138	1	1245
	44mm	281144	1	1245
	51mm	281151	1	1245
	AR White Rubber Tap Bag			
	Small 25mm	281225	1	1245
	32mm	281232	1	1245
	38mm	281238	1	1245
	AR White Rubber Tap Bag			
	Medium 25mm	281325	1	1245
	32mm	281332	1	1245
	38mm	281338	1	1245
	Black Rubber Tap Bag (for use with flange)			
	Special	382099	1	2804
	Large	382129	1	2804
	Medium	382229	1	2804
	Small	382329	1	2804
	White Rubber Tap Bag (for use with flange)			
	Large	482129	1	819
	Medium	482329	1	819
	Small	482229	1	819
	Simplicity 1 Paediatric Uri-bag			
	13mm Starter	623212	15	3219

PART IXC - STOMA APPLIANCES

UROSTOMY BAGS - cont

Manufacturer (1)	Appliance (2)		Order No (3)	Quantity (4)	List Price (5) p
Simcare	Great Ormond Street				
	Minicare Bag	Clear	WC 100-19-E	10	1483
		Opaque	WC 100-20-N	10	1483
	Rediflow Adhesive				
		19mm	WG 001-19-H	20	4607
		25mm	WG 001-25-C	20	4607
		32mm	WG 001-32-Y	20	4607
		38mm	WG 001-38-M	20	4607
		44mm	WG 001-44-G	20	4607
		51mm	WG 001-51-D	20	4607
	Mitcham, Lightweight				
		19mm	WH 002-19-U	10	2560
		25mm	WH 002-25-P	10	2560
		32mm	WH 002-32-L	10	2560
		38mm	WH 002-38-Y	10	2560
	Mini	25mm	WH 005-25-C	10	2560
		32mm	WH 005-32-Y	10	2560
	Maxi	25mm	WH 009-25-U	10	2560
		32mm	WH 009-32-R	10	2560
		38mm	WH 009-38-E	10	2560
	Standard Mitcham Bags				
	With Foam Pads	25mm	WH 012-25-U	1	447
		32mm	WH 012-32-R	1	447
		38mm	WH 012-38-E	1	447
	With Adhesive Flange				
		19mm	WH 111-19-C	10	3135
		25mm	WH 111-25-W	10	3135
		32mm	WH 111-32-T	10	3135
		38mm	WH 111-38-G	10	3135

PART IXC - STOMA APPLIANCES

UROSTOMY BAGS - cont

Manufacturer (1)	Appliance (2)		Order No (3)	Quantity (4)	List Price (5) p
Simcare	Mitcham Adhesive Bags				
	Mini	19mm	WH 116-19-Y	10	3135
		25mm	WH 116-25-T	10	3135
		32mm	WH 116-32-Q	10	3135
	Maxi	25mm	WH 119-25-G	10	3135
		32mm	WH 119-32-D	10	3135
		38mm	WH 119-38-R	10	3135
	Chiron Child's Day Bag				
	Rubber Bag		WF 221-01-D	1	1600
	Chiron Night Bag				
	White rubber	38mm	WF 211-38-X	1	2163
		44mm	WF 211-44-S	1	2163
		51mm	WF 211-51-P	1	2163
	Latex rubber	38mm	WF 213-38-G	1	2163
	Chiron Day Bag				
	White rubber	38mm	WF 201-38-S	1	1907
	Latex rubber	38mm	WF 203-38-B	1	1907

PART IXC - STOMA APPLIANCES

UROSTOMY BAGS - cont

Manufacturer (1)	Appliance (2)		Order No (3)	Quantity (4)	List Price (5) p
Simcare	Chiron Day Bag				
	Black Butyl Rubber				
		22mm	WF-205-22-T	1	2753
	Bags - Triangular				
		25mm	48-532-37	10	1538
		32mm	48-532-45	10	1538
		38mm	48-532-53	10	1538
	Oval	25mm	48-534-58	10	1538
		32mm	48-534-66	10	1538
		38mm	48-534-74	10	1538
Thackraycare (Thackray Chas F Ltd)	Raymed Butyl Night Bag				
	Screw outlet		785628	1	2310
	Tap outlet		785636	1	2390
	Stomalite Mk 2 Urostomy				
	Day Bag	1"	786136	5	2715
		1¼"	786144	5	2715
		1½"	786152	5	2715
	Night Bag	1"	786160	5	2715
		1¼"	786179	5	2715
		1½"	786209	5	2715

PART IXC – STOMA APPLIANCES

UROSTOMY SETS

Manufacturer (1)	Appliance (2)		Order No (3)	Quantity (4)	List Price (5) p
C S Bullen Ltd	The SR–U Appliance		SR–U	1	5346
	The OPR–U Appliance		OPR–U	1	7119
	The LOP–U Appliance		LOP–U	1	3413
John Drew Ltd –	Ureterostomy Appliance D½		OSTO 05	1	3557 Δ
Downs Surgical Ltd – see Simcare					
Eschmann Bros & Walsh Ltd – see Simcare					
Simcare	Chiron Ileal Bladder Apparatus		WE 202–38–P	1	6143
	Carshalton Sets				
	Oval Bag	25mm	48–503–19	1	5234
		32mm	48–503–27	1	5234
		38mm	48–503–35	1	5234
	Triang Bag	25mm	48–503–43	1	5234
		32mm	48–503–51	1	5234
		38mm	48–505–13	1	5234

PART IXC - STOMA APPLIANCES

UROSTOMY SETS - cont

Manufacturer (1)	Appliance (2)	Order No (3)	Quantity (4)	List Price (5) p

PART IXC — STOMA APPLIANCES

UROSTOMY SETS — cont

Manufacturer (1)	Appliance (2)	Order No (3)	Quantity (4)	List Price (5) p

PART IXC - STOMA APPLIANCES

CROSS REFERENCE INDEX
(STOMA APPLIANCES)

APPLIANCE RANGE	MANUFACTURER
Accordion (flange)	ConvaTec Ltd
AR	Salt & Son Ltd
Beta	Simcare
Biopore	Clinimed Ltd
Biotrol	Clinimed Ltd
Carshalton	Simcare
Cavendish	Simcare
Chiron	Simcare
Clearseal	Simcare
Clifton	Ellis, Son & Paramore Ltd
Cohesive	Salt & Son Ltd
Cohflex	Salt & Son Ltd
Colodress	ConvaTec Ltd
Coloset	Salt & Son Ltd
Combihesive	ConvaTec Ltd
Combi Micro	Cambmac Instruments Ltd
Comfeel	Coloplast Ltd
Comfort	Coloplast Ltd
Conseal	Coloplast Ltd
C & S	Cambmac Instruments Ltd
D -	John Drew Ltd
Dansac	Cambmac Instruments Ltd
D & S	Cambmac Instruments Ltd
Eakin	Salt & Son Ltd
Easy change	T J Shannon Ltd
EC1 Range	Simcare
Elite	Clinimed Ltd
Giant	Cambac Instruments Ltd
Glasgow	Simcare
Gt Ormond Street	Simcare
Hainsworth	Shaw AH & Partners Ltd
Healwell	Shaw AH & Partners Ltd
Holligard	Abbott Laboratories Ltd
Hollihesive	Abbott Laboratories Ltd
Ileo AV	Warne-Frankin
Ileo-B	Coloplast
Ileodress	ConvaTec Ltd
Ileo KAV	Warne-Frankin
Ileo S	Clinimed Ltd
Integrale	Clinimed Ltd

PART IXC — STOMA APPLIANCES

CROSS REFERENCE INDEX — cont
(STOMA APPLIANCES)

APPLIANCE RANGE	MANUFACTURER
Karayaseel	Simpla Plastics Ltd
K-Flex	Coloplast Ltd
Kombo	Salt & Son Ltd
KR	Salt & Son Ltd
Lenbul	C S Bullen Ltd
Light White	Salt & Son Ltd
Limone	Clinimed Ltd
LOP	C S Bullen Ltd
LO-Profile	Hollister
MC	Coloplast Ltd
Medena	Astra Meditec Ltd
Mitcham	Simcare
Newcastle	Simcare
New Freedom	T J Shannon Ltd
Omni	Simcare
O.P.R.	C S Bullen Ltd
Ostopore	Warne-Franklin
Perfect	Coloplast Ltd
Petit	Cambmac Instruments Ltd
Phoenix	Simpla Plastics Ltd
Preference	Clinimed Ltd
Realistic	Salt & Son Ltd
Redifit	Simcare
Rediseal	Simcare
Reliaseal	Salt & Son Ltd
Royal	Thackraycare
Salgar	Salt & Son Ltd
Saltair	Salt & Son Ltd
Sassco	Simpla Plastics Ltd
Schacht	Thackraycare
Seel-a-Peel	Simcare
SF	Salt & Son Ltd
Simplicity	Salt & Son Ltd
Skintone	Simcare
Slimline	Thackraycare
Solo	Salt & Son Ltd
SR	C S Bullen Ltd
Stomahesive	ConvaTec Ltd
Stomalite	Thackrarycare
Stomaseal	3M Health Care Ltd
Stomastar	Thackraycare
Supasac	Salt & Son Ltd
Surgicare	ConvaTec Ltd

PART IXC - STOMA APPLIANCES

CROSS REFERENCE INDEX - cont
(STOMA APPLIANCES)

APPLIANCE RANGE	MANUFACTURER
Surrey	Simcare
Symphony	Simcare
System 2	ConvaTec Ltd
Topaz	Warne-Franklin
Transacryl	Salt & Son Ltd
Translet	Warne-Franklin
Turner-Warwick	Simcare
United	Salt and Son Ltd
URO	Coloplast Ltd
Zopla Stoma Plaster	Salt and Son Ltd

PART IXC - STOMA APPLIANCES

SUPPLIERS' ADDRESSES AND TELEPHONE NUMBERS
(STOMA APPLIANCES)

Abbott Laboratories Limited - see Hollister Ltd

Astra Meditec Ltd, PO Box 13, Stroud, Gloucestershire, GL5 3DL (045-383 3377)

Bard Ltd, Forest House, Brighton Road, Crawley, West Sussex RH11 9BP (0293-27888)

C S Bullen Ltd, 3-7 Moss Street, Liverpool L6 1EY (051-207 6995/6/7/8)

Cambmac Instruments Ltd. Denny Industrial Estate, Denny End Road, Waterbeach,
   Cambridge, CB5 9PY (0223-861651)

Clinimed Ltd, Cavell House, Knaver Beech Way, Loudwater, High Wycombe, Bucks,
   HP10 9QY (0628-850100)

Coloplast Ltd, Peterborough Business Park, Peterborough, PE2 0FX (0733 239898)

ConvaTec Ltd, Reeds Lane, Moreton, Merseyside L46 1QW (051-677 2207)

Cuxson Gerrard & Co (Dressings) Ltd, 26 Fountain Lane, Oldbury, Warley, West Midlands
   B69 3BB (021-544 7117)

John Drew (London) Ltd, 433 Uxbridge Road, Ealing, London W5 3NT (081-992 0381)

Dow Corning Ltd, AVCO House, Reading, Castle Street, Berks RG1 1DZ (0734-596888)

Downs Surgical Ltd, see Simcare

Ellis, Son & Paramore Ltd, Spring Street Works, Sheffield S3 8PD (0742 738921/21269)

Eschmann Bros and Walsh Ltd, see Simcare

Francol Surgical Ltd, PO Box 2, High Wycombe, HP14 4LJ (024024-2504)

Franklin Medical Ltd - see Warne-Franklin Medical Ltd

Hollister Ltd, 43 Castle Street Reading RG1 7SN (0734 597211)(Retail Pharmacy Order
Line 0800 521392)

Kinpax and F T Mitchell Group Ltd, 631 London Road, Westcliff-on-Sea SS0 9PE
   (0702-337339)

Leyland Medical Ltd, PO Box 6, Leyland, Preston, Lancs PR5 1XR (0772 431151)

Loxley Medical, Unit 3A, Bessingby Industrial Estate, Bridlington, North Humberside
   YO16 4SJ (0262-603979)

PART IXC – STOMA APPLIANCES

SUPPLIERS' ADDRESSES AND TELEPHONE NUMBERS – cont
(STOMA APPLIANCES)

3M Health Care Ltd, 1 Morley Street, Loughborough, Leicestershire, LE11 1EP
  (0509 268181)

North West Ostomy Suppliers (Wholesale) Ltd, North West House, 62 Oakhill Trading
  Estate, Worsley, Manchester, M28 5PT (0204-709-255)

Palex Ostomy Division; Cambridge Selfcare Diagnostics Ltd, Richmond House
  Old Brewery Court, Sandyford Road, Newcastle upon Tyne, NE2 1XG (091 261 5950)

J C Peacock & Son Ltd, Friar House, Clavering Place, Newcastle Upon Tyne NE1 3NR (091-232-9917)

Donald Rose Ltd, – See Steeper (Orthopaedic) Ltd

Sallis E Ltd, Vernon Works, Waterford Street, Old Basford, Nottingham, NG6 0DH
  (0602-787841/2)

Salt and Son Ltd, Saltair House, Lord Street, Nechells, Birmingham B7 4DS (021-359-5123)

T J Shannon Ltd, 59 Bradford Street, Bolton BL2 1HT (0204-21789)

A H Shaw and Partners Ltd, Manor Road, Ossett, West Yorkshire WF5 0LF
  (0924-273474)

Simcare Peter Road, Lancing, West Sussex, BN15 8TJ
  (0903-761122).

Simpla Plastics Ltd, Phoenix Estate, Caerphilly Road, Cardiff, CF4 4XG
  (0222-621000)

Squibb Surgicare Ltd (See ConvaTec Ltd)

Steeper (Orthopaedic) Ltd, 59 North Worple Way, Mortlake, London SW14 8PS (081-878-8633)

Thackraycare (Chas F Thackray Ltd), 47 Great George Street, Leeds, LS1 3BB
  (0532-430028)

Ward Surgical Appliance Company, 57A Brightwell Avenue, Southend-on -Sea, SS1 1LU
  (0702-354064)

Warne-Franklin Medical, PO Box 138, Turnpike Road. Cressex Industrial Estate. High Wycombe,
  Bucks, HP12 3NB (0494-32761)

Welland Medical Ltd, Charlwoods Road, East Grinstead. Sussex. RH19 9LH (0342 327412)

PART IXR

APPROVED LIST OF CHEMICAL REAGENTS
See Part II, Clause 8A (page 7)

The price listed in respect of a chemical reagent specified in the following list
is the basic price [see Part II, Clause 8] on which payment will be calculated
pursuant to Part II, Clause 6A for the dispensing of that chemical reagent.

Chemical Reagent (1)		Quantity (2)	Basic Price (3) p
Nitroprusside Reagent Tablets(Acetest)		100	238
(Syn. Rothera's Tablets)			
Aminoacetic Acid anhydrous	9.0 mg		
Sodium Nitroprusside	1.0 mg		
Sodium Phosphate anhydrous	94.0 mg		
Sodium Borate anhydrous	73.0 mg		
Lactose	20.0 mg		
Starch	2.5 mg		
Magnesium Stearate	0.5 mg		
(Supplied with an instruction sheet and colour chart)			
Copper Solution Reagent Tablet (Clinitest)		36	134
Copper Sulphate anhydrous	18.75 mg		
Citric Acid anhydrous	300 mg		
Sodium Hydroxide	250 mg		
Sodium Carbonate anhydrous	62.5 mg		
Excipient			
(Supplied with an instruction sheet, analysis record and colour chart)			
Gerhardt's Reagent		25 ml	6
(Ferric Chloride Solution, 10%)			
Ammonia Solution Strong BP		500 ml	135
Compounds required for oral administration for the purpose of cholecystographic examination To be supplied in a container with instructions to patient.			
Iopanoic Acid Tablets BP 500 microgram	packet of 6		451
(Telepaque)			
Sodium Ipodate Capsules, 500 microgram	packet of 6		253
(Biloptin)			
Calcium Ipodate Sachets, 3g		1 sachet	253
(Solu–Biloptin)			

PART IXR – CHEMICAL REAGENTS

Chemical Reagent (1)	Quantity (2)	Basic Price (3) p

Detection Strips required in testing:-

A. URINE for

Glycosuria
   - Strip impregnated one end with:
   Glucose Oxidase and a peroxidase, and o–Tolidine,
      buffered (Clinistix) .... bottle of 50   218
   (Supplied with an instruction sheet, analysis record
   and colour chart)

   - Strip impregnated one end with:
   Glucose Oxidase and a perodixase, and potassium
   iodide, buffered (Diastix) .... bottle of 50   186
   (Supplied with an instruction sheet, analysis record
   and colour chart)

   - Twin zone strip impregnated one end with:-
   Glucose Oxidase/Peroxidase and Tetramethylbenzidine
   indicator (Diabur Test 5000) .... Vial of 50   186
   (Supplied with an instruction sheet, analysis record
   and colour chart)

Ketonuria (Acetonuria)
   - Strip impregnated one end with:
   Sodium Nitroprusside, Glycine, and Phosphate
   buffer (Ketostix) .... bottle of 50   186
   (Supplied with an instruction sheet and colour chart)

   - Strip impregnated one end with:
   Sodium Nitroprusside, Glycine and Akaline Buffer
   (Ketur Test) .... Vial of 50   178
   (Supplied with an instruction sheet and colour chart)

Phenylketonuria
   - Strip impregnated one end with:
   Ferric Ammonium Sulphate. Magnesium Sulphate
   and Cyclohexyl–sulphuric Acid (Phenistix) .... bottle of 50   371
   (Supplied with an instruction sheet and colour chart)

Proteinuria
   - Strip impregnated one end with:
   Tetrabromophenol Blue, and Citrate buffer
   (Albustix) .... bottle of 50   256
   (Supplied with an instruction sheet and colour chart)

   - Strips impregnated one end with+
   3', 3", 5', 5" Tetrachlorophenol 3,4,5,6
   Tetrabromosulphophthalein and Citrate Buffer
   (Albym Test) .... Vial of 50   246
   (Supplied with an instruction sheet and colour chart)

PART IXR – CHEMICAL REAGENTS

Chemical Reagent (1)	Quantity (2)	Basic Price (3) p

Detection Strips – required in testing for –

B. Blood for glucose:

Blood Glucose Testing Strips (BGTS) *
   Drug Tariff Specification 44 (Types 1–4)
                           48 (Type 5)

NB 1. * Notes on the use of BGTS are given in the Appendix to Part IXR page 278/278a

   2. For Lancets: see page 91

   3. Meters for use with BGTS are not available on general practitioner prescription
       Form FP10. See Part IX, Note 1, page 57 regarding supply arrangements.

Type 1 – ... (BM–Test 1–44) vial of   50 1138

          (previously called BM–Test Glycemie 1–44)

          Strip with twin pads at one end impregnated
          with Glucose Oxidase and peroxidase with chromagens.

          The lower test area (nearer the "handle") gives
          readings in the range 1.0–7.0 mmol/1
          (20–120 mg/100 ml)light – mid blue;

          the higher test area range is 7.0–44.0 mmol/1
          (120–800 mg/100 ml) buff – green – dark green.

          (Supplied with an instruction sheet, analysis
          record and colour chart)

Type 2 – ... (Dextrostix) bottle of   50 1134

          Strip with a single pad at one end impregnated with

          Glucose Oxidase and peroxidase with chromagens.

          The yellow test area gives readings in the range
          1.0–13.9 mmol/1 (20–200mg/100ml) grey – blue/purple.

          (Supplied with an instruction sheet, analysis
          record and colour chart)

Type 3 – ... (Glucostix) bottle of   50 1134

          Strip with twin pads at one end impregnated with

          Glucose Oxidase and peroxidase with chromagens.

          The pale green area changes to dark green
          to give readings in the range
          1.0–6.0 mmol/1 (20–110mg/100ml);
          the orange area changes to red in the range
          8–44 mmol/1 (140–800mg/100ml).

          (Supplied with an instruction sheet, analysis
          record and colour chart)

0313M/3

PART IXR – CHEMICAL REAGENTS

Chemical Reagent (1)	Quantity (2)	Basic Price (3) p

B. Blood for glucose (cont)   each

Type 4 –   ... (Hypoguard GA) container of   50 1025

Strip with twin pads at one end impregnated with

Glucose Oxidase and peroxidase with chromagens.

The yellow area (nearer the "handle") changes to
green to give readings in the range
1.1–10.0mmol/1 (20–180 mg/100 ml);
the white area changes through light to dark blue
in the range 1.1–22.2 mmol/1 (20–400 mg/100 ml).

(Supplied with an instruction sheet, analysis
record and colour chart)

Type 5 –   ... (ExacTech) container of   50 1054

Strips to be read only with the appropriate meter.

(NB This meter is not available on prescription)

The strips have a target area for the blood
sample at one end, impregnated with glucose
oxidase. This reacts with blood glucose to produce
a current proportionate to its concentration; this
is read by inserting the other end of the strip in
the meter to produce a digital reading in the range
2.2–25.0 mmol/1 (40–450 mg/100 ml).

(Supplied with an instruction sheet, analysis record,
and meter calibrator).

PART IXR - APPENDIX

NOTES ON BLOOD GLUCOSE TESTING

1.   Blood glucose testing strips (BGTS) are primarily intended for insulin-dependent diabetics who will normally have received consultant advice on their condition. One pack (50 strips) would normally be sufficient for two months. All strips should be kept in their original container and should not be cut or slit. Because of the differences in colour change in colorimetric types (1-4), strips are not interchangeable; they would normally be read by sight, but can be read using a suitable meter. Biosensor strips (type 5) can only be read with the appropriate meter. Due regard should be given to the manufacturers' instructions, and the recommendation on storage and period of use after first opening.

2.   General Practitioners should be aware that defects in colour vision may occur in diabetes and certain colorimetric BGT strips should not be prescribed for such patients for visual use. (See outline of colour changes described in each entry on pages 276/277).

3.   Misleading results, which could be hazardous if acted upon, might arise if users are inadequately trained. (Hazard Notice HN(87)(13)). It is therefore essential that patients should receive appropriate training before attempting to use BGTS for monitoring their blood glucose. The training may be given by suitably qualified health-care professionals. It should be noted that there are variations in technique between different makes. Some technical factors are given in paragraph 4 below.

4.   Reagent Strips are subject to the following limitations:

Fluoride Specimen: The strips are not to be used with blood specimens preserved with fluoride.

Serum and Plasma: The strips are not designed for use with serum or plasma.

Specimen Restrictions   Types 2, 3, 4 and 5 are not recommended for use with neonatal blood. Type 5 is also not recommended for use with grossly lipemic (fatty) specimens and for patients receiving extensive oxygen therapy; patients with elevated uric acid levels and those receiving salicylate, paracetamol, and sulphonyl ureas (such as Glibenclamide, Tolbutamide, etc) will give rise to elevated glucose level readings with this type of strip.

Haematocrit; Extremes in haematocrit levels can affect test results:

High levels ————————————> Low results
Levels above the following values can give low results
Type 1: 70%; Type 2: 55%; Type 3: 50%; Type 4: 55%; Type 5: 55%

Low levels ————————————> High results
Levels below 35% can give high results with all five types of strip.

PART IXR — APPENDIX Cont

5. At present the following types are listed in the Drug Tariff:
    Colorimetric (may be read visually):

> Type 1 .... 'BM—Test 1—44'
> Type 2 .... 'Dextrostix'
> Type 3 .... 'Glucostix'
> Type 4 .... 'Hypoguard GA'

Biosensor (appropriate meter is essential; see Note 3, page 276):

> Type 5 .... 'ExacTech'

6. Disposal of Lancets. Advice is given in a leaflet available from the Department on the safe disposal of single—use syringes and needles. Patients should be reminded of the need to exercise similar caution when disposing of used lancets. These should be placed in a tin or other strong container before disposal. (The needle clipping device listed on page 91 is not generally suitable for use with lancets).

As with single—use syringes, the arrangements outlined above are not suitable for patients where there is a risk of infection being transmitted. General Pracitioners are similarly advised that blood lancets should only be prescribed for patients who are carriers of infectious diseases where suitable arrangements have been made for the disposal of the used articles as contaminated waste. Medical Officers for environmental health can advise on these arrangements.

PART X
DOMICILIARY OXYGEN THERAPY SERVICE

A.   OXYGEN CONCENTRATOR SERVICE

EQUIPMENT WHICH MAY BE PRESCRIBED

Oxygen concentrator —
Accessories — Face mask, nasal cannula, humidifier
Emergency back—up supply (comprising regulator, tubing, administration mask
and cylinder of oxygen BP)

2.   CLAIMS FOR PAYMENT

Contractors shall despatch prescription forms together with the appropriate claim forms to the
Pricing Authority not later than the fifth day of the month following that in which the supply was
made.

3.   CONCENTRATOR SUPPLIERS

Oxygen concentrators together with face mask, nasal cannulae and humidifiers are included in the
approved list of appliances and can be obtained in the area of the Family Practitioner Committees
listed in column 1 in the table below from the suppliers listed in column 2 of that table opposite
those Committees.

Regional Groups of FPCs	Concentrator Supplier
South Western	
Avon	De Vilbiss Health Care UK Ltd
Berkshire	Airlinks
Buckinghamshire	Spitfire Way
Cornwall	Heston
Devon	Middlesex TW5 9NR
Dorset	
Gloucestershire	Telephone
Hampshire	Dial 100 and ask for
IOW	'Freephone Oxygen Concentrator'
Oxfordshire	
Somerset	
Wiltshire	
West Midlands	
Birmingham	De Vilbiss Health Care UK Ltd
Coventry	
Derbyshire	
Dudley	
Hereford & Worcester	
Leicestershire	
Northamptonshire	
Notts	

PART X - DOMICILIARY OXYGEN THERPAY SERVICE

CONCENTRATOR SUPPLIERS - cont

West Midlands - cont

Sandwell
Shropshire
Solihull
Staffs
Walsall
Warwickshire
Wolverhampton

Central and South Wales

Dyfed   De Vilbiss Health Care UK Ltd
Gwent
Mid Glamorgan
Powys
South Glamorgan
West Glamorgan

North Western and North Wales

Bolton   De Vilbiss Health Care UK Ltd
Bury
Cheshire
Clwyd
Gwynedd
Knowsley & St Helens
Lancashire
Liverpool
Manchester
Oldham
Rochdale
Salford
Sefton
Stockport
Tameside
Trafford
Wigan
Wirral

London North

Barking, Havering & Brentwood   De Vilbiss Health Care UK Ltd
Barnet
Brent & Harrow
Camden and Islington
City and E London
Enfield & Haringey
Hertfordshire
Redbridge & Waltham Forest

0313M/8

PART X - DOMICILIARY OXYGEN THERPAY SERVICE

CONTRACTOR SUPPLIERS - cont

Eastern

Bedfordshire	De Vilbiss Health Care UK Ltd
Cambridgeshire	
Essex	
Norfolk	
Sulfolk	

London South

Bromley	The Omnicare Group Ltd
Croydon	(Omnicare)
Ealing, Hammersmith and Hounslow	Technology House
E Sussex	Victoria Road
Greenwich & Bexley	Winchester
Hillingdon	SO23 7DY
Kensington, Chelsea and Westminster	
Kent	
Kingston & Richmond	
Lambeth, Southwark and Lewisham	Telephone
Merton, Sutton and Wandsworth	Dial 100 and ask for
Surrey	'Freephone Omnicare Oxygen'
W Sussex	

Yorkshire (South & West) and Humberside

Barnsley	Rimer-Alco Ltd
Bradford	Dumballs Road
Calderdale	Cardiff
Doncaster	CF1 6JE
Humberside	
Kirklees	
Leeds	
Lincolnshire	Telephone
Rotherham	Dial 0800 373580
Sheffield	
Wakefield	

Northern

Cleveland	Rimer-Alco Ltd
Cumbria	
Durham	
Gateshead	
Newcastle	
N Tyneside	
Northumberland	
N Yorkshire	
S Tyneside	
Sunderland	

PART X — DOMICILIARY OXYGEN THERPAY SERVICE

B.   OXYGEN CYLINDER SERVICE

4.   BASIS OF PAYMENT FOR SUPPLY OF APPROVED OXYGEN EQUIPMENT

a.   Set and Stand Rentals
      For sets and stands authorised by the Family Practitioner Committee
      Approved Lightweight (Single Unit) Set .... each 182p per month
      (from list on page 286), including one of either Intersurgical 010 Mask,
      28% or Ventimask Mk IV, 28% (see list on pages 286 and 287 figures 1 and
      2, page 288).
      Stand for use with 1360 litre oxygen cylinder ..... each 40p per month

b.   Basic Price
      (i)   For the supply of a mask, when prescribed after the initial, order, on a separate
      prescription form (See list of approved masks, pages 286 and 287, and illustrations, page
      288).

a.	Intersurgical 010 Mask, 28%	figure 1	97p
b.	Ventimask Mk IV, 28%	figure 2	130p
c.	Intersurgical 005 Mask	figure 3	78p
d.	MC Mask	figure 4	71p

      (ii) Oxygen BP, ... 1360 litres   525p

      Contractors are reminded of the importance of ensuring that as few empty cylinders as
      possible remain in circulation. They should be exchanged promptly and withdrawn (full or
      empty) together with other equipment should the service cease.

      (See Part X Appendix paragraph 10.7, 12.4, 12.5 and 16.2 of the tariff).

c.   Professional Fees
      Lightweight (Single Unit) Set and or Oxygen
      *Per return journey: miles each way .....

	0-3	over 3-5	over 5-10	over 10
	p	p	p	p
(i) Delivery of set and cylinders or of replacement set, return visit to check and remedy set malfunction				
a. All non-urgent deliveries	1672	2301	2475	3182
b. Deliveries between the time the premises close for dispensing and 11 pm on days other than Sundays and public holidays where the prescription form is endorsed "Urgent" by the prescriber and return visits to check and remedy set malfunction effected between these same times	2684	3313	3487	4194

	0-3 p	over 3-5 p	over 5-10 p	over 10 p
c. Deliveries between 11 pm and the time the premises open for dispensing on days other than Sundays and public holidays, and through-out Sundays and public holidays where the prescription form is endorsed "Urgent" by the prescriber; or where the prescription form, although not endorsed "Urgent" by the prescriber, has been dispensed on the day (in the case of those dispensed after midnight the day, or the day following that) on which it was written, between 11 pm and 8 am, or between 11 pm and 9 am on Sundays and public holidays, and is endorsed "dispensed urgently at ..... pm/am ..... date" by the pharmacy contractor, and signed by the patient (or his representative). Return visits to check and remedy set malfunctions between 11 pm and the time the premises open for dispensing on days other than Sundays and public holidays and throughout Sundays and public holidays	2909	3538	3712	4419
(ii) Delivery of cylinders (when not in conjunction with a set); delivery of masks (when not in conjunction with set or cylinders); delivery of replacement cylinder when original cylinder is found to be faulty; ineffective first delivery journey of set and/or cylinder				
a. All non-urgent deliveries	1505	2138	2312	3022
b. Between the time premises close for dispensing and 11 pm on days other than Sundays and public holidays, where the prescription form is endorsed "Urgent" by the prescriber.	2517	3150	3324	4034
c. Between 11 pm and the time the premises open for dispensing on days other than Sundays and public holidays, and throughout Sundays and public holidays where the prescription form is endorsed "Urgent" by the prescriber, or where the prescription form although not endorsed "Urgent" by the prescriber, has been dispensed on the day (in the case of those dispensed after midnight the day, or the day following that) on which it was written, between 11 pm and 8 am, or betweem 11 pm and 9 am on Sunday and public holidays, and is endorsed "dispensed urgently at ...... pm/am .... date" by the pharmacy contractor and signed by the patient (or his representative)	2742	3375	3549	4259
(iii) Collection of set and cylinders at the end of treatment; second journey when first was ineffective at any time	1505	2138	2312	3022

PART X – DOMICILIARY OXYGEN THERPAY SERVICE

	*Fee per form where the pharmacy contractor is normally resident on his business premises	where the pharmacy contractor is normally no resident on his business premises
	p	p

(iv) Collection at pharmacy on behalf of patient

a.   All non-urgent collections

Set and cylinders	826	826
Cylinders only (when not in conjunction with a set)	741	741
Mask only (when not in conjunction with a set or cylinders)	29	29

b.   Where the prescription form is endorsed "Urgent" by the prescriber and has been dispensed at a time when the premises are not open for dispensing (the hour, date, and where applicable "non-resident", must be endorsed by the pharmacy contractor)

(i)   Between the time the premises close for dispensing and 11 pm on days other than Sundays and public holidays

Set and cylinders	1415	2259
Cylinders only (when not in conjunction with a set)	1331	2175
Mask only (when not in conjuntion with a set or cylinders) ......,..	620	1463

(ii) Between 11 pm and the time the premises open for dispensing on days other than Sundays and public holidays and throughout Sundays and public holidays.

Set and cylinders	1584	2540
Cylinders only (when not in conjunction with a set)	1500	2456
Mask only (when not in conjunction with a set or cylinders	788	1745

PART X - DOMICILIARY OXYGEN THERPAY SERVICE

	*Fee per form	
	Where the pharmacy contractor is normally resident on his business premises p	Where the pharmacy contractor normally not resident on his business premises p

c. Where the prescription form, although not endorsed "Urgent" by the prescriber, has been dispensed, at a time when the premises are not open for dispensing, on the day (in the case of those dispensed after midnight the day, or the day following that) on which it was written, between 11 pm and 8 am, or between 11 pm and 9 am on Sundays and public holidays, and is endorsed "dispensed urgently at ...... pm/am date, and where applicable "non-resident", by the pharmacy contractor and signed by the patient (or his representative).

Set and cylinders	1584	2540
Cylinders only (when not in conjunction with a set)	1500	2456
Mask only (when not in conjunction with a set or cylinders)	788	1745

In order to qualify for the non-resident rates a pharmacy contractor who normally lives elsewhere than on his business premises will need to have left those premises and to have returned to open them to dispense an urgent prescription. In the absence of an endorsement "non-resident" payment will automatically be made at the residents' rate.

* Note: Where a doctor orders on one prescription form more than 3x1360 litre cylinders and the pharmacy contractor delivers them to the patient's home, a professional fee will be paid on the basis of one return journey for every three cylinders, or balance of an order in excesss of a multiple of three cylinders, or for the actual number of return journeys, whichever is the less. Similarly, where a patient, or his representative, collects more than 3x1360 litre cylinders a professional fee will be paid on the basis of one fee for every three cylinders, or balance of an order in excess of a multiple of three cylinders, or for the number of return journeys made by the collector, whichever is the less. For these purposes, 2x680 litres (where available) cylinders will be counted as 1x1360 litre cylinder.

PART X - DOMICILIARY OXYGEN THERPAY SERVICE

OXYGEN EQUIPMENT WHICH THE PHARMACY CONTRACTOR MAY SUPPLY ON LOAN TO THE PATIENT

5.   OXYGEN SETS

a.   The following sets* (See Specification 01A and 01B, page 289 and diagrams, pages 290 and 291) are approved for use within the Domiciliary Oxygen Therapy Service, and any one may be loaned against an order for a set:

        (i)   BOC Set (BOC 330228) ....   Specification 01A
        (ii) Medishield Domiciliary Set (MDS 240) ....   Specification 01B
        (iii) Oxylitre Set (MR 210) ....   Specification 01A
        (iv) Air Apparatus and Valve Set (D24) .... Specification 01B
        (v)   Ohmeda Domic 2/4 Set - bearing "S" stamp
              (Part No. 1550033) ....   Specification 01A

A constant performance mask (see paragraph 6a, below, and figures 1 and 2, page 288) shall be supplied by the manufacturer with each set.
When supplying an oxygen set meeting Specification 01B with a constant performance mask, the pharmacy contractor should ensure that the flow selector is at the Medium setting, ie 2 litres per minute (see diagram on page 291).

On no account should pharmacy contractor attempt to modify any oxygen set to produce a higher flow rate than that for which it has been designed. To do so could create a hazardous situation for the patient.

* Spare O-rings may be supplied by the manufacturer with the set, but these should be removed by the pharmacy contractor before the set is supplied to the patient.

6.   OXYGEN MASKS

The following masks are approved for use within the Domiciliary Oxygen Therapy Service:

a.   Constant performance masks
These masks provide a nearly constant concentration of 28% oxygen in air over a wide range of oxygen supply, and irrespective of breathing pattern. The most economic oxygen flow rate is 2 litres per minute (the Medium setting on the control head).
        (i)   Intersurgical 010 Mask 28% (figure 1, page 288)+
        The mask comprises a soft muulded plastic facepiece, an adjustable elastic headstrap and a metal nose clip to ensure a close fit across the nose. A lightweight white venturi diluter fitted to the front of the mask ensures a near constant oxygen concentration. This can be rotated to suit varying positions of the connecting tube.

Weight (less supply tube) ....   44 grams
Supplied by Intersurgical Ltd.

        (ii)   Ventimask Mk 1V 28% (figure 2, page 288) +
        The mask consists of a one piece transparent flexible moulded face-piece incorporating a lightweight rigid clear plastic venturi device that ensures near constant concentration.

        It is fitted with an adjustable elastic head-band, and has soft metal reinforcing strip to ensure a good fit over the bridge of the nose.

Weight (less supply tube) ....   66 grams
Supplied by Vickers Medical Equipment Ltd.

+ Either of these masks may be supplied with the standard set (See paragraph 11.3 and 11.4 of the appendix.

0313M/14

b.   Variable performance masks

A flow rate of 2 litres per minute is recommended for these masks, no claim being made for
the resulting oxygen concentration. They provide a variable concentration of oxygen in
air. The concentration varies with the rate of flow of oxygen supplied and the breathing
pattern of the patient.

(i)   Intersurgical 005 Mask (figure 3, page 288)

This mask comprises a soft moulded plastic face-piece, adjustable elastic headstrap
and a metal nose clip to ensure a close fit across the nose. A swivel connector on
the front of the mask, to which the oxygen tube is connected, can be rotated to suit
varying position of the connecting tube.

Weight (less supply tube) 40 grams
Supplied by Intersurgical Ltd.

(ii)   MC Mask (figure 4, page 288)

This mask comprises a clear plastic face-piece with foam edging for comfort, and a
curved connector which projects into the front of the mask to form the jet.

Weight (less connector) ....   11 grams
Supplied by Bakelite Xylonite Ltd.

7.   METHOD OF CLAIMING COMPENSATION FOR FINANCIAL LOSS IN RESPECT OF OXYGEN EQUIPMENT.

Where the pharmacy contractor suffers financial loss as a result of the act or default of a person
causing the loss of, or damage to, oxygen equipment loaned, the pharmacy contractor should
forthwith inform the Committee of such financial loss. To obtain reimbursement of the loss, the
pharmacy contractor must supply the Committee with a signed statement from the person admitting
that the damage to, or loss of, the equipment occurred while it was in his possession. The
Committee should by way of reimbursement make a payment to the pharmacy contractor based on the
value of the equipment at the date of its loss, or a payment equivalent to the cost of repairing
the said damages as the case may be.
Necessary out-of-pocket expenses incidentally involved in the repair of or replacement of the
equipment, such a postage or carriage costs, should also be met.
In this paragraph, the expression "person" means the person supplied, the patient concerned,
members of his household, or the authorities of an institution to which the equipment is
delivered, as the case may be.

PART X — DOMICILIARY OXYGEN THERPAY SERVICE

ILLUSTRATIONS OF APPROVED OXYGEN MASKS
(See list on pages 286 and 287)

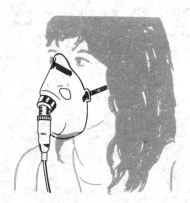

Figure 1
Inter-Surgical 010 Mask

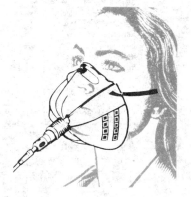

Figure 2
Ventimask Mk 4, 28%

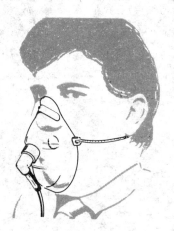

Figure 3
Inter-Surgical 005 Mask

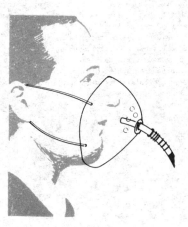

Figure 4
MC Mask

0313M/16

PART X - DOMICILIARY OXYGEN THERPAY SERVICE

ADDITIONAL SPECIFICATIONS

Lightweight (Single Unit) Oxygen Sets

SPECIFICATION 01A

The set comprises
1. The Control Head, which shall include the following features:
   a. A valve which reduces the gas cylinder pressure from 13650 k.P.a. to a pressure of 70 to 415 k.P.a.;
   b. A miniature contents (pressure) gauge, calibrated with 1/4, 1/2 and FULL markings;
   c. A cap, consisting of a two flow selector, which can be turned from the ratchet position marked OFF to ratchet positions marked MED and HIGH, these being designed to correspond to flow rates of 2 litres and 4 litres respectively per minute;
   d. An outlet, being the male portion of a bayonet type connection;
   e. A standard bull-nose cylinder adaptor designed for finger tightening, and preferably incorporating an O-ring washer;
   f. A safety device, such as a sintered filter, to prevent the spontaneous combustion of particulate material in the control head, or in the neck of the cylinder.

2. Connection Tubing: 150 cm (approximately) plastic tubing, 5 mm bore, 8mm externally (Ref. Portex 800/012/300) with at one end a bayonet fitting to the control head.

3. A Key Spanner of 100 mm to 150 mm length, for opening the oxygen cylinder valve.

4. One disposable plastic mask (figure 1 or figure 2 on page 288), in a closed plastic bag.

The set parts 1 to 3 are packed in a strong box, with full operating instructions in the lid.

The mask, being partly rigid, is packed separately and supplied with the boxed parts.

Note: Spare O-rings may be supplied by the manufacturer with the set, but these should be removed by the contractor before the set is supplied to the patient.

SPECIFICATION 01B

The set will comply with all the requirements of Specification 01A, with the exception of clause 1c, where the following clause will apply:

"A ratchet selection device to enable the gas flow to be set at predetermined positions to give flow rates of 2 litres and 4 litres per minute respectively. The positions will be clearly indicted and labelled 2L (MED) and 4L (HIGH); and a control knob which permits the flow of gas to be turned on and off. It will be suitably labelled to indicate the ON and OFF positions and the direction of rotation to turn ON ..."

SPECIFICATION 01 — cont

Lightweight (Single Unit) Set 01A

NB: Actual Shape of Control head varies with make

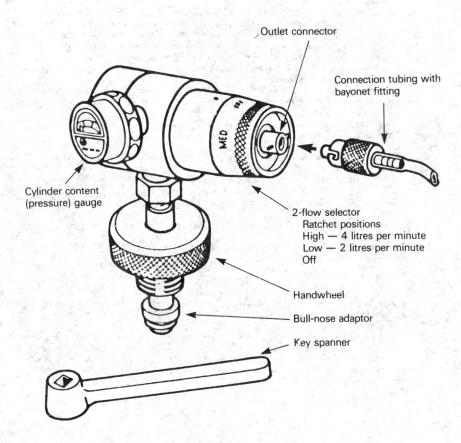

Outlet connector

Connection tubing with bayonet fitting

Cylinder content (pressure) gauge

2-flow selector
Ratchet positions
High — 4 litres per minute
Low — 2 litres per minute
Off

Handwheel

Bull-nose adaptor

Key spanner

Illustration approximately 4/10 actual size

The Set is packed in a strong box

A Constant performance mask is packed separately with the boxed parts

SPECIFICATION 01 – cont

Light Weight (Single Unit) Set 01B

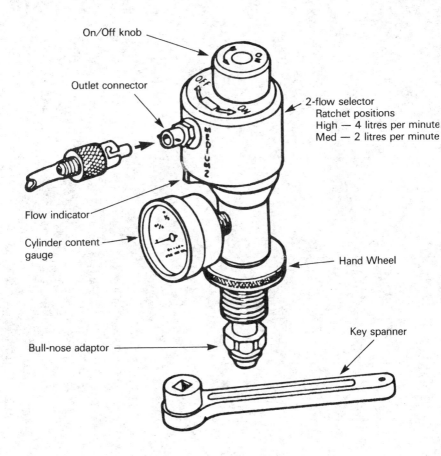

Illustration approximately 4/10 size

The Set is packed in a strong box

A Constant performance mask is packed separately and supplied with the boxed parts

PART X - APPENDIX

DOMICILIARY OXYGEN THERAPY SREVICE

Note: This Appendix contains guidance on the supply of oxygen by cylinder and concentrator.

1. DOMICILIARY OXYGEN

1.1 Oxygen should be prescribed for patients in the home only after careful evaluation and never on a placebo basis. Oxygen may be supplied in cylinders or where the quantity required justifies it, from a concentrator but in general the appropriate method of supply will depend on the type of therapy, intermittent or long term, to be prescribed.

2. INTERMITTANT THERAPY

2.1 The majority of patients will have oxygen prescribed for intermittent use in a variety of respiratory conditions. This type of therapy is used in patients with hypoxaemia of short duration, for example, asthma, when the condition is likely to recur over months or years. It may be presecribed for patients with advanced irreversible respiratory disorders to increase mobility and capacity for exercise and ease discomfort, for example in chronic obstructive bronchitis, emphysema, widespread fibrosis and primary or thromboemolic pulmonary hypertension. Such patients will usually be supplied with oxygen in cylinders.

2.2 Arrangements for the prescription and supply of cylinder oxygen to those patients who require intermittant therapy are set out at paragraph 10. GPs are asked to co-operate in an effort to make this part of the oxygen service more cost effective. If more than one or two are regularly required for a particular period, prescribing in multiples of 3 cylinders would produce savings by reducing the number of journeys. It is accepted that it will not always be possible to prescribe in this way, for example, because of the infrequency of use of oxygen or because of storage problems at the patient's home but whenever possible cylinders should be prescribed in multiples of 3.

3. LONG TERM OXYGEN THERAPY (LTOT)

3.1 Long term oxygen therapy is the provision of oxygen for 15 hours or more a day for a prolonged period and is of benefit to many patients with chronic hypoxaemia. For these patients oxygen should, where possible, be provided by a concentrator.

3.2 Since it is important to recognise that long term oxygen therapy is of benefit to a limited number of patients and that the needs of the majority of patients will continue to be met by intermittant therapy from cylinders, clinical guidelines for prescribing long term therapy have been drawn up for the benefit of general practitioners. These guidelines are set out in full below.

4. GUIDELINES FOR PRESCRIBING LONG TERM OXYGEN THERAPY (LTOT)

4.1 On present information, patients who are likely to benefit from long-term oxygen therapy will by definition have chronic hypoxaemia, but may for the purposes of these guidelines be divided into three groups:-

1. Those for whom there is an absolute indication, for which there is scientific evidence of the value of long-term oxygen therapy.

2. Those in whom there are good grounds for assuming the value of oxygen therapy, but for which there is no firm scientific evidence at present.

3. Patients in whom oxygen would have a useful palliative effect.

4.2   GPs who identify patients who might belong to any of these groups will wish to have consultant advice on the need for LTOT.

5.   INDICATIONS FOR THE USE OF LTOT

5.1   Absolute indication. Patients for whom there is clear evidence of the value of LTOT will be those with chronic obstructive airways disease, hypoxaemia and oedema. Such patients will have ankle oedema or a history of an acute exacerbation when ankle oedema was observed. It will be necessary for such patients to be seen and assessed by a respiratory physician with access to respiratory function services. Suitable patients would have a forced expiratory volume (FEV_1) of less than 1.5L, a forced vital capacity (FVC) of less than 2L, an arterial oxygen tension less than 7.3kPa (55 mm/mercury) and some elevation of arterial carbon dioxide tension ($PaCO_2$) greater than 6.0 kPa or 45 mm/mercury. These tests are the minimum requirement and they should be made in a stable phase of the condition when all reversible factors have been adequately treated eg infection, reversible airways disease, cardiac disease etc. In order to establish stability, the spirometric measurements and the arterial blood gases should be repeated at an interval of not less than three weeks. There should be variation of no more than $\pm$ 20% in the spirometric measurements and a variation of no more than $\pm$ 5 mm/mercury or 0.6 kPa in the arterial oxygen tension. If such variations are exceeded then a further three week interval should elapse before the tests are repeated again.

5.2   Other patients with chronic obstructive airways disease

The second group will include all patients with chronic obstructive airways disease having the same spirometric characteristics and the same levels of arterial oxygen tension as those described in 3.1, but in whom hypercapnia is not present and oedema has not been witnessed. Many such patients were studied in American trials of long-term domiciliary oxygen therapy and benefit was clearly shown but such patients were excluded from the British studies. However, many of these patients, including refractory asthmatics and sufferers from cystic fibrosis could be expected to benefit from long-term oxygen therapy. On present evidence long-term domiciliary oxygen therapy should not be denied but the same criteria of stability should be applied to ensure that they are established cases of chronic hypoxaemia. We hope that further studies on this group of patients can be urgently carried out.

5.3   Palliative use of oxygen

This group should include patients with other respiratory conditions associated with severe arterial hypoxaemia, but without hypercapnia, for which oxygen therapy may have a useful palliative effect, without necessarily affecting survival. Examples would be severe hypoxaemia associated with the terminal stages of fibrosing alveolitis, industrial lung fibrosis, terminal stages of emphysema, and lung infiltrations such as in sarcoidosis, lymphangitis carcinomatosa and certain collagen disorders.

5.4   Other conditions

There are other conditions in which palliation of chronic respiratory failure might be considered, for example in severe kyphoscoliosis, gross obesity and the end stages of irreversible peripheral neuropathies and muscle disorders. However, these conditions are associated with such serious disturbances of ventilatory drive that the abolition of hypoxaemia by providing additional inspired oxygen may be dangerous. There is also preliminary evidence that long-term oxygen therapy may help some children with pulmonary hypertension. For all these patients the initial assessment would have to be even more detailed than that already described for patients with chronic obstructive airways disease.

6.   POST ASSESSMENT

6.1   If LTOT is to be prescribed and used effectively it must be remembered that the treatment involves a minimum of 15 hours oxygen per day and whenever possible this should be provided by means of a concentrator. The patient must be fully acquainted with the installation, the working of the concentrator and the need to keep to the arduous therapeutic regimen. The initial flow rate of oxygen through standard nasal prongs will be 2L/min, but may need to be modified between 1.5 and 2.5 litres per minute when the arterial blood gases have been checked with the patient breathing oxygen. The aim is to elevate PAO_2, to 60 mmHg (8kPa) or more without excessive hypercapnia.

6.2   Full co-operation by the patient is essential and expert support will be necessary to enable the 15 hours daily treatment period to be achieved. Regular monitoring in the home by appropriately trained nurses or lung function technicians and follow-up in respiratory out-patients by theracic physicians will be necessary to ensure that the treatment is achieving optimum results.

7.   PATIENTS FOR WHOM LONG TERM OXYGEN THERAPY IS NOT USEFUL

7.1   It is important to stress the circumstances under which LTOT is not indicated. Patients with respiratory conditions that merely produce breathlessness without hypoxaemia should not be treated. Long term therapy is not intended for acute conditions such as lobar pneumonia and other chest infections. Patients with lesser degrees of chronic obstructive airways disease (ie not conforming to the criteria in 3.1) or reversible obstructive airways disease including those having acute exacerbations are not candidates for this form of oxygen delivery since their hypoxaemia is likely to be only of short duration.

8.   SMOKING AND LONG TERM OXYGEN THERAPY

8.1   Patients who continue to smoke are unlikely to gain much benefit from LTOT and every effort must be made to persuade them to discontinue smoking. There is also the additional hazard of fire.

9.   SUMMARY

9.1   It is anticipated that the provision of oxygen concentrators for such patients described above who have proven chronic hypoxaemia will be an additional service. It is not intended that oxygen concentrator installations will complete with intermittant oxygen therapy at present provided for patients by cylinder supplies. Patients who would benefit from LTOT from concentrators will need to be carefully selected and carefully monitored and will be relatively few in number compared with those having intermittant short burst therapy.

OXYGEN CYLINDER SERVICE

10.1 Family Practitioner Committee lists of pharmacy contractors who provide domiciliary oxygen therapy services include only those pharmacy contractors who are authorised to hold a number of light-weight single unit oxygen sets (approved sets are listed on page 280) and stands, and:

(i) regularly stock oxygen equipment, as specified in the Drug Tariff, and oxygen gas on the premises;

(ii) are prepared, when it would not be reasonable to expect that the patient's representative could safely do so or when he is unable to do so, to deliver the oxygen set and cylinders to the patient's home, to collect empty cylinders when they are being replaced, and to collect the set and cylinders when informed that treatment has been discontinued; and

(iii) are prepared to erect and explain the operation of the oxygen set and cylinders at the patient's home, particularly when a patient is having oxygen therapy for the first time.

10.2 At any time a pharmacy contractor willing to provide this service may apply to the Family Practitioner Committee for inclusion in the list.

10.3 A copy of the Family Practitioner Committee list of oxygen contractors, with details of the services being provided, is supplied to every pharmacy contractor and doctor in the area. A copy of the list for an adjacent area will be sent on application.

10.4 If a prescription for an oxygen set or cylinders is presented to a pharmacy contractor whose name is not included in the list, he should provide the patient or his representative with the name, address and telephone number of at least two pharmacy contractors who provide oxygen therapy services at the time the need arises, and who are nearest to the patient's home.

10.5 Except where, in emergency, a set has been loaned by a distant pharmacy contractor, oxygen gas shall be supplied to a patient only by the pharmacy contractor who has loaned the set. When, exceptionally, cylinder replacements are provided by a pharmacy contractor other than the one who supplied the set, he should, at the time when cylinders are supplied, satisfy himself that the patient continues to operate the equipment satisfactorily.

10.6 Delivery and collection of sets and/or cylinders is to be undertaken by the patient's representative where he is willing, providing the pharmacy contractor can fully satisfy himself that the representative is able to transport a set and/or a cylinder, carry it and secure it in position in the house, and fit the mask after the instructions provided in the set have been explained to him. In other circumstances delivery, erection and collection of sets and/or cylinders and the explanation of the operation of oxygen equipment at the patient's home, particularly at the commencement of treatment, is to be undertaken by the pharmacy contractor.

10.7 The recovery of empty cylinders from patients, and their prompt return to the supplier for refilling, is essential if adequate supplies of oxygen for the use of patients are to be maintained.

OXYGEN CYLINDER SERVICE – (CONTINUED)

11.   OXYGEN EQUIPMENT WHICH MAY BE ORDERED

11.1 The sets of equipment which may be provided by the pharmacy contractor are listed on page 284 (see also Specification 01A and 01B, page 287).

11.2 The oxygen masks which may be ordered are listed on pages 284 & 285 (See also illustrations, page 286). The type of treatment they provide is indicated in paragraph 1.

11.3 One constant performance mask (either the Intersurgical 010 Mask, 28% or the Ventimask Mk IV, 28%) is supplied as part of the set, but is packaged separately on account of bulk (see list of approved masks, pages 284 & 285 and figures 1 and 2 page 286). When a constant performance mask is supplied to a patient, the recommended flow rate is 2 litres per minute (the Medium setting on the control head, (see page 287, and diagrams on pages 288 & 289).

11.4 Where the prescriber considers that a mask different to that provided in the standard set is required for treatment, he must state which mask is to be supplied.

11.5 Every mask is supplied for the use of one patient only. All masks, therefore, are "disposable" but each is sufficiently robust to withstand usage even over a long period of treatment.

11.6 Oxygen should only be ordered in 1360 litre cylinders. When 3400 litre cylinders are prescribed, the pharmacy contractor will supply the gas in 1360 litre cylinders.

11.7 A cylinder stand may be ordered. if one is not ordered and the pharmacy contractor considers that the cylinder cannot be effectively secured to avoid the risk of accident to patient or set, a cylinder stand should be supplied on loan.

12.   PROCEDURE TO BE FOLLOWED IN LOANING EQUIPMENT, CONFIRMING CONTINUED USE AND TERMINATION OF THE FAMILY PRACTITIONER COMMITTEE'S LIABILITY

12.1 The pharmacy contractor shall on making the loan include a note with the set saying that "This Set is the property of the Pharmacy Contractor to whom it must be returned in good condition by the patient."

12.2 The pharmacy contractor shall endorse the prescription form with:

      (i)   Name of set supplied;

      (ii)   Date of commencement of loan;

      (iii) Size and number of cylinders supplied. When 3400 litre cylinders are ordered the gas is to be supplied in 1360 litre cylinders.

12.3 The pharmacy contractor shall make a monthly return on Form FP66 to the Pricing Authority, with a copy to the respective Family Practitioner Committee, showing:

      (i)   Date of loan set;

      (ii)   Date for return of set (when application) or date of notice by Family Practitioner Committee (see d. iii below); or

      (iii) Confirmation that the set is still on loan (when applicable).

OXYGEN CYLINDER SERVICE - (CONTINUED)

12.4 (i) Where the return shows that the set has been on loan at least three months and has not been returned to the pharmacy contractor, the Committee shall ascertain from the doctor whether the equipment is still required; subsequent enquiries shall be made at intervals not exceeding three months during the first year on the loan.

(ii) In cases where the equipment has been on loan to a patient for eighteen months or more, the Pricing Authority will advise the Committee where they have reason to doubt that the patient has continued need of the equipment, and the Committee should, in such cases, make special enquiries as to the circumstances of the loan.

(iii) Where the Committee are satisfied, after making enquiries, that the equipment is no longer required by the patient, or where between enquiries the doctor informs the Committee to that effect, the Committee shall notify the contractor to arrange recovery.

12.5 Where the patient fails to return the equipment the onus of collecting it rests on the pharmacy contractor.

13. OXYGEN CONCENTRATOR SERVICE

13.1 An oxygen concentrator is an electrically powered machine which separates a high proportion
of nitrogen and some other components from ambient air and thus delivers oxygen enriched gases to
patients. For the purposes of the concentrator service, England and Wales have been divided into
9 regional groups of Family Practitioner Committees and after a competitive tender exercise one
supplier has been selected to provide the service in each group. The regional groups and the
selected supplier for each one are set out in page 279. Each FPC will appoint an 'Authorised
Officer' to whom all queries relative to the concentrator service should be addressed.

13.2 Oxygen concentrator services comprise the supply, installation with full instructions to the
patient, maintenance and removal when no longer required of a concentrator and associated
equipment in a patient's home on the prescription of a general practitioner. Concentrators are
generally reliable and the risk of breakdown is low but in the event of a breakdown suppliers will
be responsible for responding to an emergency call-out within 10 hours. However, where a doctor
considers a patient to be at risk in the event of a concentrator failure, he may prescribe an
emergency back-up supply of cylinder oxygen BP which the patient could use until the concentrator
is repaired. Such back-up equipment should normally be prescribed along with the concentrator but
the GP should review the need for back-up oxygen regularly and the supply should be withdrawn if
no longer required. The emergency back-up supply will form part of the services to be provided by
the concentrator supplier. The supplier will also be responsible for the payment of patients'
electricity costs associated with concentrator usage.

14. PRESCRIBING ARRANGEMENTS FOR OXYGEN CONCENTRATORS

14.1 Concentrators will normally be prescribed when a patient requires long term oxygen therapy
(ie 15 hours or more a day over a prolonged period). However it will still be cost effective to
prescribe a concentrator for patients who require or are using the equivalent of 21 cylinders or
more per month (ie 8 hours per day). In no circumstances should a concentrator be prescribed for
patients requiring less than 8 hours oxygen per day. When a general practitioner decides that a
patient should receive long term oxygen therapy he should take the following action to obtain a
concentrator for his patient.

14.2 Using form FP10, prescribe a concentrator and any other related equipment (eg humidifier)
specifying on the form the amount of oxygen required (ie hours per day) and the flow rate. If a
back-up oxygen set and cylinder are required (see paragraph 14.8 below) these should be ordered at
the same time.

14.3 The GP should give the prescription form to the patient along with an explanation of what a
concentrator is and advise the patient that the supplier will be in touch shortly to arrange
installation. The patient should also be instructed to give the prescription form to the supplier
when he visits the patient's home.

14.4 The GP should then advise the concentrator supplier by telephone that he has prescribed a
concentrator for the patient and ask the supplier to arrange for its installation. The supplier
will acknowledge receipt of the order by sending written confirmation to the GP, the patient and
the FPC. (Details of the supplier for each region, including address and telephone number are set
out in the Drug Tariff (page 277). There is a Freephone arrangement.)

14.5 If at any time during the patient's treatment the GP wishes to order additional equipment
eg. emergency back-up set and cylinder if not previously ordered, he should follow the procedure
at paragraphs 14.2-14.4 above.

OXYGEN CONCENTRATOR SERVICE - (CONTINUED)

14.6 If for any reason the GP wishes to alter the regime he should inform the patient, complete the card which has been given to the patient by the concentrator supplier (entering the date, recommended flow rate, hours of use and his initials) and tell the patient to show it to the supplier when he next visits his home to service the machine.

14.7 It is essential that the GP notifies the FPC's Authorised Officer by telephone immediately the concentrator and/or emergency supply is no longer required by a particular patient.

14.8 Patients who are suitable for long term oxygen therapy are generally not clinically at risk if their oxygen supply is interrupted for a few hours but for those patients considered to be at risk GPs may wish to prescribe emergency back-up cylinder oxygen in case of such a breakdown. (See paragraph 13.2 above).

15. UNDER-USE OF A CONCENTRATOR

15.1 Once a patient has had a concentrator installed in his home it will be important to monitor the volume of oxygen consumption. If the patient's oxygen consumption falls below the level prescribed it may not be cost-effective for him to continue to have a concentrator. Under the terms of their contract, suppliers are required to submit to Committees a statement accompanying claims for reimbursement of patients' electricity costs, setting out in respect of each patient a comparison between the patient's average daily usage of the concentrator over the period of the claim and the daily usage as prescribed by the general practitioner. In those cases where it appears that there may have been a significant under-use of the concentrator the Committee should bring the matter to the attention of the prescriber so that he may re-consider the prescribed regime.

15.2 In those cases where the average daily usage has fallen below the specified level at which a concentrator should be prescribed (See para 14.1) prescribers should be asked specifically to confirm that the patient has been counselled and that usage of the concentrator will increase. Where no such confirmation is obtained the Committee should arrange for the concentrator to be withdrawn and for the doctor to prescribe cylinder oxygen for the patient. Similar action should be taken if, after receiving a prescriber's confirmation of a continuing need for a concentrator at the first enquiry, a further statement from the supplier indicates that usage is still below the specified level. Committees should discuss these arrangements with their Local Medical Committees in order to ensure that prescribers are absolutely clear about the interpretation.

16. TRANSFER OF EXISTING PATIENTS FROM CYLINDERS TO CONCENTRATORS

16.1 Some patients who have had cylinder oxygen prescribed for their tratment may reach a point where their oxygen requirements are such that supply would be more economical by concentrator. The Pricing Authority will identify such patients using the specified level at paragraph 14.1 and advise the Committee. The Committee will then write to each patient's general practitioner to consider whether the prescription of a concentrator would be a more appropriate form of providing oxygen therapy. If so the GP should follow the procedure at paragraph 14 of this Appendix. In such cases a close liaison between the doctor, the concentrator supplier and the patient's existing cylinder supplier will be necessary to ensure that the patient receives sufficient cylinder oxygen to meet his needs until but only until the concentrator is installed.

16.2 FPCs should ensure the oxygen cylinder contractors are aware of concentrator installations and that they withdraw their equipment and any cylinders (empty or full) from the patient's home as soon as possible after the concentrator has been installed.

OXYGEN CONCENTRATOR SERVICE – (CONTINUED)

17. <u>WITHDRAWAL OF A CONCENTRATOR AND/OR ASSOCIATED EQUIPMENT</u>

17.1 Where a GP advises the FPC that a concentrator and/or emergency supply of cylinder oxygen is no longer required for a particular patient the Committee should immediately request the supplier to arrange for removal of the equipment from the patient's home. At the same time the Committee should inform the Pricing Authority of the details and date of removal notification.

18. <u>SUPPLY OF EMERGENCY SUPPLY THROUGH OXYGEN CYLINDER CONTRACTORS</u>

18.1 When emergency back-up oxygen is prescribed it will normally be supplied by the concentrator supplier. However where exceptionally supply is made through a cylinder contrator it is important that the Committee identifies the patient and notifies the Pricing Authority so that the patient's records can be co-ordinated – FPCs should make alternative arrangements for supply to be made through the concentrator supplier as soon as possible.

PART XI - ROTA SERVICE

PART XI

ROTA SERVICE

Payment for rota service organised under Paragraph 4 of the Hours of Service Schemes shall be made by the Family Practitioner Committees direct to pharmacy contractors and is at the rate of £7.50 per hour for week day rota service, excluding early closing day and public holidays, and £17.70 per hour for rota service on early closing day, Sundays and public holidays.

No payment shall be made for any period for rota service occurring between 9.00 am and 1.00 pm on early closing days or between 9.00 am, and 6.00 pm (or 5.30 pm where the Hours of Service Scheme approved by the Family Practitioner Committee permits the closing of the pharmacy at 5.30 pm) on other week days unless they are public holidays. Payment shall not be made for more than one hour's rota service on any one day.

Claims for payment for rota service shall be submitted within six months.

PART XII

ESSENTIAL SMALL PHARMACIES SCHEME

Interpretation

1. In this Part —

    "Committee" means the Family Practitioner Committee in whose locality the premises are located;

    "contractor" means any pharmacy contractor whose name is included in a pharmaceutical list of the Committee;

    "pharmacy" means a pharmacy at premises from which the contractor supplies pharmaceutical services;

    "premises" means the premises from which the contractor provides pharmaceutical services;

    "prescriptions" means prescriptions for supply of drugs, medicines and listed appliances under pharmaceutical services.

    "year" means the period from 1 April in any one year to 31 March of the following year.

PART XII

ESSENTIAL SMALL PHARMACIES SCHEME - cont

Entitlement

2.1   Where, in any year -

a.   the pharmacy dispenses fewer than 16,000 prescriptions; and

b.   that pharmacy is more than 2 kilometres (1.24 miles) by the nearest practicable route available to the public on foot from the next nearest pharmacy or is less than 2 kilometres but previously qualified as a special consideration case and the circumstances of the pharmacy remain unchanged; and

c.   in the case of a pharmacy which has, in the year immediately preceding that year, dispensed fewer than 6,000 prescriptions, the committee certifies in writing at the beginning of that year that the pharmacy is essential to the proper provision of pharmaceutical services, the contractor shall, subject to the following sub-paragraphs, be entitled to ESPS payments calculated in accordance with paragraph 4 below. (Note. No new special consideration cases will be entertained).

2.2   A contractor shall be entitled to claim ESPS payments in any one year if,on or before 31 January in the year immediately preceding, he estimates, on the basis of the number of prescriptions dispensed in the preceding twelve months or having regard to any special circumstances, that the number of items to be dispensed in the next year will be less than 16,000.

2.3   The contractor shall apply to the Committee for ESPS payments, in the form specified (Form EPS1) for contractors on the list not less than 10 months at 31 January and Form ESPS2 for those on list less than 10 months) on or before 31 January in the year immediately preceding the year to which the claim relates.

2.4   On 1 April of the year to which the claim relates, or as soon as practicable thereafter, but before any payment is made, the contractor shall declare to the committee his estimate of the number of prescriptions dispensed by the pharmacy in the year just ended and, if the committee is satisfied that -

a.   that number is less than 16,000

b.   that the number of prescriptions to be dispensed in the year to which the claim relates is unlikely to exceed 16,000 and

c.   the conditions set out in sub-paragraphs 2.1(b) and (c) above are met,

payments shall be made by the committee in accordance with paragraph 3 below, subject to the conditions in sub-paragraphs 2.5 and 2.6 below.

2.5   The Committee, will as soon in the current financial year as they have available the Prescription Pricing Authority figure of prescriptions dispensed by the contractor during the preceding financial year compare this with the contractor's declared estimated figure (sub-paragraph 2.4 above) and if the PPA figure of prescriptions dispensed in the previous financial year is 16,000 or more, the ESPS payments made so far in the current financial year shall be recovered from the contractor in the 3 months following that in which the last ESPS payment was made.

0314M/2

PART XII

ESSENTIAL SMALL PHARMACIES SCHEME - cont

2.6   Where, at any time in any year during which ESPS payments are made to the contractor in respect of a pharmacy -

a.   the number of prescriptions dispensed by that pharmacy exceeds 16,000, the contractor shall be deemed not to have been entitled to ESPS payments for that year in respect of that pharmacy, and any such payment made to him in that year shall be recovered from the remuneration due to him in the 3 months immediately following the month in which the number of prescriptions dispensed reached 16,000;

b.   a second contractor begins to provide pharmaceutical services from a pharmacy at premises which are less than 2 kilometres (1.24 miles) by the nearest practicable route available to the public on foot from the premises of the first contractor, payment to the first contractor shall continue at the full rate during the current year and during the following year at half of the full rate but will then cease.

c.   in a case to which sub-paragraph 2.1c applies, the committee decides that the pharmacy is no longer essential, it shall notify the contractor and after the date of that notification no further ESPS payments shall be paid in that year in respect of that pharmacy.

2.7   Where the provision by the contractor of pharmaceutical services from any premises has just begun, the preceding sub-paragraphs shall be modified as follows:-

a.   the contractor may apply to the Committee for ESPS payments, in the form specified (Form ESPS2) at any time during the year;

b.   he shall be entitled to ESPS payments if -

i.   in the case of a contractor who is providing services from premises from which, immediately before the day on which he began to provide those services, those services were provided by another contractor, the number of prescriptions dispensed in the twelve months immediately preceding that day was less than 16,000;

ii.   in any other case, he estimates, and the Committee is satisfied that, less than 16,000 prescriptions will be dispensed in the first twelve months of the provision of pharmaceutical services, and

iii.   in any case the condition in sub-paragraph 2.1b is satisfied;

c.   any entitlement shall begin -

i.   if the claim is made within 3 months of the entry on to the list in question, from the date of entry;

ii.   in any other case, from the date on which the application is made.

ESSENTIAL SMALL PHARMACIES SCHEME - cont

Payments

3.1   ESPS payments shall, subject to sub-paragraph 3.3 below, be one-twelfth of the difference between the remuneration the contractor receives in the current financial year in respect of the supply of pharmaceutical services from the pharmacy, (ie Professional fees as in Part IIIA and on-cost) and £27,840 (ie the average remuneration on the same basis for the current financial year which would be paid to a pharmacy dispensing 16,000 prescriptions annually).

3.2   Payments shall be paid monthly in arrears.

3.3   The maximum monthly payment shall be £1,450.00 (the difference between one-twelfth of £10,440, the average remuneration, as determined by the Secretary of State due to a pharamcy dispensing 6,000 prescriptions annully, and one-twelfth of £27,840, the average remuneration due to a pharmacy dispensing 16,000 prescriptions annually).

3.4   Any over, or any under, ESPS payment shall be adjusted and, if necessary, corrected in the remuneration paid in the first month of the next following year.

3.5   Where a contractor normally provides pharmaceutical services at a pharmacy for less than 30 hours a week, any ESPS payment shall be calculated by reference to the following formula:-

Average hours/30 x payments appropriate to a full-time pharmacy with the same prescription volume, as determined by the Secretary of State.

PART XIII

PAYMENTS IN RESPECT OF PRE-REGISTRATION TRAINEES

A grant of £2,700 is payable to pharmacy contractors who provide the pre-registration training experience needed by pharmacy graduates and certain undergraduates for admission to the Pharmaceutical Society of Great Britain's Register of Pharmaceutical Chemists. The grants are payable at annual rates, determined annually, in respect of each pre-registration training place filled by a pharmacy graduate or an undergraduate on a sandwich course recognised by the Pharmaceutical Society of Great Britain as pre-registration training.

Pharmacy contractors who have provided pre-registration training should claim payment from the Family Practitoner Committee at the end of each 6 monthly normal training period, or in cases where the training period was shortened by unavoidable circumstances, at the end of the actual training period in which case a pro-rata grant will be calculated and paid.

NB. Claims from contractors in respect of trainees whose training periods commenced before 1 June 1990 will be paid at the former rate of £2520 per annum even if part of the training period falls after 1 June 1990.

PART XIVA

ADVICE TO RESIDENTIAL HOMES

---

1.   These arrangements will cover the provision of advice by a pharmacist who regularly supplies drugs to persons resident in a home registered under Part 1, or which is exempt from registration under Section 1 (5)(j), of the Registered Homes Act 1984. The responsibility for making suitable arrangements for the recording, safekeeping, handling and disposal of drugs will continue to rest with the manager or person in control of the home.

2.   Pharmacists who have completed a training course developed by the Royal Pharmaceutical Society of Great Britain with the support of the Pharmaceutical Services Negotiating Committee and the National Pharmaceutical Association (which is available from Radcliffe Medical Press Ltd. Oxford for England; and Dr D J Temple, UWCC, Cardiff for Wales) will be able to claim the allowances set out in paragraph 6 below. A certificate of completion of the course will be issued.

3.   A pharmacy taking part in the scheme should not normally have agreements to provide advice to more than 5 homes though the Family Practitioner Committee may accept agreements for a larger number of homes if an adequate service would not otherwise be provided. No home may have an arrangement with more than one pharmacy contractor.

4.1   Pharmacists who wish to take part in the scheme should approach the manager of a home with a view to making a written agreement to provide advice on the procedures for safekeeping and correct administration of drugs. A form of agreement between the pharmacist and the management of the home can be obtained from the Family Practitioner Committee.

4.2   When agreement has been reached with one or more homes, the pharmacy contractor should complete an application form, which is available from the Family Practitioner Committee, and send this, with a copy of the agreement completed with each home and a copy of the course completion certificate, to the Family Practitioner Committee.

4.3   Agreements with a home should run from 1 April to 31 March in the following year.

5.   Pharmacists will be required to keep a record of the name and address of each home, of the date of each visit by the pharmacist and of the nature of any advice given by him in the course of the visit, and to make these available to the Family Practitioner Committee for inspection on request.

PART XIVA

ADVICE TO RESIDENTIAL HOMES – cont

Payments

6.1   a.   For an initial visit by the pharmacist to a residential
           home and establishment of an agreement with the home for the
           provision of advice on procedures for the safekeeping and
           correct administration of medicines   –   £50

      b.   Annual fee for residential home with up to 20 places   –   £200

      c.   Annual fee for residential home with more than 20 places   –   £325

6.2   If a pharmacy contractor ceases to provide advice to a residential home and another
      pharmacy contractor enters into an agreement to provide advice under these arrangements
      an initial visit and agreement fee of £50 will be payable to the new contractor, subject
      to the Family Practitioner Committee being satisfied that it is reasonable to do so.

6.3   Payment will be for years ending on 31 March.   The initial payment will be made when
      the pharmacy contractor has satisfied the conditions of the scheme.   The continuing
      payment will be made for completed quarters (starting on 1 April, 1 July etc) in equal
      quarterly instalments in arrears, the final quarterly payment being made before the
      end of March each year.   Subject to any renewed agreement with a residential home the
      arrangement to provide services and receive appropriate payment can be transferred on
      change of ownership of a pharmacy, or on a change of pharmacist if the relevant
      training course has been completed, though in these circumstances no fee will be
      payable for the initial visit.   Payments under the scheme will cease if the service
      is discontinued.

PART XIVA

PART XIVB

PATIENT MEDICATION RECORDS

1.   These arrangements cover the keeping of records of medicines supplied to patients who are on long term medication, if they are in one of two groups:-

   a.   those who are exempt from prescription charges having reached pensionable age: women age 60 or men age 65;

   b.   others whom the pharmacist considers may have difficulty in understanding the nature and dosage of the drug supplied and the times at which it is to be taken.

Each record should cover all the drugs supplied to one patient. It will be eligible for inclusion in these arrangements only if the circumstances and nature of one or more of the drugs which are being or have been supplied by the pharmacist to the patient are such that in the opinion of the pharmacist supplying them, the same or a similar drug is likely to be prescribed for that person regularly on future occasions.

2.   The record keeping system should be suitable for the purpose of the arrangements and provide appropriate levels of confidentiality. It may be computer based or use a manual recording system. It must provide as a minimum a record of the name and address of the person to whom the drug is supplied, the name, quantity and dosage of the drug supplied and the date on which it is supplied. Pharmacy contractors taking part in the scheme will be responsible for any necessary registration under the Data Protection Act 1984.

3.   Pharmacists who have completed a training course developed by the Royal Pharmaceutical Society of Great Britain, with the support of the Pharmaceutical Services Negotiating Committee and the National Pharmaceutical Association (which is available from Radcliffe Medical Press Ltd. Oxford for England; and Dr D J Temple, UWCC, Cardiff for Wales) will be able to claim the allowances set out in paragraph 6 below. A certificate of completion of the course will be issued.

4.   Pharmacy contractors who wish to take part in the scheme should apply to the Family Practitioner Committee confirming that the minimum number of medication records has been reached. Application forms are available from the Family Practitioner Committee. The completed application form should be returned to the Family Practitioner Committee with a copy of the course completion certificate.

5.   Pharmacists will be required to make all records kept as part of these arrangements available to the Family Practitioner Committee for inspection on request.

PART XIVB

PATIENT MEDICATION RECORDS – cont

Payments

6.1 To qualify for payment the record keeping system shall contain records for a minimum of 100 patients. In the case of a pharmacy which qualifies for support under the Essential Small Pharmacy Scheme the minimum number of records shall be for 50 patients.

6.2 For systems which meet the minimum requirements before 31 March 1991, there will be a fee for setting up the record keeping system of £165.

6.3 For maintaining a record system there will be an annual fee of £110.

6.4 Payment will be for years ending on 31 March. The initial payment will be made when the pharmacy contractor has satisfied the conditions of the scheme. The continuing payment will be made for completed quarters (starting on 1 April, 1 July etc) in equal quarterly instalments in arrears, the final quarterly payment being made before the end of March each year. A record keeping system can be transferred on change of ownership of a pharmacy, or on a change of pharmacist if the appropriate training course has been completed, but payment will cease if the service is discontinued.

PART XIVB

PART XV

BORDERLINE SUBSTANCES

LIST A

This is an alphabetical index of products which the ACBS has recommended for the management of the conditions shown under each product.

"General Practitioners are reminded that the ACBS recommends products on the basis that they may be regarded as drugs for the treatment of specified conditions. Doctors should satisfy themselves that the products can safely be prescribed, that patients are adequately monitored and that, where necessary, expert hospital supervision is available."

† "The Committee has defined lactose or sucrose intolerance as follows:-

> Proven lactose or sucrose intolerance is a condition of intolerance to an intake of the relevant disaccharide confirmed by:

> i.   a demonstrated clinical benefit of the effectiveness of the disaccharide free diet; and

> ii.   the presence of reducing substances and/or excessive acid (100pH) in the stools, a low concentration of the correspondent disaccharidase enzyme on intestinal biopsy, or by breath tests or lactose tolerance tests."

AGLUTELLA AZETA CREAM FILLED WAFERS

See: Low Protein products.

AGLUTELLA GLUTEN – FREE LOW PROTEIN SPAGHETTI, SPAGHETTI RINGS, MACARONI, PASTA SPIRALS, TAGLIATELLE AND SEMOLINA

See: Gluten-free; Low Protein products.

† ALIIO (NESTLE)

Proven lactose intolerance in pre-school children, galactosaemia and galactokinase dificiency.

ALBUMAID COMPLETE

Malabsorption states where there is failure to hydrolyse and/or absorb protein.

ALBUMAID RVHB X METHIONINE
ALBUMAID RVHB COMPLETE X METHIONINE

Homocystinuria

ALBUMID XP
ALBUMAID XP CONCENTRATE

Phenylketonuria

ALCOHOLIC BEVERAGES (SEE RECTIFIED SPIRIT)

ALEMBICOL-D (MCT OIL)

Steatorrhoea associated with cystic fibrosis of the pancreas, intestinal lymphangiectasia, surgery of the intestine, chronic liver disease, liver cirrhosis, other proven malabsorption syndromes and in a ketogenic diet in the management of epilepsy.

ALFARE

Proven whole protein sensitivity. (The ACBS has defined this as "intolerance to whole protein, proven by at least two withdrawal and challenge tests, as suggested by an accurate dietary history".)

0315M/1

LIST A — cont

ALMAY TOTAL SUN BLOCK CREAM
ALMAY TOTAL BLOCK LIP PROTECTOR

Protection of skin from UV radiation in photodermatosis including those resulting from radiotherapy.

ALPHOSYL

Psoriasis and other scaly disorders of the scalp.

† AMINEX

Phenylketonuria, similar amino acid abnormalities, liver cirrhosis, chronic renal failure and lactose with sucrose intolerance.

AMINOGRAN FOOD SUPPLEMENT

Phenylketonuria

AMINOGRAN MINERAL MIXTURE

Phenylketonuria and as a mineral supplement in synthetic diets.

ANALOG XP

Phenylketonuria

ANALOG RVHB

Hypermethioninaemia, Homocystinuria

ANALOG XPHEN TYR

Tyrosinaemia

ANALOG XMET THRE VAL ISOLEU

Methylmalonic acidaemia, Propionic acidaemia

ANALOG MSUD

Maple Syrup Urine Disease

APROTEN (ANELLINI, BISCUITS, CRISPBREAD, DITALINI, FLOUR, LOW PROTEIN AND GLUTEN—FREE BREAD AND CAKE MIXES, RIGATINI, TAGLIATELLE)

See: Gluten free; Low Protein products.

AVEENO OILATED AND AVEENO REGULAR SACHETS

Endogenous and exogenous eczema, xerodernea, ichthyosis and senile pruritus associated with dry skin.

BETADINE SKIN CLEANSERS:

Infective conditions of the skin — Shampoo: only for seborrhoeic conditions of the scalp associated with excessive dandruff, pruritic scaling, seborrhoeic dermatitis, pityriasis capitis, infected lesions of the scalp, pyodermas (recurrent furunculosis, infective folliculities, impetigo).

BI—AGLUT GLUTEN FREE PRODUCTS

See: Gluten—free products.

BOOTS COVERING CREAM

See: Covering Creams.

LIST A — cont

CALOGEN

Renal failure and other conditions requiring a high energy, low—fluid, low—electrolyte diet, disorders of amino acid metabolism or carbohydrate absorption, in a ketogenic diet in the management of epilepsy.

CALONUTRIN/CALOREEN:

Renal failure, liver cirrhosis, disaccharide intolerance (without isomaltose intolerance), disorders of amino acid metabolism (and other similar disorders) and/or whole protein intolerance, malabsorption states and other conditions, including proven hypoglycaemia, requiring a high energy, low fluid intake, whether or not sodium and/or potassium restriction is essential.

CAPITOL

Pityriasis capitis and seborrhoeic dermatitis of the scalp.

CASILAN

Biochemically proven hypoproteinaemia.

CEANEL CONCENTRATE

Psoriasis or seborrhoeic conditions.

CETAVLON PC

Seborrhoea capitis and seborrheoic dermatitis.

CLINIFEED

Short bowel syndrome, intractable malabsorption, pre—operative preparation of patients who are undernourished, treatment for those with proven inflammatory bowel disease, treatment following total gastrectomy, dysphagia, bowel fistulae, anorexia nervosa and neoplasia related (associated) cachexia (anorexia). Not to be prescribed for any child under one year, unsuitable as a sole source of nutrition for young children up to five years of age.

CLINIFEED FAVOUR

Short bowel syndrome, intractable malabsorption, pre—operative preparation of patients who are undernourished, treatment for those with proven inflammatory bowel disease, treatment following total gastrectomy, dysphagia, bowel fistulae, anorexia nervosa and neoplasia related (associated) cachexia (anorexia). Not to be prescribed for any child under one year, unsuitable as a sole source of nutrition for young children up to five years of age.

COMMINUTED CHICKEN MEAT (COW AND GATE)

Carbohydrate intolerance in association with possible or proven intolerance of milk, glucose and galactose intolerance.

COPPERTONE SUNSTICK 15
COPPERTONE SUPERSHADE 15
COPPERTONE ULTRASHADE 23

Protection of skin from U—V radiation in photodermatoses including those resulting from radiotherapy.

CORN FLOUR AND CORN STARCH

Hypoglycaemia associated with glycogen storage disease.

CORN OIL

Familial hypercholesterolaemia.

0315M/3

LIST A — Cont

COVERING CREAMS AND CONCEALMENT OF BIRTH MARKS:

The following listed products:

Boots Covering Cream	Covermark Finishing Powder
Covermark Covering Cream	Dermacolor Camouflage Cream
Covermark Spotstick	Dermacolor Fixing Powder
Covermark Rouge Cream	Keromask Masking Cream
Covermark Shading Cream	Keromask Finishing Powder
Covermark Grey Toner	Veil Cover Cream

For post operative scars and other deformaties and as adjunctive therapy in the relief of emotional disturbance due to mutilating skin disease.

COVERMARK PRODUCTS

See: Covering creams

DELIAL 10

Protection of skin from U–V radiation in photodermatoses including those resulting from radiotherapy.

DERMACOLOR CAMOUFLAGE SYSTEM

See: Covering Creams

DEXTROSE

Glycogen storage disease and sucrose/isomaltose intolerance.

DIALAMINE

Oral feeding where essential amino acid supplements are required, for example chronic renal failure, hypoproteinaemia, wound fistula leakage with excessive protein loss, conditions requiring a controlled nitrogen intake and haemodialysis.

DISINFECTANTS (ANTISEPTICS)

May be prescribed on FP10 only when ordered in such quantities and with such directions as are appropriate for the treatment of patients, but not if ordered for general hygienic purposes.

dp LOW PROTEIN BUTTERSCOTCH FLAVOURED CHIP COOKIES AND dp LOW PROTEIN CHOCOLATE FLAVOURED CHIP COOKIES

See: Low protein products.

SUPER SOLUABLE DUOCAL AND LIQUID DUOCAL

Renal failure, liver cirrhosis, disaccharide intolerance (without isomaltose intolerance), disorders of amino acid metabolism (and other similar disorders) and/or whole protein intolerance, malabsorption states and other conditions, requiring a high energy, low fluid intake, whether or not sodium and/or potassium restriction is essential.

LIST A – Cont

ELEMENTAL 028 ELEMENTAL 028 ORANGE

Short bowel syndrome, intractable malabsorption, pre-operative preparation of patients who are
undernourished, treatment for those with proven inflammatory bowel disease, treatment following
gastrectomy, dysphagia, bowel fistulae and neoplasia related (associated) cachexia (anorexia).
Not to be prescribed for any child under one year, unsuitable as a sole source of nutrition for
young children up to five years of age.

ENER-G PRODUCTS

See: Gluten-free products

ENRICH

Short bowel syndrome, intractable malabsorption, pre-operative preparation of patients who are
under nourished, treatment for those with proven inflammatory bowel disease, treatment following
total gastrectomy, dysphagia, bowel fistulae, anorexia nervosa and neoplasia related
(associated) cachexia (anorexia). Not to be prescribed for any child under one year, unsuitable
as a sole source of nutrition for young children up to five years of age.

ENSURE, (ASPARAGUS, CHICKEN, CHOCOLATE, COFFEE, EGGNOG, MUSHROOM, NUT AND VANILLA FLAVOURS) ENSURE
PLUS AND ENSURE POWDER

Short bowel syndrome, intractable malabsorption, pre-operative preparation of patients who are
undernourished, treatment for those with proven inflammatory bowel disease, treatment following
total gastrectomy, dysphagia, bowel fistulae, anorexia nervosa and neoplasia related
(associated) cachexia (anorexia). Not to be prescribed for any child under one year, unsuitable
as a sole source of nutrition for young children up to five years of age.

FARLEY'S GLUTEN-FREE BISCUITS

See: Gluten-free Products.

FLEXICAL

Short bowel syndrome, intractable malabsorption, pre-operative preparation of patients who are
undernourished, treatment following total gastrectomy, bowel fistulae, anorexia nervosa and
neoplasia related (associated) cachexia (anorexia). Not to be prescribed for any child under
one year, unsuitable as a sole source of nutrition for young children up to five years of age.

FORCEVAL PROTEIN

Biochemically proven hypoprotinaemia.

FORMULA MCT (1) POWDER (COW & GATE)

Steatorrhoea associated with cystic fibrosis of the pancreas, intestinal lymphangiectasia,
chronic liver disease, and surgery of the intestine.

† FORMULA 'S' SOYA FOOD

Proven lactose and sucrose intolerance in pre-school children, galactolinase deficiency,
galactasaemia and proven whole cows milk sensitivity.

PART XV - BORDERLINE SUBSTANCES

LIST A - Cont

FORTICAL (NEUTRAL, APPLE, APRICOT, BLACKCURRANT, LEMON AND ORANGE FLAVOURS)

Renal failure, liver cirrhosis or other conditions requiring a high energy, low fluid, low electrolyte diet.

FORTISIP BANANA, MUSHROOM, NEUTRAL, ORANGE, TROPICAL FRUIT AND VANILLA FLAVOURS

Short bowel syndrome, intractable malabsorption, pre-operative preparation of patients who are undernourished, treatment for those with proven inflammatory bowel disease, treatment following total gastrectomy, dysphagia, bowel fistulae, anorexia nervosa and neoplasia related (associated) cachexia (anorexia). Not to be prescribed for any child under one year, unsuitable as a sole source of nutrition for young children up to five years of age.

† FORTISON SOYA

Milk intolerance and lactose intolerance. Not to be prescribed for any child under one year, unsuitable as a sole source of nutrition for young children up to five years of age.

FORTISON ENERGY-PLUS AND FORTISON STANDARD

Short bowel syndrome, intractable malabsorption, pre-operative preparation of patients who are undernourished, treatment for those with proven inflammatory bowel disease, treatment following total gastrectomy, dysphagia, bowel fistulae, anorexia nervosa and neoplasia related (associated) cachexia (anorexia). Not to be prescribed for any child under one year, unsuitable as a sole source of nutrition for young children up to five years of age.

FRESUBIN LIQUID AND SIP FEEDS (VANILLA, MOCHA, NUT, PEACH, CHOCOLATE FLAVOURS)
FRESUIN PLUS F (VEGETABLE SOUP AND MUESLI FLAVOURS)

Short bowel syndrome, intractable malabsorption, pre-operative preparation of patients who are undernourished, treatment for those with proven inflamatory bowel disease, treatment following gastrectomy, bowel fistulae, dysphagia and anorexia nervosa and neoplasia related (associated) cachexia (anorexia). Not to be prescribed for any child under one year, unsuitable as a sole source of nutrition for young children up to five years of age.

FRUCTOSE

Proven glucose/galactose intolerance.

† GALACTOMIN 17 (NEW FORMULA)

Proven lactose intolerance in pre-school children, galactosaemia and galactokinase deficiency.

GALACTOMIN 19 (FRUCTOSE FORMULA)

Glucose plus galactose intolerance.

GELCOTAR

Psoriasis of the scalp, saborrhoeic dermatitis and dandruff.

GENISOL

Psoriasis, eczema and scaling of the scalp (psoriasis, dandruff or eczema).

LIST A - Cont

G F DIETARY GLUTEN FREE BISCUITS
G F DIETARY GLUTEN FREE CRACKERS

See: Gluten-free Products.

GLUCOSE

Glycogen storage disease and sucrose/isomaltose intolerance.

GLUTENEX (LIGA)

See: Gluten-free Products.

GLUTEN FREE PRODUCTS:

Not necessarily low-protein, lactose or sucrose free.

Aglutella gluten-free - low protein spaghetti, spaghetti rings, macaroni, pasta spirals, tagliatelle and semolina.

Aproten Products   - anellini, biscuits, crispbread, ditalini, flour, low protein and gluten-free bread and cake mixes, rigatini, tagliatelle.

Bi-Aglut biscuits
Bi-Aglut gluten-free flour
Bi-Aglut gluten-free toast
Ener G brown rice bread
Farley's gluten-free biscuits
GF Dietary Gluten-free crackers
Glutenex (Liga)
Juvela gluten-free corn mix
Juvela gluten-free loaf (sliced and unsliced)
Juvela gluten-free fibre mix
Juvela gluten-free high fibre loaf (sliced and unsliced)
Juvela gluten-free flour mix
Juvela low-protein loaf (sliced and unsliced)
Juvela low protein flour mix
Liga gluten-free rusks (Cow and Gate)
Nutricia Gluten free biscuits
Polial gluten-free biscuits
Rite-Diet gluten-free high fibre crackers
Rite-Diet gluten-free bread mix
Rite-Diet gluten-free white bread mix
Rite-Diet gluten-free brown bread mix
Rite-Diet gluten-free high fibre bread (with added soya bran)
Rite-Diet gluten-free bread with soya bran (dispensed in tin) 280g.
Rite-Diet gluten-free flour mix 500g.
Rite-Diet gluten-free savoury biscuits 125g
Rite-Diet gluten-free digestive biscuits 150g
Rite-Diet gluten-free sweet biscuits (without chocolate or sultanas) 150g
Rite-Diet gluten-free tea biscuits
Rite-Diet gluten-free white bread (400g).
Rite-Diet baking mix
Rite-Diet low protein bread (dispensed in tin) with or without salt 227g.
Rite-Diet low protein gluten-free biscuits
Rite-Diet low protein gluten-free crackers
Rite-Diet low protein macaroni
Rite-Diet low protein spaghetti (short cut)
Rite-Diet low protein spaghetti rings
Rite-Diet low protein flour mix 400g

LIST A - Cont

Tritamyl gluten-free flour
Tritamyl PK flour
Trufree special dietary flour no.1
Trufree special dietary flour no.2 with rice bran
Trufree special dietary flour no.3 for cantabread
Trufree special dietary flour no.4 white
Trufree special dietary flour no.5 brown
Trufree special dietary flour no.6 plain
Trufree special dietary flour no.7 self-raising
See also certain low-protein products

Gluten-sensitive enteropathies including steatorrhoea due to gluten-sensitivity, coeliac disease and dermatitis herpetiformis.

HEPATIC AID II

For patients with chronic Liver disease and/or porto-hepatic encephalopathy.

HYCAL

Renal failure, liver cirrhosis or other conditions requiring a high energy, low fluid, low electrolyte diet.

INSTANT CAROBEL

Thickening feeds in the treatment of vomiting.

IONAX SCRUB

Control and hygiene of acne and the cleaning of the skin prior to acne treatment.

IONIL T

Seborrhoeic dermatitis of the scalp.

ISOCAL

Short bowel syndrome, intractable malabsorption, pre-operative preparation of patients who are undernourished, treatment for those with proven inflammatory bowel disease, treatment following total gastrectomy, dysphagia, bowel fistulae, anorexia nervosa and neoplasia related (associated) cachexia (anorexia). Not to be prescribed for any child under one year; unsuitable as a sole source of nutrition for young children up to five years of age.

† ISOMIL POWDER

Proven lactose intolerance in pre-school children, galactokinase deficiency, galactasaemia and proven whole cows milk sensitivity.

JUVELA GLUTEN-FREE PRODUCTS

See: Gluten-free products.

LIST A - Cont

JUVELA LOW PROTEIN PRODUCTS

See: Gluten-free; low-protein products.

KEROMASK

See: Covering creams.

LIGA GLUTEN FREE RUSKS (COW AND GATE)

See: Gluten free products.

LIQUID MAXIJUL AND LIQUID MAXIJUL (ORANGE)

Renal failure, liver cirrhosis, disaccharide intolerance (without isomaltose intolerance), disorders of amino acid metabolism (and other similar disorders) and/or whole protein intolerance, malabsorption states and other conditions, including proven hypoglycaemia, requiring a high energy low fluid intake.

LIQUIGEN

Steatorrhoea associated with cystic fibrosis of the pancreas, intestinal lymphangiectasia, surgery of the intestine, chronic liver disease, liver cirrhosis, other proven malabsorption syndromes, a ketogenic diet in the management of epilepsy and in type 1 hyperlipoproteinaemia.

LIQUISORB

Short bowel syndrome, intractable malabsorption, pre-operative preparation of patients who are undernourished, treatment for those with proven inflammatory bowel disease, treatment following total gastrectomy, dysphagia, bowel fistulae, and anoraxia nervosa and neoplasia related (associated) cachexia (anorexia). Not to be prescribed for any child under one year, unsuitable as a sole source of nutrition for young children up to five years of age.

LIQUISORB (HIGH FIBRE) TUBE FEED AND DRINK (BANANA, CHOCOLATE, NEUTRAL, STRAWBERRY, VANILLA AND VEGETABLE FLAVOURS)

Intractable malabsorption, pre-operative preparation of patients who are undernourished, treatment of those with proven inflammatory bowel disease, dyspagia and anorexia nervosa and neoplasia related (associated) cachexia (anorexia). Not to be prescribed for any child under one year, unsuitable as a sole source of nutrition for young children up to five years of age.

LIQUISORBON MCT

Short bowel syndrome, intractable malabsorption, pre-operative preparation of patients who are undernourished, treatment for those with proven inflammatory bowel disease, treatment following total gastrectomy, dysphagia, bowel fistulae and anorexia nervosa and neoplasia related (associated) cachexia (anorexia). Not to be prescribed for any child under one year, unsuitable as a sole source of nutrition for young children up to five years of age.

LOCASOL AND LOCASOL NEW FORMULA

Intolerance to calcium.

PART XV - BORDERLINE SUBSTANCES

LIST A - Cont

LOFENALAC

Phenylketonuria.

LOW-PROTEIN PRODUCTS

Aglutella Azeta cream filled wafers (except for those conditions marked*).
Aglutella gluten-free low-protein spaghetti, spaghetti rings, macaroni,
                pasta spirals, tagliatelle and semolina.
Aminex - (except for those conditions marked*).
Aproten Products - anellini, biscuits, crispbread, ditalini, flour, low-protein and
                gluten-free bread and cake mixes, rigatini, tagliatelle.
dp Low Protein Butterscotch Flavoured Chip Cookies (except for those conditions marked*).
dp Low Protein Chocolate Flavoured Chip Cookies (except for those conditions marked*).
Juvela gluten-free low protein chocolate chip, orange and cinnamon flavour cookies (except for
those conditions marked)*
Juvela low-protein loaf. (Sliced and unsliced)
Juvela low-protein flour mix.
Rite-Diet gluten-free low-protein bread (dispensed in tin) with and without salt.
Rite-Diet baking mix.
Rite-Diet low-protein cream filled biscuits - chocolate flavour (except for those conditions
marked*).
Rite-Diet low-protein cream filled wafers-vanilla orange and chocolate flavour (except for those
conditions marked*).
Rite-Diet low-protein flour mix
Rite-Diet low-protein gluten-free biscuits
Rite-Diet low-protein gluten free crackers.
Rite-Diet low-protein macaroni
Rite-Diet low-protein spaghetti (short cut)
Rite-Diet low-protein spaghetti rings
Rite-Diet low-protein sweet biscuits (except for those conditions marked*).
Rite-Diet low-protein white bread (with added fibre)
Tritamyl PK flour
Phenylketonuria; similar amino acid abnormalities; renal failure; liver failure; liver
cirrhosis; gluten-sensitive enteropathies including steatorrhoea due to gluten-sensitivity*;
coeliac disease*; dermatitis herpetiformis*.

MAXAMAID XP AND MAXAMAID XP ORANGE

Phenylketonuria

MAXAMUM XP

Phenylketanuria. Not to be prescribed for children under 8 years old.

MAXIJUL LE

As for super soluble Maxijul where sodium and/or potassium restriction is essential.

MAXIPRO (INSTANT) AND MAXIPRO HBV

Biochemically proven hypoproteinaemia.

LIST A - Cont

MEDIUM-CHAIN TRIGLYCERIDE OIL (MCT)

Steatorrhoea associated with cystic fibrosis of the pancreas, intestinal lymphangiectasia, surgery of the intestine, chronic liver disease, liver cirrhosis, other proven malabsorption syndromes, in a ketogenic diet in the management of epilepsy and in type 1 hyperlipoproteinaemia.

METABOLIC MINERAL MIXTURE

Mineral supplement in synthetic diets.

MILUPA lpd

Inherited disorders of amigo acid metabolism in childhood.

MINAFEN

Phenylketonuria.

MSUD AID

Maple syrup urine disease.

NESTARGEL

Thickening feeds in the treatment of vomiting.

† NUTRAMIGEN

Infants over 3 months and children with galactokinase deficiency, galactosaemia, proven lactose and/or sucrose intolerance, in pre-school children, proven sensitivity to whole protein. (The ACBS has defined this as "intolerance to whole protein, proven by at least two withdrawal and challenge tests, as suggested by an accurate dietary history").

NUTRICIA GLUTEN FREE BISCUITS

See: Gluten free products

OSMOLITE

Short bowel syndrome, intractable malabsorption, pre-operative preparation of patients who are undernourished, treatment for those with proven inflammatory bowel disease, treatment following total gastrectomy, dysphagia, bowel fistulae, anorexia nervosa and neoplasia related (associated) cachexia (anorexia). Not to be prescribed for any child under one year, unsuitable as a sole source of nutrition for young children up to five years of age.

† OSTERSOY

Proven lactose and sucrose intolerance in pre-school children, galactokinase deficiency, galactosaemia and proven whole cows milk protein sensitivity.

PAEDIASURE

Short bowel syndrome, intractable malabsorption, pre-operative preparation of patients who are undernourished, treatment for those with proven inflammatory bowel disease, dysphagia, bowel fistulae, cystic fibrosis and neoplasia related (associated) cachexia (anorexia). Not to be prescribed for any child under one year.

0315M/11

LIST A - Cont

PEPTAMEN

Short bowel syndrome, intractable malabsorption, pre-operative preparation of patients who are undernourished, treatment for those with proven inflammatory bowel disease, treatment following total gastrectomy, dysphagia, bowel fistulae, anorexia nervosa and neoplasia related (associated) cachexia (anorexia). Not to be prescribed for any child under one year, unsuitable as a sole source of nutrition for young childred up to five years of age.

PEPTI - 2000 LF

Intractable malabsorption, bowel fistulae, treatment following total gastrectomy and neoplasia related (associated) cachexia (anorexia). Not to be prescribed for any child under one year, unsuitable as a sole source of nutrition for young children up to five years of age.

PEPTI - JUNIOR

Proven lactose and/or associated sucrose intolerance in association with proven whole protein intolerance, steatorrhoea associated with cystic fibrosis and other proven malabsorption syndromes.

(The ACBS has defined proven whole protein sensitivity as "intolerance to whole protein, proven by at least two withdrawal and challenge tests, as suggested by an accurate dietary history").

PEPTISORB

Intractable malabsorption, bowel fistulae, treatment following total gastrectomy and neoplasia related (associated) cachexia (anorexia). For adult use only.

PEPTISORBON

Intractable malabsorption, bowel fistulae, treatment following total gastrectomy and neoplasia related (associated) cachexia (anorexia). Not to be given to children.

PIZ BUIN CREME SPF NO 12

Protection of skin from U-V radiation in photodermatoses including those resulting from radiotherapy.

PK AID 1 (SCIENTIFIC HOSPITAL SUPPLIES LTD)

Phenylketonuria.

PKU 2 (MILUPA)

Phenyleketonuria

PKU 3 (MILUPA)

Phenyleketonuria (not normally to be prescribed for a child below about 8 months old.)

PKU DRINK GF DIETARY

Phenyketonuria

POLIAL GLUTEN FREE BISCUITS

See: Gluten free products.

POLYCAL

Renal failure, liver cirrhosis, disaccharide intolerance (without isomaltose intolerance), disorders of amino acid metabolism (and other similar disorders) and/or whole protein intolerance, malabsorption states and other conditions, including proven hypoglycaemia, requiring a high energy, low fluid intake, whether or not sodium and/or potassium restriction is essential.

LIST A - Cont

POLYCOSE LIQUID AND POWDER

Renal failure, liver cirrhosis, disaccharide intolerance (without isomaltose intolerance) disorders of amino acid metabolism (and other similar disorders) and/or whole protein intolerance, malabsorption states and other conditions, including proven hypoglycaemia, requiring a high energy, low fluid intake, whether or not sodium and/or potassium restriction is essential.

POLYTAR EMOLLIENT

Psoriasis, eczema, atopic and pruritic dermatoses.

POLYTAR LIQUID

Psoriasis, eczema, scaling of the scalp (psoriasis, dandruff and eczema).

POLYTAR PLUS

Scalp disorders such as scaling (psoriasis, dandruff and eczema), pruritus and in the removal of pastes and pomades used in the treatment of psoriasis.

† PORTAGEN

Lactose intolerance without sucrose intolerance but requiring MCT, malabsorption associated with cystic fibrosis of the pancreas intestinal lymphangiectasia, surgery of the intestine, chronic liver disease, liver cirrhosis and other proven malabsorption syndromes, and neoplosia related (associated) cachexia (anorexia).

† PREGESTIMIL

Sucrose and/or lactose intolerance in association with whole protein intolerance or where amino acids and peptides are indicated in conjunction with MCT. Also for proven malabsorption syndromes in which a reduced fat diet is indicated such as steatorrhoea associated with cystic fibrosis and surgery of the intestine, galactosaemia and galactokinase deficiency and neoplosia related (associated) cachexia (anorexia).

† PREJOMIN (MILUPA)

Proven lactose and sucrose intolerance in pre-school children, fructose intolerance, galactosaemiagalactokinase deficiency, and proven sensitivity to whole protein. (The ACBS has defined proven whole protein sensitivity as "intolerance to whole protein, proven by at least two withdrawal and challenge tests, as suggested by an accurate dietary history".)

PRO-MOD

Biochemically proven hypoproteinaemia.

† PROSOBEE LIQUID AND POWDER

Proven lactose and associated sucrose introlerance in pre-school children, glactokinase deficiency, galactosaemia and proven whole cows milk sensitivity.

PROTIFAR

Biochemically proven hypoproteinaemia.

LIST A — Cont

REABILAN

Short bowel syndrome, intractable malabsorption, pre—operative preparation of patients who are undernourished, treatment for those with proven inflammatory bowel disease, treatment following total gastrectomy, dysphagia and bowel fistulae and neoplasia related (associated) cachexia (anorexia). Not to be prescribed for any child under one year, unsuitable as a sole source of nutrition for young children up to five years of age.

RECTIFIED SPIRIT

Where the therapeutic qualities of alcohol are required rectified spirit (suitably flavoured and diluted) should be prescribed.

RITE—DIET LOW SODIUM BREAD

For conditions in which a low sodium diet is indicated.

RITE—DIET PRODUCTS

See: Gluten—free and low protein products.

ROC OPAQUE TOTAL SUNBLOCK CREAM SPF 15 A&B (COLOURLESS/TINTED)
ROC TOTAL SUNBLOCK CREAM 10 (COLOURLESS)

Protection of skin from UV radiation in photodermatoses including those resulting from radiotherapy.

SPECTRABAN 15

Protection of skin from UV radiation in photodermatoses including those resulting from radiotherapy.

STER—ZAC BATH CONCENTRATE

Staphylococcal skin infections.

SUNFLOWER OIL

Familial hypercholesterolanaemia (Non—drug for multiple sclerosis).

SUPER SOLUBLE DUOCAL

See: Duocal.

SUPER SOLUBLE MAXIJUL

Renal failure, liver cirrhosis, disaccharide intolerance (without isomaltose intolerance), disorders of amino acid metabolism (and other similar disorders) and/or whole protein intolerance, malabsorption states and other conditions, including proven hypoglycaemia, requiring a high energy low fluid intake.

TETMOSOL

Control of scabies.

LIST A - Cont

T GEL SHAMPOO

Psoriasis, eczema, scaling of the scalp (psoriasis, dandruff and eczema).

TRIOSORBON

Short bowel syndrome, intractable malabsorption, pre-operative preparation of patients who are undernourished, treatment for those with proven inflammatory bowel disease, treatment following total gastrectomy, dysphagia, bowel fistulae, anorexia nervosa and neoplasia related (associated) cachexia (anorexia). Not to be prescribed for any child under one year, unsuitable as a sole source of nutrition for young children up to five years of age.

TRITAMYL GLUTEN FREE FLOUR

See: Gluten-free Products.

TRITAMYL PK FLOUR

See: Gluten free and low Protein Products.

TRUFREE PRODUCTS

See: Gluten-free products.

UVISTAT SUN CREAM (FACTOR 10)
UVISTAT WATER RESISTANT SUN CREAM (FACTOR 8)

Protection of skin from UV radiation in photodermatoses including those resulting from radiotherapy.

VEIL COVER CREAM

See: Covering Creams

VITAMIN PREPARATIONS

Only when used in the management of actual or potential vitamin deficiency.

WYETH STANDARD ENTERAL FEED

Short bowel syndrome, intractable malabsorption, pre-operative preparation of pateints who are undernourished, treatment for those with proven inflammatory bowel disease, treatment following total gastrectomy, dysphagia, bowel fistulae. anorexia nervosa and neoplasia related (associated) cachexia (anorexia). Not to be prescribed for any child under on year, unsuitable as a sole source of nutrition for young children up to five years of age.

† WYSOY

Proven lactose intolerance in pre-school children, galactokinase deficiency, galactosaemia and proven whole cows milk sensitivity.

LIST B

This is a cross index listing clinical conditions and the products which the ACBS has approved for the management of those conditions. It is essential to consult LIST A for more precise guidance.

ACNE

    Ionex scrub

AMINO ACID METABOLIC DISORDERS AND SIMILAR PROTEIN DISORDERS

See: Milupa lpd
See: Phenylketonuria
    Histidinaemia
    Homocystinuria
    Maple syrup urine disease
    Synthetic diets
    Low protein products

ANOREXIA NERVOSA

    Clinifeed
    Enrich
    Ensure
    Ensure Plus
    Ensure Powder
    Fortisip
    Fortison Energy-Plus
    Fortison Standard
    Fresubin Liquid and Sip Feeds
    Isocal
    Liquisorb
    Liquisorb (High Fibre) Tube Feed and Drink
    Liquisorbon MCT
    Osmolite
    Peptamen
    Triosorbon
    Wyeth Standard Enteral Feed

BIRTHMARKS

See: Disfiguring skin lesions

BOWEL FISTULAE

    Clinifeed
    Elemental 028
    Elemental 028 Orange
    Enrich
    Ensure
    Ensure Plus
    Ensure Powder
    Flexical
    Forceval Protein
    Fortisip

This is a cross index listing clinical conditions and the products which the ACBS has approved for the management of those conditions. It is essential to consult LIST A for more precise guidance.

LIST B –Cont

    Fortison Energy–Plus
    Fortison Standard
    Fresubin Liquid and Sip Feeds
    Fresubin Plus F
    Isocal
    Liquisorb
    Liquisorbon MCT
    Maxipro HBV
    Maxipro Instant
    Nutranel
    Osmolite
    Paediasure
    Peptamen
    Pepti – 2000 LF
    Peptisorb
    Peptisorbon
    Reabilan
    Triosorbon
    Wyeth Standard Enteral Feed

CALCIUM INTOLERANCE

    Locasol and Locasol New Formula

CARBOHYDRATE MALABSORPTION

    Calogen
See: Synthetic diets
    Malabsorption states

    <u>Disaccharide intolerance</u> (without isomaltose intolerance)

        Calonutrin
        Caloreen
        Liquid Duocal, Super Soluble Duocal
        Liquid Maxijul
        Liquid Maxijul (orange)
        Maxijul LE
        Polycal
        Polycose Liquid and Powder
        Super Soluble Maxijul
    See: Lactose intolerance,
        Lactose with Sucrose intolerance

    <u>Isomaltose intolerance</u>

        Glucose

    <u>Glucose + galactose intolerance</u>

        Comminuted Chicken Meat (Cow & Gate)
        Fructose
        Galactomin 19 (Fructose Formula)

This is a cross index listing clinical conditions and the products which the ACBS has approved for the management of those conditions. It is essential to consult LIST A for more precise guidance.

LIST B - Cont

† Lactose intolerance

ALII0 (Nestle)
Aminex
Comminuted Chicken Meat (Cow & Gate)
Formula S Soya Food
Fortison Soya
Galactomin 17 (New Formula)
Isomil Powder
Nutramigen
Ostersoy
Portagen
Pregestimil
Prejomin
Prosobee liquid and powder
Prosparol
Wysoy

† Lactose with associated sucrose intolerance

Aminex
Comminuted Chicken Meat (Cow & Gate)
Formula 'S' Soya Food
Galactomin 17 (New Formula)
Nutramigen
Ostersoy
Pepti-Junior
Pregestimil
Prejomin (Milupa)
Prosobee liquid and powder

† Sucrose intolerance

Glucose "For Oral use" (dextrose)
see: Synthetic diets
Malabsorption
Lactose with sucrose intolerance

CIRRHOSIS OF THE LIVER AND CHRONIC LIVER DISEASE:

See: Liver Disease

† "The Committee has defined lactose or sucrose intolerance as:

Proven lactose or sucrose intolerance is a condition of intolerance to an intake of the relevant disaccharide confirmed by:

i. a demonstrated clinical benefit of the effectiveness of the disaccharide free diet; and

ii. the presence of reducing substances and/or excessive acid(100pH) in the stools, a low concentration of the correspondent disaccharidase enzyme on intestinal biopsy, or by breath tests or lactose tolerance tests".

COELIAC DISEASE:

See: Gluten sensitive enteropathies

This is a cross index listing clinical conditions and the products which the ACBS has approved for the management of those conditions. It is essential to consult LIST A for more precise guidance.

LIST B - Cont

CYSTIC FIBROSIS

See: Malabsorption

DERMATITIS (INCLUDES CONTACT,ATOPIC AND INFECTIVE DERMATOSES, ECZEMA AND PRURITIC DERMATOSES

Aveeno Oilated Sachets
Aveeno Regular Sachets
Betadine skin cleanser and foam
Genisol
Polytar emollient
Polytar plus
Polytar liquid
Ster-Zac bath concentrate
T Gel Shampoo

DERMATITIS HERPETIFORMIS

See: Gluten-sensitive enteropathies.

DISACCHARIDE INTOLERANCE

See: Carbohydrate malabsorption

DISFIGURING SKIN LESIONS (BIRTHMARKS, MUTILATING LESIONS AND SCARS)

Boots Covering Cream
Covermark Products
Dermacolor Camouflage System
Keromask Masking Cream and Keromask Finishing Powder
Veil Covering Cream

DYSPHAGIA

Clinifeed
Elemental 028
Elemental 028 Orange
Enrich
Ensure
Ensure Plus
Ensure Powder
Forceval Protein
Fortisip
Fortison Energy-Plus
Fortison Standard
Fresubin Liquid and Sip Feeds
Fresubin Plus F
Isocal
Liquisorb
Liquisorb (High Fibre Tube Feed Drink)
Liquisorbon MCT
Maxipro Instant
Osmolite
Paediasure
Peptamen
Reabilan

This is a cross index listing clinical conditions and the products which the ACBS has approved for the management of those conditions. It is essential to consult LIST A for more precise guidance.

LIST B — Cont

Triosorbon
Wyeth Standard Enteral Feed

(The ACBS has defined Dysphagia as that associated with:

Intrinsic disease of the Oesophagus eg Oesophagtitis;
Neuromuscular disorders, eg Multiple Sclerosis and Motor Neurone Disease;
Major surgery and/or radiotherapy for cancer of the upper digestive tract;
Protracted severe inflammatory disease of the upper digestive tract, eg
Stevens—Johnson Syndrome and Epidermolysis Bullosa).

ECZEMA   (See: Dermatitis)

EPILEPSY (Ketogenic Diet in)

Alembicol D
Calogen
Liquigen
Medium—chain triglyceride oil (MCT)

GALACTOKINASE DEFICIENCY AND GALACTOSAEMIA

ALIIO (Nestle)
Alfare
Formula S Soya Food
Galactomin 17 (New Formula)
Isomil Powder
Nutramigen
Ostersoy
Pregestimil
Prejomin (Milupa)
Prosobee liquid and powder
Wysoy

GASTRECTOMY (TOTAL)

Clinifeed
ELemental 028
Elemental 028 Orange
Enrich
Ensure
Ensure Plus
Ensure Powder
Flexical
Forceval protein
Fortisip
Fortison Energy—Plus
Fortison Standard
Fresubin Liquid and Sip Feeds
Fresubin plus F
Isocal
Liquisorb
Liquisorbon MCT

This is a cross index listing clinical conditions and the products which the ACBS has approved for
the management of those conditions. It is essential to consult LIST A for more precise guidance.

PART XV - BORDERLINE SUBSTANCES

LIST B - Cont

  Maxipro Instant
  Osmolite
  Peptamen
  Pepti-2000 LF
  Peptisorb
  Peptisorbon
  Reabilan
  Triosorbon
  Wyeth Standard Enteral Feed

GLUCOSE/GALACTOSE INTOLERANCE

See: Carbohydrate Malabsorption

  Comminuted Chicken Meat (Cow and Gate)

GLUTEN-SENSITIVE ENTEROPATHIES

  Aglutella gluten-free low protein spaghetti, spaghetti rings, macaroni, pasta
            spirals, tagliatelle and semolina.
  Aproten Products - anellini, biscuits, crispbread, ditalini, flour, low protein
            and gluten-free bread and cake mixes, rigatini,tagliatelle
  Bi-Aglut biscuits
  Bi-Aglut gluten - free flour
  Bi-Aglut gluten-free toast
  Ener G brown rice bread
  Farley's gluten-free biscuits
  G F Dietary gluten-free biscuits
  G F Dietary gluten-free crackers
  Glutenex (Liga)
  Juvela gluten-free corn mix
  Juvela gluten-free loaf (sliced and unsliced)
  Juvela gluten-free high fibre loaf (sliced and unsliced)
  Juvela gluten-free fibre mix
  Juvela gluten-free flour mix
  Juvela low-protein loaf (sliced and unsliced)
  Juvela low-protein flour mix
  Liga glute-free rusks (Cow + Gate)
  Nutricia gluten-free tea biscuits
  Polial gluten-free biscuits
  Rite-Diet gluten-free high fibre crackers
  Rite-Diet gluten-free bread mix
  Rite-Diet gluten-free white bread mix
  Rite-Diet gluten-free brown bread mix
  Rite-Diet gluten-free high fibre bread (with added soya bran) 400g
  Rite-Diet gluten-tree low-protein bread with soya bran (dispensed in tin) 280g
  Rite-Diet gluten-free flour
  Rite-Diet gluten-free flour mix 500g
  Rite-Diet gluten-free digestive biscuits 150g
  Rite-Diet gluten-free low protein bread (dispensed in tin) with or without salt 227g
  Rite-Diet gluten-free low-protein flour
  Rite-Diet gluten-free sweet biscuits (without chocolate or sultanas) 150g
  Rite-Diet gluten-free savoury biscuits 125g

This is a cross index listing clinical conditions and the products which the ACBS has approved for
the management of those conditions. It is essential to consult LIST A for more precise guidance.

LIST B - Cont

    Rite-Diet gluten-free tea biscuits
    Rite-Diet gluten-free white bread 400g
    Rite-Diet baking mix
    Rite-Diet low-protein gluten-free biscuits
    Rite-Diet low-protein gluten-free crackers
    Rite-Diet low-protein macaroni
    Rite-Diet low-protein spaghetti (short cut)
    Rite-Diet low-protein spaghetti rings
    Tritamyl gluten-free flour
    Tritamyl PK flour
    Trufree special dietary flour No 1
    Trufree special dietary flour No 2 with rice bran
    Trufree special dietary flour No 3 for cantabread
    Trufree special dietary flour No 4 white
    Trufree special dietary flour No 5 brown
    Trufree special dietary flour No 6 plain
    Trufree special dietary flour No 7 self-raising

GLYCOGEN STORAGE DISEASE

    Calonutrin
    Caloreen
    Corn Flour or Corn Starch
    Dextrose
    Glucose
    Liquid Maxijul
    Liquid Maxijul (Orange)
    Maxijul LE
    Polycal
    Polycose Liquid and Powder
    Super Soluble Maxijul

HISTIDINAEMIA

see: Low Protein products
            Synthetic diets

HOMOCYSTINURIA

    Albumaid RVHB X Methionine
    Albumaid RVHB Complete X Methionine
see: Low Protein products
            Synthetic diets.

HYPERCHOLESTEROLAEMIA (FAMILIAL)

    Corn oil
    Sunflower oil

HYPERLIPOPROTEINAEMIA TYPE 1

    Liquigen
    Medium chain triglyceride oil

This is a cross index listing clinical conditions and the products which the ACBS has approved for
the management of those conditions. It is essential to consult LIST A for more precise guidance.

LIST B - Cont

HYPOGLYCAEMIA

    Calonutrin
    Caloreen
    Corn Flour or Corn Starch
    Liquid Maxijul
    Liquid Maxijul (Orange)
    Maxijul LE
    Polycal
    Polycose Liquid and Powder
    Super Soluble Maxijul
see: Glycogen storage disease

HYPOPROTEINAEMIA

    Casilan
    Dialamine
    Forceval protein
    Maxipro HBV
    Maxipro Instant
    Pro-Mod
    Protifar

INTESTINAL LYMPHANGIECTASIA (SEE MALABSORPTION)

INTESTINAL SURGERY (SEE MALABSORPTION)

ISOMALTOSE INTOLERANCE (SEE CARBOHYDRATE MALABSORPTION)

LACTOSE INTOLERANCE (SEE CARBOHYDRATE MALABSORPTION)

LIVER DISEASE (i.e. CHRONIC LIVER DISEASE, CIRRHOSIS):

    Aglutella Azeta cream filled wafers
    Aglutella gluten-free low protein spaghetti, spaghetti rings, macaroni,
                    pasta spirals, taglitelle and semolina.
    Alembicol D
    Aminex
    Aproten Products - anellini, biscuits, crispbread, ditalini, flour, low protein and
                  gluten-free bread and cake mixes, rigatini, tagliatelle.
    Calonutrin
    Caloreen
    dp Low-Protein butterscotch flavoured chip cookies
    dp Low-Protein chocolate flavoured chip cookies
    Formula MCT (1) Powder
    Fortical
    Hepatic Aid II
    Hycal
    Juvela gluten-free low protein chocolate chip, orange and cinnamen flavour cookies
    Juvela low-protein loaf (sliced and unsliced)
    Juvela low-protein mix
    Liquid Duocal, Super Soluble Duocal
    Liquid Maxijul

This is a cross index listing clinical conditions and the products which the ACBS has approved for the management of those conditions. It is essential to consult LIST A for more precise guidance.

PART XV – BORDERLINE SUBSTANCES

LIST B– Cont

    Liquid Maxijul (orange)
    Liquigen
    Maxijul LE
    Medium chain triglyceride oil
    Polycal
    Polycose Liquid and Powder
    Portagen
    Rite-Diet gluten-free low-protein bread (dispensed in tin)
    Rite-Diet baking mix
    Rite-Diet low-protein flour mix 400g
    Rite-Diet low-protein cream filled biscuits – chocolate flavour
    Rite-Diet low-protein gluten-free biscuits
    Rite-Diet low-protein macaroni
    Rite-Diet low-protein spaghetti (short cut)
    Rite-Diet low-protein spaghetti rings
    Rite-Diet low-protein sweet biscuits 150g
    Rite-Diet low-protein cream filled wafers-vanilla orange and chocolate flavour
    Rite-Diet low-protein white bread (with added fibre)
    Super Soluble Maxijul
    Tritamyl PK flour

LOW-PROTEIN PRODUCTS

    Aglutella Azeta cream filled wafers (except for those conditions marked*).
    Aglutella gluten-free low-protein spaghetti, spaghetti rings, macaroni, pasta
           spirals, tagliatelle and semolina.
    Aminex – (except for those conditions marked*).
    Aproten Products – anellini, biscuits, crispbread, ditalini, flour, low-protein
        * and gluten-free bread and cake mixes, rigatini, tagliatelle.
    dp Low Protein Butterscotch Flavoured Chip Cookies (except for those conditions marked*).
    dp Low Protein Chocolate Flavoured Chip Cookies (except for those conditions marked*).
    Juvela glute-free low protein chocolate chip, orange and cinnamon flavour
              cookies (except those conditions marked*)
    Juvela low-protein loaf. (Sliced and Unsliced)
    Juvela low-protein mix.
    Rite-Diet gluten-free low-protein bread (dispensed in tin) with and without salt
    Rite-Diet baking mix
    Rite-Diet low-protein cream filled biscuits – chocolate flavour
            (except for those conditions marked*).
    Rite-Diet low-protein cream filled wafers-vanilla, orange and chocolate
            flavour (except for those conditions marked*).
    Rite-Diet low-protein flour mix.
    Rite-Diet low-protein gluten-free biscuits
    Rite-Diet low-protein gluten-free crackers
    Rite-Diet low-protein macaroni
    Rite-Diet low-protein spaghetti (short cut)
    Rite-Diet low-protein spaghetti rings
    Rite-Diet low-protein sweet biscuits (except for those conditions marked*).
    Rite-Diet low-protein white bread (with added fibre)
    Tritamyl PK flour

    Phenylketonuria, similar amino acid abnormalities, renal failure, liver failure, liver
    cirrhosis, gluten-sensitive enteropathies including steatorrhoea due to gluten-sensitivity*,
    coeliac disease*, dermatitis herpetiformis*.

This is a cross index listing clinical conditions and the products which the ACBS has approved for
the management of those conditions. It is essential to consult LIST A for more precise guidance.

LIST B – Cont

MALABSORPTION STATES

(See also: gluten-sensitive enteropathies, liver disease, carbohydrate malabsorption, intestinal lymphangiectasia, milk intolerance and synthetic diets)

    a.   Protein sources

        Albumaid Complete
        Comminuted Chicken Meat (Cow & Gate)
        Forceval Protein
        Liquid Duocal and Super Soluble Duocal
        Maxipro Instant

    b.   Fat sources

        Alembicol D
        Calogen
        Liquigen
        Medium chain triglyceride oil

    c.   Carbohydrate:

        Calonutrin
        Caloreen
        Fortical
        Hycal
        Liquid Maxijul
        Liquid Maxijul (Orange)
        Maxijul LE
        Maxijul Super
        Polycal
        Polycose Liquid and Powder
        Super Soluble Maxijul

    d.   Complete Feeds

        Clinifeed and Clinifeed Favour
        Elemental 028
        Elemental 028 Orange
        Enrich
        Ensure
        Ensure Plus
        Ensure Powder
        Flexical
        Formula MCT (1) Powder
         (with appropriate vitamin and mineral supplements)
        Fortisip
        Fortison Energy-Plus
        Fortison Standard
        Fresubin Liquid and Sip Feeds
        Fresubin Plus F
        Isocal

This is a cross index listing clinical conditions and the products which the ACBS has approved for the management of those conditions. It is essential to consult LIST A for more precise guidance.

LIST B – Cont

  Liquisorb
  Liquisorb (High Fibre) Tube Feed and Drink
  Liquisorbon MCT
  Osmolite
  Paediasure
  Peptamen
  Pepti – 2000 LF
  Pepti – Junior
  Pepisorb
  Peptisorbon
  Portagen
  Pregestimil
  Reabilan
  Triosorbon
  Wyeth Standard Enteral Feed

  e. Minerals

  Aminogran Mineral Mixture
  Metabolic Mineral Mixture

  f. Vitamins – as appropriate

  see: Synthetic diets

MAPLE SYRUP URINE DISEASE

  Analog MSUD
  MSUD Aid
see: Low Protein Products Synthetic diets

METHYLMALONIC ACIDAEMIA AND PROPIONIC ACIDAEMIA

  Analog XMET, THRE, VAL, ISOLEU

MILK PROTEIN SENSITIVITY

  Comminuted Chicken meat (Cow & Gate)
  Formula S Soya Food
  Fortison Soya
  Isomil Powder
  Nutramigen
  Ostersoy
  Pregestimil
  Prosobee liquid and powder
  Wysoy

see: Synthetic diets.

NEOPLASIA RELATED (ASSOCIATED)

CACHEXIA (ANOREXIA)

  Clinifeed and Clinifeed Favour
  Elemental 028
  Elemental 028 Orange
  Enrich
  Ensure
  Ensure Plus

This is a cross index listing clinical conditions and the products which the ACBS has approved for the management of those conditions. It is essential to consult LIST A for more precise guidance.

0317M/11

LIST B - Cont

> Ensure Powder
> Flexical
> Fortisip
> Fortison Energy-Plus
> Fortison Standard
> Fresubin Liquid and Sip Feeds
> Fresubin Plus F
> Isocal
> Liquisorb
> Liquisorb (High Fibre) Tube Feed and Drink
> Liquisorbon MCT
> Osmolite
> Paediasure
> Peptamen
> Pepti-2000 LF
> Peptisorb
> Peptisorbon
> Portagen
> Pregestimil
> Reabilan
> Triosorbon
> Wyeth Standard Enteral Feed

NUTRITIONAL SUPPORT FOR ADULTS (for precise conditions for which these products have been approved see the product listing in List A)

A. a. Nutritionally complete feeds (chemically defined diets whole protein based) - for oral, sip or tube feeding.

> i. Gluten Free
>
>> Clinifeed and Clinifeed Favour
>> Fortisip
>> Fortison Energy-Plus
>> Fortison Standard
>> Fresubin Liquid and Sip Feeds
>> Fresubin Plus F (Vegetable Soup Flavour only)
>> Liquisorb
>> Liquisorb (High Fibre) Tube and Feed Drink
>> Liquisorbon MCT
>> Peptamen
>> Peptisorb
>> Peptisorbon
>> Triosorbon
>
> ii. Lactose and Gluten Free
>
>> Enrich
>> Ensure
>> Ensure Plus
>> Ensure Powder

This is a cross index listing clinical conditions and the products which the ACBS has approved for the management of those conditions. It is essential to consult LIST A for more precise guidance.

LIST B — Cont

Formula MCT (i) Powder (with appropriate vitamin and mineral supplements)
Isocal
Osmolite
Portagen
Reabilan
Wyeth Standard Enteral Feed

b.   Elemental and Low Lactose

Flexical
Peptison powder

B.   Nutritional Source Supplements

See: Synthetic Diets
Malabsorption States.

a.   Carbohydrates — lactose free and gluten free

Calonutrin
Caloreen*
Fortical*
Hycal*
Liquid Duocal, Super Soluble Duocal*
Liquid Maxijul
Liquid Maxijul (Orange)
Maxijul LE*
Polycal
Polycose Liquid and Powder
Super Soluble Maxijul
* Have low electrolyte content

b.   Fat

Alembicol D
Calogen
Liquigen
MCT Oil

This is a cross index listing clinical conditions and the products which the ACBS has approved for the management of those conditions. It is essential to consult LIST A for more precise guidance.

LIST B - Cont

   c.   Nitrogen Sources

          Albumaid complete   (hydrolysed protein based)
          Casilan   (whole protein based, low sodium)
          Forceval protein (whole protein based, low sodium)
          Maxipro Instant
          Pro-Mod   (whey protein based, low sodium)

   d.   Minerals

          Aminogran mineral mixture
          Metabolic mineral mixture

PHENYLKETONURIA

     Aglutella Azeta cream filled wafers
     Aglutella gluten-free low-protein spaghetti, spaghetti rings, macaroni,
         pasta spirals, tagliatelle and semolina
     Albumaid XP
     Albumaid XP Concentrate
     Aminex
     Aminogran food supplement
     Aminogran mineral mixture
     Analog XP
     Aproten Products - anellini, biscuits, crispbread, ditalini, flour,
         low-protein and gluten-free bread and cake mixes, rigatini,tagliatelle
     Calonutrin
     Calogen
     Caloreen
     dp low protein butterscotch flavoured chip cookies
     dp low protein chocolate flavoured chip cookies
     Juvela gluten-free low protein chocolate chip; orange and cinnamon flavour cookies
     Juvela low-protein loaf (sliced and unsliced)
     Juvela low-protein flour mix
     Lofenalac
     Maxamaid XP
     Maximaid XP Orange
     Metabolic Mineral Mixture
     Minafen
     PK Aid 1
     PKU Drink (GF Dietary)
     PKU 2 (Milupa)
     PKU 3 (Milupa)
     Polycal
     Polycose Liquid and Powder
     Rite-Diet gluten-free low-protein bread (dispensed in tin) with and without salt
     Rite-Diet baking mix
     Rite-Diet low-protein cream filled biscuits-chocolate flavour
     Rite-Diet low-protein flour mix 400g
     Rite-Diet low-protein gluten free biscuits
     Rite-Diet low-protein gluten free crackers
     Rite-Diet low-protein macaroni
     Rite-Diet low-protein spaghetti (short cut)

This is a cross index listing clinical conditions and the products which the ACBS has approved for the management of those conditions. It is essential to consult LIST A for more precise guidance.

PART XV - BORDERLINE SUBSTANCES

LIST B - Cont

    Rite-Diet low-protein spaghetti rings
    Rite-Diet low-protein sweet biscuits
    Rite-Diet low-protein cream filled wafers-vanilla, orange and chocolate flavour
    Rite-Diet low-protein white bread (with added fibre)
    Tritamyl PK Flour
    and see: Low Protein Products and Synthetic Diets

PHOTODERMATOSES (SKIN PROTECTION)

    Almay Total Sun Block Cream
    Almay Total Block Lip Protector
    Coppertone Sunstick 15
    Coppertone Supershade 15
    Coppertone Supershade 23
    Delial 10
    Piz Buin Creme SPF No.12
    RoC Opaque Total Sunblock Cream SPF 15 A&B (Colourless and Tinted)
    RoC Total Sunblock Cream 10 (Colourless)
    Spectraban 15
    Uvistat Sun Cream (Factor 10)
    Uvistat Water Resistant Sun Cream (Factor 8)

PROTEIN INTOLERANCE

    See: Amino acid metabolic disorders
           Low protein products
           Milk protein sensitivity
           Synthetic diets
           Whole protein sensitivity

PRURITUS (See: Dermatitis)
PSORIASIS (See: Scaling of the Scalp)

RENAL FAILURE

    Aglutella Azeta cream filled wafers
    Aglutella gluten-free low-protein spaghetti, spaghetti rings, macaroni, pasta spirals,
        tagliatelle and semolina
    Aminex
    Aproten Products - anellini, biscuits, crispbread, ditalini, flour, low-protein
        and gluten-free bread and cake mixes, rigatini, tagliatelle
    Calogen
    Calonutrin
    Caloreen
    Dialamine
    dp low-protein butterscotch flavoured chip cookies
    dp low-protein chocolate flavoured chip cookies
    Fortical
    Hycal
    Juvela, gluten-free low protein chocolate chip, orange and cinnamon flavour cookies
    Juvela low-protein loaf (sliced and unsliced)
    Juvela low-protein flour mix
    Liquid Duocal and Super Soluble Duocal

This is a cross index listing clinical conditions and the products which the ACBS has approved for the management of those conditions. It is essential to consult LIST A for more precise guidance.

LIST B - Cont

Liquid Maxijul
Liquid Maxijul (orange)
Maxijul LE
Polycal
Polycose Liquid and Powder
Rite-Diet baking mix
Rite-Diet gluten-free low-protein bread (dispensed in tin) with or without salt
Rite-Diet low-protein cream filled biscuits-chocolate flavour
Rite-Diet low-protein flour mix
Rite-Diet low-protein gluten-free biscuits
Rite-Diet low-protein gluten-free crackers
Rite-Diet low-protein pasta macaroni
Rite-Diet low-protein spaghetti (short cut)
Rite-Diet low-protein spaghetti rings
Rite-Diet low-protein sweet biscuits
Rite-Diet low-protein cream filled wafers-vanilla, orange and chocolate flavour
Rite-Diet low sodium bread
Rite-Diet low-protein white bread (with added fibre)
Super Soluble Maxijul
Tritamyl PK flour

SCABIES

Tetmosol

SCALING OF THE SCALP (PSORIASIS, DANDRUFF, ECZEMA)

Alphosyl
Betadine
Capitol
Ceanal concentrate
Cetavlon PC
Gelcotar
Genisol
Ionil T
Polytar emollient
Polytar liquid
Polytar plus
T Gel Shampoo

SHORT BOWEL SYNDROME (See: Malabsorption)

SODIUM DIETARY REDUCTION

Rite-Diet low sodium bread

SODIUM INTOLERANCE (See: Carbohydrate Malabsorption)

This is a cross index listing clinical conditions and the products which the ACBS has approved for
the management of those conditions. It is essential to consult LIST A for more precise guidance.

LIST B — Cont

SYNTHETIC DIETS (for precise conditions for which these products have been approved see the product listing in List A)

a.   Fat

> Alembicol D
> Calogen
> Liquigen
> Medium Chain Triglyceride oil

b.   Carbohydrate

> Calonutrin
> Caloreen
> Fortical
> Hycal
> Liquid Maxijul
> Liquid Maxijul (Orange)
> Maxijul LE
> Polycal
> Polycose Liquid and Powder
> Super Soluble Maxijul

c.   Minerals

> Aminogran Mineral Mixture
> Metabolic Mineral Mixture

d.   Protein Sources

> See: Malabsorption states
>   Complete feeds

e.   Vitamins — as appropriate

> see: Malabsorption States
>   Nutritional Support for Adults

TYROSINAEMIA

> Analog XPHEN, TYR

VOMITING IN INFANCY

> Instant Carobel
> Nestargel

WHOLE PROTEIN SENSITIVITY

> Defined as "Intolerance to whole protein, proven by at least two withdrawal and challenge tests, as suggested by an accurate dietary history"
>
> Alfare
> Nutramigen
> Pepti — Junior
> Prejomin

This is a cross index listing clinical conditions and the products which the ACBS has approved for the management of those conditions. It is essential to consult LIST A for more precise guidance.

LIST C

The products which have been considered by the ACBS and may not be prescribed on Form FP10, are now included in Part XVIIIA (page 353 to 371).

PART XVI – NOTES ON CHARGES

PART XVI

NOTES ON CHARGES FOR DRUGS AND APPLIANCES PAYABLE UNDER
REGULATIONS MADE UNDER SECTION 77(1) OF THE NATIONAL HEALTH
SERVICE ACT 1977

(N.B: Information is also given on the counting of prescriptions for pricing purposes in para H
(page 333) with examples of the application of the prescription charge arrangements in para 1
(page 334).)

A. CHARGES PAYABLE

£3.05 for each prescription item, preparation or type of appliance including each anklet, legging,
knee–cap, below–knee, above–knee or thigh stocking. £3.05 for each month (or part thereof) during
which a patient is provided with oxygen concentrator services under the FPS.

B. PHARMACY, APPLIANCE AND DRUG STORE CONTRACTORS

Unless a completed declaration of entitlement to exemption is received (see "Exemptions" page 331)
a charge is payable for each drug or appliance supplied, including each piece of elastic hosiery.
The charges are collected and retained by the pharmacy, appliance and drug store contractor, whose
remuneration is adjusted accordingly. In order to secure exemption from prescription charges when
presenting a prescription form to a pharmacy, appliance and drug store contractor, the patient, or
a person on his behalf, must complete the declaration on the back of the prescription form.

C. DISPENSING DOCTORS

Unless the patient declares that he is entitled to exemption (see "Exemptions" page 331), the
charges set out at (A) above are payable in respect of each item supplied by a dispensing doctor.
The charges are collected and paid over by the doctor to the Family Practitioner Committee. Where
the drug or appliance is being supplied by a dispensing doctor, the patient, or person on his
behalf, should make an oral or written declaration to the doctor that he is in one of the
categories listed.

PART XVI - NOTES ON CHARGES

D.   EXEMPTIONS

Provided that the appropriate declaration is received, a charge is not payable to the contractor
or dispensing doctor for drugs or appliances, including elastic hosiery, supplied for:

    Children under 16
    Students under 19 in full-time education
    Men aged 65 and over
    Women aged 60 and over

People holding Family Practitioner Committee exemption certificates, which are issued to:

    Expectant mothers;
    Women who have borne a child in the last 12 months;
    People suffering from the following specified medical conditions -

    (i)   Permanent fistula (including Caecostomy, Colostomy, Ileostomy or Laryngostomy)
    requiring continuous surgical dressing or an appliance.

    (ii)   Forms of hypoadrenalism (including Addison's disease) for which specific substitution
            therapy is essential.
            Diabetes insipidus and other forms of hypopituitarism
            Diabetes mellitus except where treatment is by diet alone
            Hypoparathyroidism
            Myasthenia gravis
            Myxoedema (Hypothyroidism)

    (iii)   Epilepsy requiring continuous anti-convulsive therapy.

    (iv)   A continuing physical disability which prevents the patient leaving his residence
    except with the help of another person (this does not mean a temporary disability even if it
    is likely to last a few months).

People holding DHSS exemption certificates, which are issued to:

    War and service pensioners (for prescriptions needed for treating their accepted
    disablement);

    People receiving income support or family credit;*

    Anyone aged 16 or over (exept students under 19 in full-time education) whose income is not
    much above income support level.

    (Young people can apply for an exemption certificate on their own income, whether or not
    they are in work and irrespective of their parent's circumstances).

People who have purchased a prepayment certificate (FP96) from the Family Practitioner Committee.

(*these certificates also cover dependants)

Full details of the exemption arrangements are contained in Leaflet P11, stocks of which are
obtainable from the Family Practitioner Committee. The Leaflet includes claim forms and guidance
for patients to apply for exemption certificates.

PART XVI - NOTES ON CHARGES

E.   PREPAYMENT CERTIFICATES (Season Tickets)

Doctors and contractors could greatly assist any patient who makes frequent payments for prescriptions by drawing attention to the availability of prepayment certificates, ("Season tickets"). These Certificates cost £43.50 for one year or £15.80 for four months.

They are worthwhile for anyone requiring more than 14 items on prescription in a year or 5 items in four months. An application form FP95 can be obtained from the Post Office, NHS Family Practitioner Committee, local Social Security Office, or Pharmacies.

F.   BULK PRESCRIPTIONS

Charges are not payable in respect of "bulk" prescriptions for schools or institutions supplied in accordance with the Regulations (See Note 6, Part VIII, page 33).

G.   CONTRACEPTIVE SERVICES

No charge is payable for contraceptive substances and listed contraceptive appliances for women prescribed on FP10 or any of its variants.

The great majority of family planning prescriptions will be for contraceptive devices (See Part IXA page 70) spermicidal gels, creams, films, pessaries and aerosols; or those systemic drugs promoted as contraceptives which are listed below: prescriptions for those products will not be specially marked and a prescription charge should not be levied.

Prescriptions for other drugs - If the prescription is for contraceptive purposes the prescriber may mark the item with the symbol ♀ and a prescription charge should not be levied for any items so marked. In the absence of the symbol ♀ the normal prescription charge arrangements will apply to that item.

Where a dispensing doctor paid on the Drug Tariff basis supplies for contraceptive purposes a drug which is not on the list he should mark the item with the symbol ♀ on the prescription form before it is submitted for pricing.

List of Contraceptive Drugs to be Dispensed Free of Charge

Progestogen only	50 Micrograms of Oestrogen		Under 50 micrograms of Oestrogen	
Femulen	Eugynon 50		Bi Novum	Microgynon 30
Micronor	Minilyn	†	Brevinor	Minulet
Microval	Norinyl-1		Conova 30	Neocon 1/35
Neogest	Ortho-Novin 1/50		Eugynon 30	Norimin
Norgeston	Ovran		Femodene	Ovran 30
Noriday	PC4		Femodene ED	Ovranette
			Loestrin 20	Ovysmen
			Loestrin 30	Synphase
			Logynon	Trinordiol
			Logynon ED	Trinovum
			Marvelon	Trinovum ED
			Mercilon	

† to be deleted 1 October 1990

H.   NOTES ON CHARGES PAYABLE

(i)   SINGLE PRESCRIPTION CHARGE PAYABLE
Unless the patient claims exemption or the prescription is covered by the provisions at (E) and
(F) a single prescription charge is payable where:

- (a)   The same drug or preparation is supplied in more than one container.
- (b)   Different strengths of the same drug are ordered as separate prescriptions at the
         same time.
- (c)   More than one appliance of the same type (other than elastic hosiery*) is supplied.
- (d)   A set of parts making up a complete appliance is supplied.
- (e)   Drugs are supplied in powder form with the solvent separate for subsequent admixing.
- (f)   A drug is supplied with a dropper, throat brush, or vaginal applicator.
- (g)   Several flavours of the same preparation are supplied.

(ii)   MULTIPLE PRESCRIPTION CHARGES PAYABLE
More than one prescription charge is payable where:

- (a)   Different drugs, types of dressings or appliances are supplied.
- (b)   Different formulations or presentations of the same drug or preparation are supplied.
- (c)   Additional parts are supplied together with a complete set of apparatus or additional
         dressing(s) together with a dressing pack.
- (d)   More than one piece of elastic hosiery* is supplied.

(iii) "NO CHARGE" ITEMS
The number of "no charge" items (ie items which are counted as prescriptions for pricing purposes
but which do not carry a prescription charge) should be included on the invoice submitted with the
prescription forms to the Pricing Authority.

*(Anklet, legging, knee-cap; below-knee, above-knee or thigh stocking)

PART XVI — NOTES ON CHARGES

I.   EXAMPLES OF APPLICATION OF PRESCRIPTION CHARGE ARRANGEMENTS

	Professional Fees	Number of Prescription Charges	No Charge Prescriptions
(i) LIQUIDS — Required by the prescriber to be supplied in more than one container. Certain preparations, if extemporaneously dispensed, may be subject to additional fees, (see part IIIA page 11).			
Ammonium Chloride Mixture 300ml x 3	1	1	—
Boric Acid Eye Lotion 100ml x 2	1	1	—
Chloramphenicol Ear Drops 10ml x 2	1	1	—
Ferric Chloride Gargle 200ml x 2	1	1	—
Hydrogen Peroxide Ear Drops 10ml x 3	1	1	—
Lead Lotion 200ml x 2	1	1	—
Sulphacetamide Sodium Eye Drops 10ml x 2	1	1	—
(ii) INJECTIONS			
(a) Sets containing graded strength of the same drug			
Allpyral G — sets of 3 graduated strength vials	1	1	—
Migen — set of 6 graded strength unit-dose syringes	1	1	—
(b) Same injection, different strength			
Deca–Durabolin 25mg x 3) Deca–Duralolin 100mg x 3)	1	1	—
(c) Dispensed in powder form with solvent			
Streptomycin Sulphate 1g x 10) Water for Injection 2ml x 10)	2	1	1
Digoxin Amps 0.5mg x 10) Normal Saline Amps 5ml x 10)	2	1	1
(d) Influenza Vaccine (2 different strains in separate ampoules)	2	1	1
(iii) TABLETS, CAPSULES, etc. — Different strengths of the same drug ordered as separate prescriptions at the same time			
Phenindione Tabs 50mg one three times daily, 90 Phenindione Tabs 10mg, one three times daily, 90	2	1	1
Phenindione Tabs 50mg, one in the morning, 30 Phenindione Tabs 10mg, three at night, 90	2	1	1
Prednisolone Tabs 5mg, one in the morning, 28 Prednisolone Tabs 1mg, one in the morning, 28	2	1	1
Sulphacetamide Eye Drops 10% Sulphacetamide Eye Drops 30%	2	1	1

0318M/5

PART XVI – NOTES ON CHARGES

I.   EXAMPLES OF APPLICATION OF PRESCRIPTION CHARGE ARRANGEMENTS – cont.

	Professional Fees	Number of Prescription Charges	No Charge Prescriptions
(iv) TABLETS, CAPSULES, etc.			
(a) Different formulations or presentation of the same drug ordered as separate prescriptions			
Dioralyte Plain ⎫ Dioralyte Cherry ⎭	2	1	1
Indocid Caps ⎫ Indocid R Caps ⎭	2	2	–
Isordil Tabs ⎫ Isordil Sublingual Tabs ⎭	2	2	–
Achromycin Caps 250mg ⎫ Achromycin Tabs 250mg ⎭	2	2	–
Camcolit 250 Tabs ⎫ Camcolit 400 Tabs sustained release ⎭	2	2	–
Bezalip Tabs 200mg ⎫ Bezalip Mono Tabs ⎭	2	2	–
Prednisolone Tabs 1mg ⎫ Prednesol Tabs 5mg (ie Prednisolone Sodium Phosphate) ⎭	2	2	–
Prednisolone Tabs 1mg ⎫ Prednisolone Tabs 2.5mg enteric coated ⎭	2	2	–
Ronicol Tabs ⎫ Ronicol Timespan Tabs ⎭	2	2	–
Trasicor Tabs ⎫ Slow Trasicor Tabs ⎭	2	2	–
(b) Strength ordered not listed – must be dispensed and priced by a combination of two different strengths and/or presentations.			
Diabinese Tabs – 350mg x 60 Contractor endorses – 100mg x 60 ⎫ 250mg x 60 ⎭	2	1	1
Prothiaden – 100mg x 100 Contractor endorses – Caps 25mg x 100 ⎫ Tabs 75mg x 100 ⎭	2	1	1

0318M/6

PART XVI - NOTES ON CHARGES

I.   EXAMPLES OF APPLICATION OF PRESCRIPTION CHARGE ARRANGEMENTS - cont.

	Professional Fees	Number of Prescription Charges	No Charge Prescriptions
(v) COMBINATION PACKS			
Becloforte-VM	2	2	-
Canestan Duo Pack	2	2	-
Cyclo-Progynova Tabs 1 mg or 2 mg	2	2	-
Cyclo-Progynova Tabs 1mg } Cyclo-Progynova Tabs 2mg } prescribed together	4	3	1
Daktarin Twin Pack	2	2	-
Ecostatin Twin Pack	2	2	-
Estrapak 50 } Estraderm 100 mg } prescribed together	3	2	1
Flagyl Compak	2	2	-
Frusemide/Kloref Treatment Pack	2	2	-
Gyno-Daktarin Combipack	2	2	-
Gyno-Pevaryl 150 Combipack	2	2	-
Hypovase BD Starter Pack	2	1	-
Ismo Starter Pack	2	1	-
Lasix + K	2	2	-
Migraleve Duo Pack	2	2	-
Nystan Triple Pack	3	3	-
Prempak - C 0.625	2	2	-
Prempak - C 1.25	2	2	-
Synphase	2	-	2
Syntex Menophase	6	2	4
Trisequens	3	2	1
Ultraproct Combipack	2	2	-
(vi) MULTIPLES OF SAME APPLIANCES OF SAME OR DIFFERING SIZE			
Becotide Rotahaler } prescribed together Ventolin Rotahaler }	2	2	-
Crepe Bandages 2 x 5 cm	1	1	-
Open-Wove Bandages 1 x 2.5 cm } 1 x 5 cm } 1 x 7.5 cm }	1	1	-
Polythene Occulusive Dressings } Gloves - Polythene 100 gauge }	1	1	-
Arm Sleeve - Polythene 150 gauge } Leg Sleeve - Polythene 150 gauge } Foot Bag - Polythene 150 gauge }* Torso Vest - Polythene 150 gauge }	4	1	3
Shorts - Polythene 150 gauge	1	1	-
Trousers - Polythene 150 gauge	1	1	-

(*Arm Sleeves, leg sleeves, foot bags and
torso vest are all regarded as plastics sleeves).

0318M/7

PART XVI – NOTES ON CHARGES

I. EXAMPLES OF APPLICATION OF PRESCRIPTION CHARGE ARRANGEMENTS – cont.

	Professional Fees	Number of Prescription Charges	No Charge Prescriptions
(vii) SET OF APPLIANCES OR DRESSINGS			
Atomizer	1	1	–
Douche	1	1	–
Hypodermic Syringe	1	1	–
Multiple Pack Dressing No.1	1	1	–
Multiple Pack Dressing No.2	1	1	–
Portable Urinal	1	1	–
Suprapubic Belt	1	1	–
Higginson's Enema Syringe	1	1	–
(viii) SETS OF APPLIANCES ORDERED WITH EXTRA PARTS			
Hypodermic Syringe } Hypodermic Needles }	2	2	–
Multiple Pack Dressing No.2 } Absorbent Cotton 25g }	2	2	–
Portable Urinal } Spare Sheaths 2 }	1	1	–
(ix) DIFFERENT APPLIANCES			
Lint 25g } Absorbent Cotton 25g } Gauze 90cm x 1m }	3	3	–
(x) DRUGS ORDERED WITH DRUG TARIFF APPLIANCES			
Brovon Inhalant } Brovon Inhaler }	2	2	–
Clinitest Set and extra } Clinitest Tablets }	2	1	1
Intal Spincaps } Spinhaler }	2	2	–
Rynacrom Capsules } Rynacrom Insufflator }	2	2	–
Pig Iod Co 25ml } Iodine Brush }	2	1	1
Ventolin Tablets } Ventolin Inhaler }	2	2	–

I.   EXAMPLES OF APPLICATION OF PRESCRIPTION CHARGE ARRANGEMENTS - cont.

	Professional Fees	Number of Prescription Charges	No Charge Prescriptions
(xi) DRUGS PACKED WITH NON DRUG TARIFF APPLIANCES*			
(including metered aerosols with refills)			
Alupent Inhaler }	1	1	-
Alupent Refill(s) }			
Betadine Vaginal Preparations:-			
Gel (with applicator)	1	1	-
Pessaries (with applicator)	1	1	-
V.C. Kit	1	1	-
Syntaris Nasal Spray	1	1	-
Verrugon Ointment (Composite Pack)	1	1	-
* (These appliances are being allowed because			
they are packed with drug/preparation).			
(xii) ELASTIC HOSIERY			
1 pr Knee-caps - One Way Stretch	1	2	-
1 pr Thigh Stockings - Class II	1	2	-
1 pr spare Suspenders	1	1	-
1 Suspender Belt	1	1	-
(xiii) MISCELLANEOUS			
(a) Preparations supplied as separate parts			
for admixing as required for use			
Chlorhexidine 0.2% Aqueous Solution 400ml }	2	1	1
Sodium Fluoride 2% Aqueous Solution 400ml }			
(b) Preparations having various flavours			
Hycal assorted flavours. Mitte 3	3	1	2
Hycal assorted flavours. Mitte 8	4	1	3
(At present 4 flavours available)			
Rite-Diet Gluten Free Biscuits Sweet }	2	1	1
Rite-Diet Gluten Free Biscuits Savoury)			
(c) Different but related preparations			
Aminogran Food Supplement	1	1	-
Aminogran Mineral Mixture	1	1	-
Brasivol-fine, medium and coarse	3	1	2
Parentrovite IM Maintenance	2	2	-
Parentrovite IV High Potency	2	2	-
Parentrovite IM High Potency	2	2	-

PART XVI - NOTES ON CHARGES

I.   EXAMPLES OF APPLICATION OF PRESCRIPTION CHARGE ARRANGEMENTS - cont.

	Professional Fees	Number of Prescription Charges	No Charge Prescriptions
Rite-Diet Gluten Free Flour Rite-Diet Gluten Free Bread Mix }	2	2	-
Migraleve Tabs, yellow	1	1	-
Migraleve Tabs, pink	1	1	-
Migraleve Tabs, yellow and pink	2	2	-
Migraleve Duo Pack with additional tablets (yellow and/or pink)	2	2	-
Triptafen-M Triptafen }	2	2	-

I.   EXAMPLES OF APPLICATION OF PRESCRIPTION CHARGE ARRANGEMENTS – cont.

	Professional Fees	Number of Prescription Charges	No Charge Prescriptions
(xiii) MISCELLANEOUS – cont.			
(d) Eye, Ear and Nasal Drops (Supplied in dropper bottles, or with a separate dropper where appropriate. See Part IV.Containers – page 24).	1	1	–
(e) A drug in powder form together with a solvent in the same packs (Treatment Pack) (2 vials of powder and 2 vials of solvent) Actinac	2	1	1
(f) Oxygen Oxygen Therapy Set with cylinder(s)	1	1	–
Oxygen Cylinders (See Part X, Domiciliary Oxygen Therapy Service, page 282).	1	1	–
(g) Trusses Spring Truss } Inguinal – Single }	1	1	–
Elastic Band Truss } Scrotal–Double }	1	1	–
(h) Vaginal Creams and Applicators* Duracreme } Vaginal Applicator – Type 2 }	2	–	2
Ortho Creme } Vaginal Applicator – Type 1 }	2	–	2
Sultrin (Triple Sulfa) Cream } Vaginal Applicator – Type 1 }	2	1	1
Vaginal Applicator (See page 58) Type 1 (Ortho)	1	–	1
type 2 (Durex)	1	–	1

* (No attempt should be made to determine whether or not the applicator is required for use with a contraceptive)

List of Preparations approved by the Secretary of State which may be prescribed on form FP14 by Dentists for National Health Service patients

Acyclovir Cream, DPF
Acyclovir Suspension, DPF
Acyclovir Tablets, DPF
Amoxycillin Capsules, BP
Amoxycillin Injection, DPF
Amoxycillin Mixture, BP
    (Syn: Amoxycillin Oral Suspension;
      Amoxycillin Syrup)
    (includes sugar-free formulation)
Amoxycillin Oral Powder, DPF
Amoxycillin Tablets, Dispersible, DPF
Amphotericin Lozenges, BP
Amphotericin Mixture, DPF
Amphotericin Ointment, DPF
Amphotericin Tablets, DPF
Ampicillin Capsules, BP
Ampicillin Mixture, BP
    (Syn: Ampicillin Oral Suspension;
      Ampicillin Syrup)
Ampicillin Tablets, Paediatric, BP
Artificial Saliva, DPF
Ascorbic Acid Tablets, BP
Aspirin, Paracetamol Codeine Tablets, DPF
Aspirin Tablets, BP
*Aspirin Tablets, Dispersible, BP
(Aspirin Tablets, Soluble)

Benzocaine Lozenges, DPF
Benzydamine Mouth-wash, DPF
Benzydamine Oral Spray, DPF
Benzylpenicillin Injection, BP

Carbamazepine Tablets, BP
Carmellose Gelatin Paste, DPF
Cephalexin Capsules, BP
Cephalexin Mixture, DPF
Cephalexin Tablets, BP
Cephradine Capsules, BP
Cephradine Elixir, DPF
Cephradine Injection, DPF
Chlorhexidine Gluconate Gels
    containing at least 1 per cent
Chlorhexidine Mouth-wash, DPF
Chlorpheniramine Tablets, BP
Choline Salicylate Dental Gel, BP
    (formerly: Choline Salicylate
    Dental Paste, DPF)

Clindamycin Capsules, BP
Clindamycin Injection, DPF
Clindamycin Mixture, Paediatric, DPF
Co-codamol Tablets, DPF
    (formerly: Codeine and
    Paracetamol Tablets)
Co-codamol Tablets Dispersible, DPF
    (formerly: Codeine and
    Paracetamol Dispersible Tablets)
Co-codaprin Tablets Dispersible, BP
    (Syn: Aspirin and Codeine Tablets
    Dispersible)
Co-dydramol Tablets, DPF
    (formerly: Dihydrocodeine and
    Paracetamol Tablets)
Co-trimoxazole Mixture, BP
    (Syn: Co-trimoxazole Oral Suspension)
Co-trimoxazole Mixture, Paediatric, BP
    (Syn: Co-trimoxazole Oral Suspension
    Paediatric)
Co-trimoxazole Tablets, BP, 80/400
Co-trimoxazole Tablets, Dispersible, BP, 80/400
Co-trimoxazole Tablets BP,
    Double Strength, 160/800
Co-trimoxazole Tablets Dispersible BP,
    Double Strength, 160/800
Co-trimoxazole Tablets, Paediatric, BP, 20/100

Diazepam Capsules, BP
Diazepam Elixir, BP 2 mg/5ml
    (Syn: Diazepam Oral Solution)
Diazepam Tablets, BP
Diflunisal Tablets, BP
Dihydrocodeine Tablets, BP

Ephedrine Nasal Drops, BPC
Erythromycin Ethylsuccinate Mixture, DPF
Erythromycin Ethylsuccinate Mixture,
    Paediatric, DPF
Erythromycin Ethylsuccinate Oral Powder,
    DPF
Erythromycin Ethylsuccinate Tablets, DPF
Erythromycin Lactobionate Injection, DPF
Erythromycin Stearate Tablets, BP
Erythromycin Tablets, BP

*This entry differs from that given in the DPF 1988/90.

Hydrocortisone Cream, BP
Hydrocortisone Lozenges, BPC
Hydrocortisone and Miconazole Cream DPF
Hydrocortisone and Miconazole Ointment DPF
Hydrogen Peroxide Mouth-wash, DPF

Ibuprofen Tablets, BP
Idoxuridine 5% in Dimethyl Sulphoxide,
    DPF

Lignocaine 5% Ointment, DPF

Mefenamic Acid Capsules, BP
Menthol and Eucalyptus Inhalation, BP 1980
Metronidazole Mixture, DPF
Metronidazole Tablets, BP
Miconazole Oral Gel, DPF
Mouth-wash Solution Tablets, DPF

Nitrazepam Tablets, BP
Nystatin Mixture, BP
    (Syn: Nystatin Oral Suspension)
    (includes sugar-free formulation)
Nystatin Ointment, BP
Nystatin Pastilles, DPF
Nystatin Tablets, BP

Oxytetracycline Capsules, BP
Oxytetracycline Tablets, BP

Paracetamol Oral Suspension, BP,
    Paediatric, (120mg/5ml)
Paracetamol Tablets, BP
Penicillin Triple Injection, BPC
Pentazocine Tablets, BP
Pethidine Tablets, BP
Phenoxymethylpenicillin Capsules BP
    (Syn: Penicillin VK Capsules)
Phenoxymethylpenicillin Elixir, BP
    (Syn: Phenoxymethylpenicillin
    Oral Solution)
    (Formerly: Pencillin V Elixir)
Phenoxymethylpenicillin Tablets BP
    (Syn: Penicillin VK Tablets)
Povidone-iodine Mouth-wash, DPF
Procaine Penicillin Injection, BP
Promethazine Hydrochloride Elixir, BP
    (Syn: Promethazine Oral Solution)
Promethazine Hydrochloride Tablets, BP

Sodium Chloride Mouth-wash, Compound, BP
Sodium Fusidate Ointment, BP
    (formerly: Fusidic Acid Ointment, DPF)
Sodium Perborate Mouth-wash, Buffered, DPF

Temazepam Capsules, DPF
Temazepam Elixir, DPF
Temazepam Tablets, DPF
Tetracycline Capsules, BP
Tetracycline Mixture, BP
    (Syn: Tetracycline Oral Suspension)
Tetracycline Tablets, BP
Thymol Glycerin, Compound, BP
Triamcinolone Dental Paste, BP

Vitamin B Tablets, Compound, Strong, BPC

Zinc Sulphate Mouth-wash, DPF

PART XVIIIA

DRUGS AND OTHER SUBSTANCES NOT TO BE PRESCRIBED UNDER
THE NATIONAL HEALTH SERVICE PHARMACEUTICAL SERVICES

10 Day Slimmer Tablets
10 Hour Capsules
10.10 Cleaning and Disinfecting Solution
10.10 Rinsing and Neutralising Solution
Abidec Capsules
Acne Aid Bar
Actal Suspension
Actal Tablets
Actifed Compound Linctus
Actifed Expectorant
Actifed Linctus with Codeine
Actified Syrup
Actifed Tablets
Actonorm Gel
Actonorm Powder
Actonorm Tablets
Actron Tablets
Adexolin Vitamin Drops
Adult Cough Balsam (Cupal)
Adult Meltus Cough & Catarrh Linctus
Adult Tonic Mixture (Thornton & Ross)
Afrazine Nasal Drops
Afrazine Nasal Spray
Afrazine Paediatric Nasal Drops
Agarol Emulsion
Agiolax Granules
Airbal Breathe Easy Vapour Inhaler
AL Tablets
Alagbin Tablets
Alcin Tablets
Aletres Cordial (Potters)
Alexitol Sodium Suspension 360 mg/5 ml
Alexitol Sodium Tablets
Algipan Tablets
Alka-Donna Suspension
Alka-Donna Tablets
Alka-Donna P Mixture
Alka-Donna P Tablets
Alka Mints
Alka-Seltzer Tablets
Alket Powders
All Fours Cough Mixture (Harwood)
All Fours Mixture (Glynwed
    Wholesale Chemists)
All Fours Mixture (Roberts Laboratories)
Allbee with C Capsules
Allbee with C Elixir
Almasilate Tablets 500 mg
Almazine Tablets 1 mg
Almazine Tablets 2.5 mg
Aloin Tablets 40 mg
Alophen Pills

Alpine Tea
Alprazolam Tablets 0.25 mg
Alprazolam Tablets 0.5 mg
Alprazolam Tablets 1 mg
Altacaps
Altacite Suspension
Altacite Plus Tablets
Altacite Tablets
Aludrox Gel
Aludrox Suspension
Aludrox M H Suspension
Aludrox S A Suspension
Aludrox Tablets
Aluhyde Tablets
Aluminium Hydroxide & Silicone
    Suspension
Aluminium Phosphate Gel
Aluminium Phosphate Tablets 400 mg
Alupent Expectorant Mixture
Alupent Expectorant Tablets
Aluphos Gel
Aluphos Tablets
Alupram Tablets 2 mg
Alupram Tablets 5 mg
Alupram Tablets 10 mg
Aluzyme Tablet
Alzed Tablets
Amisyn Tablets
Ami – 10 Rinsing and Storage Solution
Amiclear Contact Lens Cleanser Tablets
Amidose Saline Solution 30 ml
Amin-Aid
Ammonia and Ipecacuanha Mixture BP
Ammonium Chloride and Morphine
    Mixture BP
Anadin Analgesic Capsules Maximum
    Strength
Anadin Analgesic Tablets
Anadin Extra Analgesic Tablets
Anadin Paracetamol Tablets
Anadin Tablets Soluble
Andrews Liver Salts Effervescent Powder
Andrews Liver Salts (Diabetic Formula)
    Effervescent Powder
Andursil Liquid
Andursil Tablets
Anestan Bronchial Tablets
Aneurone Mixture
Angiers Junior Aspirin Tablets
Angiers Junior Paracematol Tablets
Anorvit Tablets
Antasil Liquid

0319M/5

Antasil Tablets
Antistin-Privine Nasal Drops
Antistin-Privine Nasal Spray
Antitussive Linctus (Cox)
Antoin Tablets
Antussin Liquid (Sterling Winthrop)
Anxon Capsules 15 mg
Anxon Capsules 30 mg
Anxon Capsules 45 mg
Aperient Tablets (Brome & Schimmer)
Aperient Tablets (Kerbina)
Apodorm Tablets 2.5 mg
Apodorm Tablets 5 mg
APP Stomach Powder
APP Stomach Tablets
Arocin Capsules
Ascorbef Tablets
Ascorbic Acid & Hesperidin Capsules
    (Regent Laboratories)
Asilone Tablets 250 mg
Asilone Orange Tablets
Askit Powders
Askit Tablets
Aspergum Chewing Gum Tablets 227 mg
Aspirin Chewing-Gum Tablets 277mg
Aspirin Tablets, Effervescent, 300mg
Aspirin Tablets, Effervescent Soluble
Aspirin Tablets, Slow
    (Micro-Encapsulated) 648mg
Aspro Clear Tablets
Aspro Clear Extra Tablets
Aspro Extra Strength Tablets 500 mg
Aspro Junior Tablets
Aspro Microfined Tablets
Asthma Tablets (Cathay)
Astroplast Analgesic Capsules
Atensine Tablets 2 mg
Atensine Tablets 5 mg
Atensine Tablets 10 mg
Ativan Tablets 1 mg
Ativan Tablets 2.5 mg
Atrixo
Aveeno Bar
Aveeno Bar Oilated
Ayrtons Macleans Formula Tablets

B Complex Capsules (Rodale)
B Complex Super Capsules (Rodale)
B Extra Tablets (British
    Chemotherapeutic Products)
Babezone Syrup
Baby Chest Rub Ointment (Cupal)
Babylix Syrup
Babysafe Tablets
Badedas Bath Gelee
Balm of Gilead (Robinsons)

Balm of Gilead Cough Mixture (Wicker
    Herbal Stores)
Balm of Gilead Liquid (Culpeper)
Balm of Gilead Mixture (Potters)
Banfi Hungarian Hair Tonic
Banimax Tablets
Barker's Liquid of Life Solution
Barker's Liquid of Life Tablets
Barkoff Cough Syrup
Barnes - Hind Cleaning and Soaking Solution
Barnes - Hind Intensive Cleaner
Barnes - Hind No 4 Cleaner
Barnes - Hind Wetting and Soaking Solution
Bausch and Lomb Cleaning Tablets
Bausch and Lomb Daily Lens Cleaner
Bausch and Lomb Saline Solution
Bayer Aspirin Tablets 300 mg
BC500 Tablets
BC500 with Iron Tablets
BC500 Vitamin Sachets effervescent
Becosym Forte Tablets
Becosym Syrup
Becosym Tablets
Becotab Tablets
Beechams Day Nurse Capsules
Beechams Day Nurse Syrup
Beechams Catarrh Capsules
Beechams Pills
Beechams Powders
Beechams Powders Tablet Form
Beechams Powders Mentholated
Beehive Balsam
Bekovit Tablets
Belladonna and Ephedrine Mixture,
    Paediatric, BPC
Bellocarb Tablets
Benadon Tablets 20 mg
Benadon Tablets 50 mg
Benafed Linctus
Benerva Compound Tablets
Benerva Injection 25 mg/ml
Benerva Injection 100 mg/ml
Benerva Tablets 3 mg
Benerva Tablets 10 mg
Benerva Tablets 25 mg
Benerva Tablets 50 mg
Benerva Tablets 100 mg
Benerva Tablets 300 mg
Bengers Food
Bengue's Balsam
Benylin Chesty Cough Linctus
Benylin Childrens Cough Linctus
Benylin Day & Night Cold Treatment
Benylin Decongestant Linctus
Benylin Dry Cough Linctus
Benylin Expectorant
Benylin Fortified Linctus

Benylin Mentholated Cough &
   Decongestant Linctus
Benylin Paediatric
Benylin with Codeine
Benzedrex Inhaler
Benzoin Inhalation BP
Bepro Cough Syrup
Bergasol Ultra Protection Tanning Lotion
Biactol Anti-Bacterial Face Wash
Bile Beans Formula 1 Pill
Bioflavonoid C Capsules
Bioscal Hair Formula
Bio-Strath Drops
Bio-Strath Elixir
Biovital Liquid
Biovital Tablets
Birley's Antacid Powder
Bis-Mag Lozenge
Bis-Peps Tablets
Bisma-Calna Cream
Bisma-Rex Powder
Bisma-Rex Tablets
Bismag Antacid Powder
Bismag Tablets
Bismuth Compound Lozenges BPC
Bismuth Dyspepsia Lozenges
Bismuth Pepsin and Pancreatin Tablets
Bismuth, Soda and Pepsin Mixture
Bisodol Antacid Powder
Bisodol Tablets
Bisolvomycin Capsules
Bisolvon Elixir
Bisolvon Tablets
Blackcurrant Cough Elixir
   (Thornton & Ross)
Blackcurrant Syrup Compound (Beben)
Blandax Suspension
Blavig Tablets
Blood Tonic Mixture (Thompsons)
Boldolaxine Tablets
Bonemeal Calfos, Vit A Ester, Vit D
   Tablets
Bonomint Chewing Gum
Bonomint Tablets
Booth's Cough & Catarrh Elixir
Boots Baby Oil
Boots Cold Relief Powder for Solution
Boots Compound Laxative Syrup of Figs
Boots Cough Relief for Adults
Boots Glycerin & Blackcurrant Soothing
   Cough Relief
Boots Hard Lens Wetting Solution
Boots Health Salts
Boots Indigestion Plus Mixture
Boots Indigestion Powder
Boots Orange Drink
Boots Soft Lens Comfort Solution

Boots Soft Lens Soaking Solution
Boots Soya Milk
Boots Vapour Rub Ointment
Boston Lens Cleaning Solution
Boston Lens Wetting and Soaking Solution
Box's Balm of Gilead Cough Mixture
Bravit Capsules
Bravit Tablets
Breoprin Tablets 648 mg
Brewers Yeast Tablets (3M Health Care)
Brewers Yeast-Super B Tablets (Rodale)
Brewers Yeast Tablets (Phillips Yeast
   Products)
Bricanyl Compound Tablets
Bricanyl Expectorant
Brogans Cough Mixture
Brogans Cough Syrup
Bromazepam Tablets 1.5 mg
Bromazepam Tablets 3 mg
Bromazepam Tablets 6 mg
Bromhexine Hydrochloride Elixir
   6 mg/5 ml
Bromhexine Hydrochloride Tablets 8 mg
Bronalin Expectorant
Bronalin Paediatric Cough Syrup
Bronchial & Cough Mixture
   (Worthington Walter)
Bronchial Balsam (Cox)
Bronchial Catarrh Syrup (Rusco)
Bronchial Cough Mixture (Evans Medical)
Bronchial Emulsion (Three Flasks)
   (Thornton & Ross)
Bronchial Emulsion AS Extra Strong
   (Ayrton Saunders)
Bronchial Mixture (Rusco)
Bronchial Mixture Extra Strong (Cox)
Bronchial Mixture Sure Shield Brand
Bronchial Tablets (Leoren)
Bronchialis Mist Liquid (Industrial
   Pharmaceutical Services)
Bronchialis Mist Nig Double Strength
   (Phillip Harris Medical)
Bronchisan Childrens Cough Syrup
Bronchisan Cough Syrup
Broncholia Mixture
Bronchotone Solution
Bronkure Cough & Bronchitis Mixture
   (Jacksons)
Brontus Syrup
Brontus Syrup for Children
Brontussin Cough Suppressant Mixture
Brooklax Tablets
Brotizolam Tablets 0.125 mg
Brotizolam Tablets 0.25 mg
Bufferin Tablets
Buttercup Baby Cough Linctus
Buttercup Syrup

Cabdrivers Adult Linctus
Cabdrivers Diabetic Linctus
Cabdrivers Nasal Decongestant Tablets
Cadbury's Coffee Compliment
Cafadol Tablets
Caffeine & Dextrose Tablets
Calamage
Calcimax Syrup
Calcinate Tablets
Calcium Syrup (Berk Pharmaceuticals)
California Syrup of Figs
Calpol Six Plus Suspension
Calpol Tablets
Calsalettes Sugar Coated Tablets
Calsalettes Uncoated Tablets
Camfortix Linctus Pl
Cantaflour
Capramin Tablets
Carbellon Tablets
Carisoma Compound Tablets
Carnation Coffeemate
Carnation Instant Build-Up
Carnation Slender Meal Replacement (All Flavours)
Carrzone Powder
Carters Little Pills
Cascara Evacuant Liquid Mixture
Cascara Tablets BP
Castellan No 10 Cough Mixture
Catarrh & Bronchial Syrup (Thornton & Ross)
Catarrh Cough Syrup (Boots)
Catarrh-Ex Tablets
Catarrh Mixture (Herbal Laboratories)
Catarrh Syrup for Children (Boots)
Catarrh Tablets (Cathay)
Ce-Cobalin Syrup
Ceeyees Tablets
Celaton Rejuvenation Tablets
Celaton CH3 Strong & Calm Tablets
Celaton CH3 Triplus Tablets
Celaton CH3 + Ease & Vitality Tablets
Celaton Whole Wheat Germ Capsules
Celavit 1 Powder
Celavit 2 Powder
Celavit 3 Powder
Celevac Granules
Centrax Tablets 10 mg
Cephos Powders
Cephos Tablets
Charabs Tablets
Charvita Tablets
Cheroline Cough Linctus
Cherry Bark Cough Syrup Childrens
    (Loveridge)
Cherry Bark Linctus Adults (Loveridge)
Cherry Cough Balsam (Herbal
    Laboratories)
Cherry Cough Linctus (Savory & Moore)

Cherry Cough Mixture (Rusco)
Cherry Flavoured Extract of Malt
    (Distillers)
Chest & Cough Tablets (Brome &
    Schimmer)
Chest & Cough Tablets (Kerbina)
Chest & Throat Tablets No 8,000
    (English Grains)
Chest Pills (Brome & Schimmer)
Chest Tablets (Kerbina)
Chesty Cough Syrup (Scott & Bowne)
Chilblain Tablets (Boots)
Child's Cherry Flavoured Linctus
    (Cupal)
Children's Blackcurrant Cough Syrup
    (Rusco)
Children's Cherry Cough Syrup
    (Thornton & Ross)
Children's Cough Linctus (Ransoms)
Children's Cough Mixture (Beecham)
Children's Cough Mixture (Loveridge)
Children's Cough Syrup (Ayrton
    Saunders)
Children's Cough Syrup (Cox)
Children's Cough Syrup (Evans Medical)
Children's Cough Syrup (Thornbers)
Children's Medicine Liquid (Hall's)
Children's Phensic Tablets
Children's Wild Cherry Cough Linctus
    (Evans Medical)
Chilvax Tablets
Chocolate Laxative Tablets (Isola)
Chocovite Tablets
Cidal
Cinnamon Essence Medicinal Mixture
    (Langdale)
Cinnamon Tablets Medicinal (Langdale)
Cinota Drops
Citrosan Powder
Claradin Effervescent Tablets
Clarkes Blood Mixture
Clean and Soak
Cleansing Herb Dried (Potters)
Cleansing Herbs (Brome & Schimmer)
Cleansing Herbs Powder (Dorwest)
Clorazepate Dipotassium Capsules
    7.5 mg
Clorazepate Dipotassium Capsules
    15 mg
Clorazepate Dipotassium Tablets 15 mg
Co-op Aspirin Tablets BP 300 mg
Co-op Bronchial Mixture
Co-op Halibut Liver Oil Capsules BP
Co-op Paracetamol Tablets BP 500 mg
Co-op Soluble Aspirin Tablets BP 300 mg
Cobalin H Injection 250 mcg/ml
Cobalin H Injection 1000 mcg/ml

Cobalin Injection 100 mcg/ml
Cobalin Injection 250 mcg/ml
Cobalin Injection 500 mcg/ml
Cobalin Injection 1000 mcg/ml
Cod Liver Oil & Creosote Capsules
(5 Oval) (R P Scherer)
Cod Liver Oil & Creosote Capsules
(10 Oval) (R P Scherer)
Cod Liver Oil Caps 10 Minims
(Woodward)
Cod Liver Oil High Potency Capsules
(R P Scherer)
Cod Liver Oil with Malt Extract &
Hypophosphite Syrup (Distillers)
Cod Liver Oil 0.3 ml Capsules
(R P Scherer)
Cod Liver Oil 0.6 ml Capsules
(R P Scherer)
Coda - Med Tablets
Codanin Analgesic Tablets
Codis Soluble Tablets
Codural Tablets
Cojene Tablets
Cold & Influenza Capsules (Regent
Laboratories)
Cold & Influenza Mixture (Boots)
Cold & Influenza Mixture (Davidson)
Cold & Influenza Mixture (Rusco)
Cold & Influenza Mixture (Thornton &
Ross)
Cold Relief Capsules (Scott & Bowne)
Cold Relief (Blackcurrant Flavour)
Granular Powder (Boots)
Cold Relief Tablets (Boots)
Cold Tablets (Roberts)
Coldrex Powder
Coldrex Tablets
Colgard Emergency Essence (Lane
Health Products)
Colgate Disclosing Tablets
Collins Elixir
Colocynth & Jalap Tablets Compound
BPC 1963
Colocynth Compound Pills BPC 1963
Cologel Liquid
Complan
Comploment Continus Tablets
Compound Fig Elixir BP
Compound Rhubarb Oral Powder BP
Compound Rhubarb Tincture BP
Compound Syrup of Glycerophosphates
BPC 1963
Compound Syrup of Hypophosphites
BPC 1963
Comtrex Capsules
Comtrex Liquid
Concavit Capsules
Concavit Drops

Comtrex Tablets
Concavit Injection
Concavit Syrup
Congreves Balsamic Elixir
Constipation Herb Dried (Potters)
Constipation Herbs (Hall's)
Constipation Herbs (Mixed Herbs)
(Brome & Schimmer)
Constipation Mixture No 105 (Potters)
Contac 400 Capsules
Contactaclean Cleaning Solution
Contactasoak Disinfecting and Soaking Solution
Contactasol 02 Care Solution
Contactasol Complete Care all-in-one Solution
Contactasol Wetting Solution
Copholco Cough Syrup
Corrective Tablets (Ayrton Saunders)
Correctol Tablets
Cosalgesic Tablets
Cosylan Syrup
Coterpin Syrup
Cough & Bronchitis Mixture (Davidson)
Cough & Cold Mixture (Beecham)
Cough Balsam (Abernethy's)
Cough Balsam (Thornbers)
Cough Expectorant Elixir (Regent
Laboratories)
Cough Linctus (Sanderson's)
Cough Linctus Alcoholic (Thomas Guest)
Cough Linctus for Children (Boots)
Cough Medicine for Infants & Children
Solution (Boots)
Cough Mixture (Tingles)
Cough Mixture Adults (Thornton &
Ross)
Cough Mixture Adults (Wicker Herbal
Stores)
Cough Syrup Best (Diopharm)
Cough Tablets (Kerbina)
Covermark Removing Cream
Covonia Bronchial Balsam Linctus
Cow & Gate Babymeals Stage One
Cow & Gate Baby Milk Plus
Cow & Gate Premium Baby Food
Cox Pain Tablets
Crampex Tablets
Cream of Magnesia Tablets 300 mg
Cremaffin Emulsion
Creosote Bronchial Mixture (Loveridge)
Crookes One-a-Day Multivitamins with Iron
Crookes One-a-Day Multivitamins
without Iron
Croupline Cough Syrup (Roberts)
Cupal Health Salts
Cupal Nail Bite Lotion
Cuticura Medicated Foam Bath
Cyanocobalamin Solution (any strength)
Cyanocobalamin Tablets (any strength)

Cytacon Liquid
Cytacon Tablets
Cytamen 250 Injection
Cytamen 1000 Injection

Dakin's Golden Vitamin Malt Syrup
Dalivit Capsules
Dalivit Syrup
Dalmane Capsules 15 mg
Dalmane Capsules 30 mg
Dansac Skin Lotion
Davenol Linctus
Daxaids Tablets
Day-Vits Multivitamin & Mineral Tablets
Dayovite
De Witt's Analgesic Pills
De Witt's Antacid Powder
De Witt's Antacid Tablets
De Witt's Baby Cough Syrup
De Witt's Cough Syrup
De Witt's PL Pills
Deakin & Hughes Cough & Cold Healer
    Mixture
Deakin's Fever & Inflammation Remedy
    Mixture
Delax Emulsion
Delimon
Dentakit Toothache First Aid Kit
Derbac Soap
Dermacolor Cleansing Cream
Dermacolor Cleansing Lotion
Dermacolor Cleansing Milk
Desiccated Liver Tablets
Desiccated Liver USNF Tablets
Detox Tablets (Hursdrex)
Dextrogesic Tablets
Dextromethorphan Hydrobromide
    Solution 3.75 mg/5 ml
Dextromethorphan Hydrobromide
    Solution 7.5 mg/5 ml
Dextromethorphan Hydrobromide
    Syrup 6.6 mg/5 ml
Dextromethorphan Hydrobromide
    Syrup 13.5 mg/5 ml
Dextropropoxyphene & Paracetamol
    Dispersible Tablets
Dextropropoxyphene & Paracetamol
    Soluble Tablets
DF 118 Elixir
DF 118 Injection
DF 118 Tablets
DGL 1 Suspension
DGL 2 Suspension
DGT 1 Tablets
DGT 2 Tablets
Diabetic Bronal Syrup
Dialar Forte Syrup 5 mg/5 ml

Dialar Syrup 2 mg/5 ml
Dialume Capsules 500 mg
Diazepam Capsules, Slow 10 mg
Diazepam Elixir 5 mg/5 ml
Digesprin Antacid Tablets
Digestells Lozenges
Dihydroxyaluminium Sodium Carbonate
    Tablets
Dijex Liquid
Dijex Tablets
Dimotane Expectorant
Dimotane Expectorant DC
Dimotane with Codeine Elixir
Dimotane with Codeine Paediatric Elixir
Dimotapp Elixir
Dimotapp Elixir Paediatric
Dimotapp LA Tablets
Dimotapp P Tablets
Dimyril Linctus
Dinnefords Gripe Mixture
Disprin Tablets
Disprinex Tablets
Disprol Tablets
Distalgesic Soluble Tablets
Distalgesic Tablets
Do-Do Linctus
Do-Do Tablets
Dolasan Tablets
Doloxene Capsules
Doloxene Compound Pulvules
Dolvan Tablets
Dorbanex Capsules
Dorbanex Liquid
Dorbanex Liquid Forte
Dormonoct Tablets 1 mg
Dr Brandreth's Pills
Dr D E Jongh's Cod Liver Oil with Malt
    Extract & Vitamins Fortified Syrup
Dr William's Pink Pills
Drastin Tablets
Dristan Decongestant Tablets with
    Antihistamine
Dristan Nasal Spray
Droxalin Tablets
Dry Cough Linctus (Scott & Bowne)
Dual-Lax Extra Strong Tablets
Dual-Lax Tablets
Dulca Tablets
Dulcodos Tablets
Dulcolax Suppositories
Dulcolax Tablets
Duo-Gastritis Mixture (Baldwin's)
Duphalac Syrup
Duralin Capsules Extra Strength
Duralin Tablets
Duttons Cough Mixture
Dynese Aqueous Suspension
Dynese Tablets

D001 Capsules
D002 Capsules
D004 Capsules
D006 Capsules
D007 Capsules
D009 Capsules
D010 Capsules
D011 Capsules
D012 Capsules
D013 Capsules
D014 Capsules
D017 Capsules
D018 Capsules
D019 Capsules
D020 Capsules
D021 Capsules
D024 Capsules
D029 Capsules
D030 Capsules
D031 Capsules
D032 Capsules
D033 Capsules
D034 Capsules
D036 Capsules

Ecdilyn Syrup
Educol Tablets
Efamol
Efamol Capsules
Effer-C Tablets
Effico Syrup
Eldermint Cough Mixture (Herbal
    Laboratories)
Elizabeth Arden Flawless Finish
Elizabeth Arden Sunblock Cream Factor 15
Elizabeth Arden Sunscience-Superblock
    Cream opf 34
Elkamol Tablets
Endet Powders
Ener-G Gluten-free and Soya-free Macaroon Cookies
Ener-G Gluten-free Rice and Peanut-Butter Cookies
Ener-G Gluten-free Rice Walnut Cookies
Ener-G Low-Protection and Gluten-free Egg Replacer
Energen Starch Reduced Crispbread
Engran HP Tablets
Engran Tablets
Eno Fruit Salts
EP Tablets
Equagesic Tablets
Eskornade Spansule Capsules
Eskornade Syrup
Eso-Col Cold Treatment Tablets
Euhypnos Capsules 10 mg
Euhypnos Elixir 10 mg/5 ml
Euhypnos Forte Capsules 20 mg
Evacalm Tablets 2 mg
Evacalm Tablets 5 mg

Evans Cough Balsam
Evening Primrose Oil
Evident Disclosing Cream
Ex-Lax Chocolate Laxative Tablets
Ex-Lax Pills
Expectorant Cough Mixtures (Beecham)
Expulin Cough Linctus
Expulin Paediatric Cough Linctus
Expurhin Paediatric Decongestant
Extil Compound Linctus
Extravite Tablets
Extren Tablets
Exyphen Elixir
E001 Capsules
E015 Capsules
E018 Capsules
E021 Capsules
E031 Capsules
E032 Caspules

Fabrol Granules
Fairy Household Liquid
Falcodyl Linctus
Falkamin
Fam Lax Tablets
Famel Expectorant
Famel Linctus
Famel Original Linctus
Family Cherry Flavoured Linctus (Cupal)
Family Herbal Pills
Farex Fingers
Farleys Rusks
Father Pierre's Monastery Herbs
Fe-Cap C Capsules
Feac Tablets
Feen-a-Mint Tablets
Fefol-Vit Spansules
Femerital Tablets
Feminax Tablets
Fendamin Tablets
Fennings Adult Powders
Fennings Children's Cooling Powders
Fennings Little Healers Pills
Fennings Mixture
Fennings Soluble Junior Aspirin Tablets
Fenox Nasal Drops
Fenox Nasal Spray
Ferfolic Tablets
Fergluvite Tablets
Ferraplex B Tablets
Ferrlecit Tablets/Dragees
Ferrograd C Tablets
Ferrol
Ferrol Compound Mixture
Ferromyn B Elixir
Ferromyn B Tablets
Ferrous Gluconate Compound Tablets

Fesovit Spansules
Fesovit Z Spansules
Fiberform
Fibre Biscuits
Fine Fare Aspirin Tablets 300 mg
Fine Fare Hot Lemon Powders
Flar Capsules
Flavelix Syrup
Flexcare Soft Lens Solution
Flexsol Solution
Flora Margarine
Floradix Formula Liquid
Floradix Tablets
Floral Arbour Tablets (Cathay)
Flu-Rex Tablets
Flucaps
Flunitrazepam Tablets 1 mg
Fluralar Capsules 15 mg
Fluralar Capsules 30 mg
Flurazepam Capsules 15 mg
Flurazepam Capsules 30 mg
Flurazepam Hydrochloride Capsules
   15 mg
Flurazepam Hydrochloride Capsules
   30 mg
Folped
Forceval Capsules
Forceval Junior Capsules
Forprin Tablets
Fortagesic Tablets
Fortimel
Fortison Low Sodium
Fortral Capsules 50 mg
Fortral Injection
Fortral Suppositories
Fortral Tablets 25 mg
Fortral Tablets 50 mg
Fortris Solution
Fosfor Syrup
Franol Expectorant
Franolyn Sed Liquid
Fresubin 750
Frisium Capsules 5 mg
Frisium Capsules 10 mg
Frisium Capsules 20 mg
Fybranta Tablets
Fynnon Calcium Aspirin Tablets
Fynnon Salt

G Brand Linctus
Galake Tablets
Galfer-Vit Capsules
Galloway's Baby Cough Linctus
Galloway's Bronchial Expectorant
Galloway's Cough Syrup
Gamophen
Gastalar Tablets

Gastric Ulcer Tablets no 1001
Gastrils Pastiles
Gastritabs
Gastrovite Tablets
Gatinar Syrup
Gaviscon Granules
Gelusil Lac Powder
Gelusil Tablets
Genasprin Tablets
Genatosan
Gentian Acid Mixture with Nux Vomica
Gentian Alkaline Mixture with Nux Vomica
Gentian & Rhubarb Mixture BPC
Georges Vapour Rub Ointment
Geriplex Capsules
Gevral Capsules
GF Brand Chocolate Nut Cookies
GF Brand Fruit Bran Biscuits
GF Brand Ginger Cookies
GF Brand Gluten-free Coconut Cookies
GF Brand Gluten-free Maize Biscuits
   with Chocolate
GF Brand Gluten-Free Maize Biscuits
   with Hazel-Nut
GF Brand Gluten-Free Pastry Mix
GF Brand Gluten-Free Thin Wafer Bread
GF Brand Muesli
GF Brand Muesli Fruit Biscuits
GF Dietary Low Protein Pizza Mix with
   Tomato Topping Mix and Baking Dish
GF Dietary Low Protein Vegetable in
   low protein sauce
GF Dietary Low Protein
   Vegetable Cassarole
Givitol Capsules
Gladlax Tablets
Glemony Balsam (Baldwin's)
Glenco Elixir
Gluca-Seltzer Effervescent Powder
Glucodin
Glycerin Honey & Lemon Cough
   Mixture (Isola)
Glycerin Honey & Lemon Linctus
   (Boots)
Glycerin Honey & Lemon Linctus with
   Ipecacuanha (Boots)
Glycerin Lemon & Honey and
   Ipecacuanha (Thomas Guest)
Glycerin Lemon & Honey Linctus
   (Rusco)
Glycerin Lemon & Honey Syrup (Cupal)
Glycerin Lemon & Honey Syrup (Thomas
   Guest)
Glycerin Lemon & Honey Syrup
   (Waterhouse)
Glycerin Lemon & Ipecacuanha Cough
   Mixture (Isola)
Glykola Elixir

Glykola Infants Elixi
Golden Age Vitamin & Mineral Capsules
Golden Health Tablets (Kerbina)
Golden Health Tablets (Brome &
    Schimmer)
Gon Tablets
Gonfalcon Tablets
Grangewood Insomnia Tablets
Granogen
Granoton Emulsion
Granose Liquid Soya Milk
Gregovite C Tablets
GS Tablets
Guaiphenesin Syrup (any strength)
Guanor Expectorant

H-Pantoten Tablets
Hactos Chest & Cough Mixture
    (Thomas Hubert)
Halaurant Syrup
Halcion Tablets 0.125 mg
Halcion Tablets 0.25 mg
Haliborange Syrup
Haliborange Tablets
Halibut Liver Oil A & D Capsules
    (Rodale)
Halin Tablets
Halocaps Inhalant Capsules
Halycitrol Emulsion
Hayphryn Nasal Spray
Head and Shoulders Shampoo
Health Salts (Wicker Herbal Stores)
Health Tonic Mixture (Hall's)
Healtheries Rice Crispbread
Heart Shape Indigestion Tablets
Hedamol Capsules
Hedex Plus Capsules
Hedex Seltzer Granules
Hedex Soluble Granules
Hedex Tablets
Hemingways Catarrh Syrup
Hemoplex Injection
Hepacon B12 Injection
Hepacon Liver Extract Injection
Hepacon-Plex
Hepacon B-Forte Injection
Hepanorm Tablets
Herbal Aperient Tablets (Cathay)
Herbal Aperient Tablets (Kerbina)
Herbal Bronchial Cough Tablets (English
    Grains)
Herbal Laxative Naturtabs
Herbal Pile Tablets
Herbal Quiet Nite Sleep Naturtabs
Herbal Syrup (Baldwin's)
Herbalene Herbs
Hermesetas (blue)

Hermesetas Gold
Hermesetas Light
Hermesetas Liquid Sweetener
Hermesetas Sprinkle Sweet
Hexidin Solution
Hi-g-ah Tea
Hi-pro Liver Tablets
Hill's Bronchial Balsam
Hill's Junior Balsam
Hip C Rose Hip Syrup
Histalix Expectorant
Honey & Molasses Cough Mixture (Lane
    Health Products)
Hot Blackcurrant Cold Remedy (Beechmans)
Hot Lemon Cold Remedy   (Beechmans)
Hot Lemon Cold Treatment (Scott &
    Bowne)
Hot Measure Solution (Reckitt & Colman)
Hydrocare Boiling/Rinsing Solution
Hydrocare Cleaning and Soaking Solution
Hydrocare Preserved Saline Solution
Hydrocare Protein Remover Tablets
Hydroclean Solution
Hydron Europe Cleaning Solution
Hydron Europe Comfort Soaking Solution
Hydron European Solusal
Hydron Europe Solution Comfort
Hydrosoak Disinfecting and Soaking Solution
Hydrosol Comfort Solution
Hypon Tablets

Iberet 500 Tablets
Iberol Tablets
ICC Analgesic Tablets
Iliadin Mini Nasal Drops
Iliadin Mini Paediatric Nasal Drops
Imarale Agba Suspension
Imarale Omode Suspendion
Inabrin Tablets 200 mg
Indian Brandy Solution
Indigestion Mixture (Boots)
Indigestion Mixture (Thornton & Ross)
Indigestion Mixture (William Ransom)
Indigo Indigestion Lozenges
Infa-Care Baby Bath
Influenza and Cold Mixture 2315
    (Wright Layman & Umney)
Inhalit liquid Inhalation
Innoxa Finishing Touch Loose Powder
Innoxa Moisturised Liquid Make-up
Iodinated Glycerol Elixir 60 mg/5 ml
Iodo-Ephedrine Mixture
Iodised Vitamin Capsules
Ipecacuanha Pills 20 mg
Ipecacuanha & Morphine Mixture BP
Ipecacuanha & Squill Linctus
    Paediatric BPC

Ipsel Hygienic Babysalve
Irofol C
Iron & Brewers Yeast Tablets
    (3M Health Care)
Iron & Vitamin Tablets (Davidson)
Iron Formula Tablets (Rodale)
Iron Jelloids Tablets
Iron Tonic Tablets (Boots)
Ironorm Capsules
Ironorm Tonic
Ironplan Capsules
Ivy Tablets (Ayrton Saunders)

Jaap's Health Salts
Jacksons All Fours Cough Mixture
Jacksons Febrifuge
Jambomins Tablets
Jenners Suspension
Jenners Tablets
Johnson & Johnson Baby Bath
Johnson & Johnson Baby Cream
Johnson & Johnson Baby Lotion
Johnson & Johnson Baby Oil
Johnson & Johnson Baby Powder
Johnson & Johnson Baby Shampoo
Jordans Crunchy Bar
Junamac
Jung Junipah Tablets
Junior Cabdrivers Linctus
Junior Disprin Tablets
Junior Disprol Suspension
Junior Disprol Tablets
Junior Ex-Lax Chocolate Tablets
Junior Lemsip Powder
Junior Meltus Cough & Catarrh Linctus
Junior Mucron Liquid
Junior Paraclear Tablets
Junior Tablets (Rodale)
Juno-Junipah Mineral Salts
Juvel Elixir
Juvel Tablets

Karvol Capsules
Kelsoak 2 Solution
Kelvinol 2 Wetting Solution
Kendales Adult Cough Syrup
Kendales Cherry Linctus
Kest Tablets
Ketazolam Capsules 15 mg
Ketazolam Capsules 30 mg
Ketazolam Capsules 45 mg
Keybells Linctus of Glycerine, Lemon &
    Ipecacuanha
Kingo Cough Syrup
Koladex Tablets
Kolanticon Tablets

Kolanticon Wafers
Kolantyl Gel
Krauses Cough Linctus
Kruschen Salts
Kuralax Herbs

Labiton Kola Tonic
Laboprin Tablets
Lac Bismuth Mixture
Lactaid Lactase enzyme for milk drops
Lactaid Lactase enzyme tablets
Lactaid Lactose reduced skimmed and whole milk
Lacto Calamine
Laevoral
Lance B & C Tablets
Lane's Cut-a-Cough
Lane's Laxative Herb Tablets
Lane's Sage and Garlic Catarrh Remedy
Lantigen B
Laxaliver Pills
Laxatabs Leoren
Laxipurg Tablets
Laxoberal Elixir
LC 65 Cleaning Solution
Lederplex Capsules
Lederplex Liquid
Lejfibre Biscuit
Lem-Plus Hot Lemon Drink
Lemeze Cough Syrup
Lemon Eno Powder
Lemon Flu-Cold Concentrated Syrup
Lemon Glycerine & Honey Cough Syrup
    Compound (Carter Bond)
Lemon Glycerine & Honey Lung
    Mixture (Whitehall Laboratories)
Lemon Glycerine & Ipecac Cough Syrup
    Compound (Carter Bond)
Lemon Juice, Glycerine & Honey A S
    Syrup (Ayrton Saunders)
Lemon Linctus 1-472
Lemsip Powder
Lendormin Tablets 0.125 mg
Lendormin Tablets 0.25 mg
Lensept Solution
Lensine 5 All in One Solution
Lensplus Sterile Saline Spray
Lensrins Solution
Leoren Tonic Tablets
Lexotan Tablets 1.5 mg
Lexotan Tablets 3 mg
Lexotan Tablets 6 mg
Libraxin Tablets
Librium Capsules 5 mg
Librium Capsules 10 mg
Librium Tablets 5 mg
Librium Tablets 10 mg
Librium Tablets 25 mg

Librofem Tablets
Lightning Cough Remedy Solution
    (Potters)
Limbitrol Capsules "5"
Limbitrol Capsules "10"
Linctified Expectorant
Linctified Expectorant Paediatric
Linctoid C
Linituss
Linoleic Acid
Linus Vitamin C Powder
Lipoflavonoid Capsules
Lipotriad Capsules
Lipotriad Liquid
Liquifruta Blackcurrant Cough Medicine
Liquifilm Wetting Solution
Liquifruta Honey & Lemon Cough
    Medicine
Liquifruta Medica
Liquifruta Medica Garlic Flavoured
    Cough Medicine
Liquid Formula (Food Concentrate)
    (Rodale)
Liquid Paraffin & Phenolphthalein
    Emulsion BP
Liquid Paraffin Emulsion with Cascara
    BPC
Listerine Antiseptic Mouthwash
Listermint Mouthwash
Liver Herbs (Hall's)
Livibron Mixture
Loasid Tablets
Lobak Tablets
Lofthouse's Original Fisherman's Friend
    Honey Cough Syrup
Loramet Capsules 1 mg
Loramet Tablets 0.5 mg
Loramet Tablets 1 mg
Lotussin Cough Syrup
Locozade
Luma Bath Salts
Lung Balsam (Rusco)
Lypsyl Lemon
Lypsyl Mint
Lypsyl Original
Lysaldin

M & B Children's Cough Linctus
Maalox Concentrate Suspension
Maalox Plus Tablets
Mackenzies Smelling Salts
Maclean Indigestion Powder
Maclean Indigestion Tablets
Magaldrate Tablets
Mainstay Pure Cod Liver Oil
Male Gland Double Strength Supplement
    Tablets

Male Sex Hormone Tablets (Diopharm)
Malinal Plus Tablets
Malinal Suspension 500 mg/5 ml
Malinal Tablets 500 mg
Malt Extract with Cod Liver Oil &
    Chemical Food (Distillers)
Malt Extract with Cod Liver Oil BPC &
    Hypophosphites (Distillers)
Malt Extract with Cod Liver Oil BPC
    Soft Extract (Jeffreys Miller)
Malt Extract with Haemoglobin &
    Vitamins Syrup (Distillers)
Malt Extract with Halibut Liver-Oil
    Syrup (Distillers)
Mandarin Tablets
Manna Herbal Rheumapainaway Tablets
Marvel
Matthew Cough Mixture
Maturaplus Tablets
Max Factor Face Powder
Max Factor Pan-Stik
Maxisorb
Maxivits Tablets
Medathlon Aspirin Tablets 300 mg
Medazepam Capsules 5 mg
Medazepam Capsules 10 mg
Medex Elixir
Mediclean Soft lens Solutions
Medilax Tablets
Medipain Tablets
Medised Suspension
Medised tablets
Medisoak Soft Lens Solution
Meditus Syrup
Medocodene Tablets
Meggeson Dyspepsia Tablets
Melissin Syrup
Melo Brand Glycerin Lemon & Honey
    with Ipecac
Meloids Lozenges
Menthacol Liquid
Menthells Pellet/Pill
Menthol & Benzoin Inhalation BP
Menthol & Eucalyptus (M in P) Pastilles
    (Thomas Guest)
Menthol Inhalation
Mentholated Balsam (Loveridge)
Mentholated Balsam (Savory & Moore)
Mentholated Balsam (Wright Layman & Umney)
Mentholated Balsam Mixture (Pilsworth
    Manufacturing)
Mentholatum Balm
Mentholatum Nasal Inhaler
Metatone
Methylcisteine Tablets 100 mg
Midro-Tea Powder
Milgard Baby Cleansing Milk
Milk of Magnesia Tablets

Mil-Par Suspension
Milupa Aptamil Baby Milk
Milupa Camomile Infant Drink
Milupa 7 Cereal Breakfast
Milupa Fennel Variety Infant Drink
Milupa Modified Yoghurt
Milupa Special Formula HN25
Minadex Syrup
Minamino Syrup
Minivits Tablets
Minoxidil Cream
Minoxidil Lotion
Minoxidil Ointment
Minoxidil Solution (for external use)
Mira Flow Soft Lens Solution
Mira Soak Lens Soaking Solution
Mira Sol Soft Lens Solution
Modifast Nutritionally Complete
    Supplemented Fasting Formula
Mogadon Capsules 5 mg
Mogadon Tablets 5 mg
Moorland Indigestion Tablets
Morning Glory Tablets
Morny Lavender Talc
Mrs Cullen's Lemsoothe Powder
Mrs Cullen's Powders
Mu-Cron Tablets
Mucodyne Capsules
Mucodyne Syrup
Mucodyne Forte Syrup
Mucodyne Forte Tablets
Mucodyne Paediatric Syrup
Mucofalk Sachets
Mucolex Syrup
Mucolex Tablets
Mucron Liquid
Muflin Linctus
Multi-Vitamin Tablets (English Grains)
Multivitamin Capsules (Regent
    Laboratories)
Multivitamin Tablets
    (Approved Prescription Services)
Multivitamin Tablets (Chemipharm)
Multivitamin Tablets (Evans Medical)
Multivitamin Tablets (UAC
    International)
Multivitamin with Mineral Capsules
    (Potters)
Multivitamin with Minerals Tablets
    (Chemipharm)
Multivite Pellets
Multone Tablets
My Baby Cough Syrup
Mycolactine Tablets
Mylanta Liquid
Mylanta Tablets
Myolgin Tablets

N Tonic Syrup (Cupal)
N-300 Capsules
Napoloids Tablets
Napsalgesic Tablets
Natex 12A Tablets
Natural Bran
Natural Herb Laxative Tablets (Kerbina)
Natural Herb Laxative Tablets (Brome &
    Schimmer)
Natural Herb Tablet (Kerbina)
Natural Herb Tablets (Dorwest)
Natural Herb Tablets (Lane)
Naturavite Tablets
Naudicelle
Neo-Cytamen Injection 250 mcg/ml
Neo-Cytamen Injection 1000 mcg/ml
Neoklenz Powder
Neophyrn Nasal Drops
Neophyrn Nasal Spray
Nethaprin Expectorant
Neuro Phosphates
Neurodyne Capsules
Neutradonna Powder
Neutradonna Sed Powder
Neutradonna Sed Tablets
Neutradonna Tablets
Neutragena Soap
Neutrolactis Tablets
New Formula Beechams Powders
    Capsules
New Life Herbs
New Life Tablets
Newton's Children's Cough Treatment
Newton's Cough Mixture for Adults
Nezcaam Syrup
Nicobrevin
Nicorette
Night Nurse Capsules
Night Nurse Cold Remedy
Nirolex Expectorant Linctus
Nitrados Tablets 5 mg
Nitrazepam Capsules 5 mg
Nivea
No 177 Tablets (Leoren)
Nobrium Capsules 5 mg
Nobrium Capsules 10 mg
Nocold Tablets
Noctamid Tablets 0.5 mg
Noctamid Tablets 1 mg
Noctesed Tablets 5 mg
Noradran Bronchial Syrup
Norgesic Tablets
Normacol Antispasmodic
Normax Capsules
Normison Capsules 10 mg
Normison Capsules 20 mg
Norvits Syrup
Noscapine Linctus BP

Novasil Antacid Tablets
Novasil Antacid Viscous Suspension
Nucross Coconut Oil
Nulacin Tablets
Nurodol Tablets
Nurofen Tablets 200 mg
Nurse Sykes Powders
Nurse Sykes Bronchial Balsam
Nu-Soft Baby Oil
Nux Vomica Acid Mixture
Nux Vomica Alkaline Mixture
Nux Vomica Elixir BPC
Nylax Tablets

Octovit Tablets
Oilatum Bar
Olbas Oil
Omeiri Iron Tonic Tablets
Omilcaf Suspension
Onadox 118 Tablets
One Gram C Capsule
Opas Powder
Opas Tablets
Opobly Bailey Pills
Oral B Plaque Check Disclosing Tablets
Orange & Halibut Vitamins (Kirby
    Warrick Pharmaceuticals)
Organidin Elixir
Organidin Solution
Organidin Tablets
Original Indigestion Tablets (Boots)
Orovite Elixir
Orovite Tablets
Orovite 7
Orthoxicol Syrup
Ostermilk Complete Formula
Ostermilk Two Milk Powder
Otrivine Nasal Drops 0.05%
Otrivine Nasal Drops 0.1%
Otrivine Nasal Spray 0.1%
Otrivine-Antistin Nasal Drops
Otrivine-Antistin Nasal Spray
Overnight Bedtime Cold Medicine
Owbridge's Cough Mixture
Oxanid Tablets 10 mg
Oxanid Tablets 15 mg
Oxanid Tablets 30 mg
Oxymetazoline Hydrochloride Nasal
    Drops 0.025%
Oxymetazoline Hydrochloride Nasal
    Drops 0.05%
Oxymetazoline Hydrochloride Nasal
    Spray 0.05%

Pacidal Tablets
Paedo-Sed Syrup
Pain Relief Tablets (Cox)
Pain Relief Tablets (Davidson)
Pameton Tablets
Panacron Nasal Spray
Panacron Tablets
Panadeine Co Tablets
Panadeine Forte Tablets
Panadeine Soluble Effervescent Tablets
Panadeine Tablets
Panadol Caplets
Panadol Junior Sachets
Panadol Soluble Tablets
Panadol Tablets
Panaleve Junior
Panasorb Tablets
Panets Tablets
Pango Pain Paracetamol Codeine Tablets
    (Cupal)
Papain Compound Tablets
Paprika Tablets (Kerbina)
Para-Seltzer Effervescent Tablets
Paracetamol & Caffeine Capsules
Paracetamol & Caffeine Tablets
Paracetamol DC Tablets
Paracetamol Tablets Soluble (Boots)
Paracetamol Tablets, Sorbitol Basis
    500 mg
Paracets Tablets 500 mg
Paraclear Tablets
Paracodol Capsules
Paracodol Tablets
Paradeine R Tablets
Paragesic Effervescent Tablets
Parahypon Tablets
Parake Tablets
Paralgin Tablets
Paramin Capsules
Paramol Tablets
Paranorm Cough Syrup
Pardale Tablets
Parenamps Intramuscular Injection
Pastilaids Pastilles
Pavacol Cough Syrup
Paxadon Tablets
Paxalgesic Tablets
Paxidal Tablets
Paynocil Tablets
PEM Linctus
Penetrol Inhalant
Pentazocine-Aspirin Compound Tablets
Peplax Peppermint Flavoured Laxative
    Tablets
Peppermint Indigestion Tablets (Boots)
Pepto-Bismol Suspension
Pernivit Tablets
Persomnia Tablets

Petrolagar Emulsion Plain
Petrolagar Emulsion with
    Phenolphthalein
PF Plus Tablets
Pharmacin Capsules
Pharmacin Effervescent Plus C Tablets
Pharmacin Effervescent Tablets 325 mg
Pharmaton Capsules
Pharmidone Tablets
Phenergan Compound Expectorant
    Linctus
Phenolphthalein Tablets BP
Phenolphthalein Compound Tablets BPC
    1963
Phenolphthalein Compound Pills BPC
Phensedyl Cough Linctus
Phensic Tablets
Phensic 2 Tablets
Phenylephrine Hydrochloride Nasal
    Drops 0.25%
Phenylephrine Hydrochloride Nasal
    Spray 0.5%
Phillips Iron Tonic Tablets
Phillips Tonic Yeast Tablets
Phillips Toothpaste
Phisoderm
Pholcolix Syrup
Pholcomed Diabetic Forte Linctus
Pholcomed Expectorant
Pholcomed Forte Linctus
Pholcomed Linctus
Pholtex Syrup
Pholtussa Mixture
Phosferine Liquid
Phosferine Multi-Vitamin Liquid
Phosferine Tablets
Phyllosan Tablets
Physeptone Linctus
Pile Mixture (Ayrton Saunders)
Pile Tablets (Ayrton Saunders)
Pine Catarrh Drops Lozenges
Piz Buin Children's Balm SPF 8
Piz Buin Creme factor 6
Piz Buin Creme factor 8
Piz Buin Lip Protection Stick SPF 8
Piz Buin SPF 6 Lotion
Piz Buin SPF 8 Lotion
Plenamin Super
Plenivite with Iron Tablets
Pliagel Soft lens Solution
Plurivite M Tablets
Plurivite Tablets
Polyalk Gel
Polyalk Tablets
Polyvite Capsules
Potaba + 6 Capsules
Potaba + 6 Tablets

Potassium Bromide & Nux Vomica
    Mixture BPC 1963
Powdered Bran Tablets 2 g
Powder Plus Super Multivitamin and
    Mineral Capsules
Powerin Tablets
PP Tablets
PR Tablets
Prazepam Tablets 10 mg
PRD 200 Tablets   600 mg
Preflex Solution
Pregnadon Tablets
Pregnavite Forte Tablets
Premit Tablets 20 mg
Prenatal Dri-Kaps Capsules
Prenatol Anti Stretch Mark Cream
Primes Premiums Tablets
Priory Cleansing Herbs Powder
Procol Capsules
Proctofibe Tablets
Prodexin Tablets
Proflex Tablets 200 mg
Propain Tablets
Pro-Plus He-Vite Elixir
Proteolised Liver Tablets
Pro-Vitamin A Capsules (Rodale)
Pru Sen Tablet Bar
Pulmo Bailly Liquid
Purgoids Tablets
Purgoids Tablets
Pyridoxine Tablets, Slow 100 mg

Quick Action Cough Cure (Brian C Spencer)
Quiet Life Tablets

Rabenhorst Tomato Juice
Raspberry Tablets No B039
Rayglo Chest Rub Ointment
Rayglo Laxative Tablets
Reactivan Tablets
Red Catarrh Pastilles (Baldwin)
Redelan Effervescent Tablets
Redoxon Adult Multivitamin Tablets
Redoxon C Effervescent Tablets 1 g
Redoxon C Tablets 25 mg
Redoxon C Tablets 50 mg
Redoxon C Tablets 200 mg
Redoxon C Tablets 250 mg
Redoxon C Tablets 500 mg
Redoxon Childrens Multivitamin Tablets
Redoxon Effervescent Tablets 1 g
Regaine
Reg-U-Lett Tablets
Relanium Tablets 2 mg
Relanium Tablets 5 mg
Relanium Tablets 10 mg

Relcol Tablets
Remnos Tablets 5 mg
Remnos Tablets 10 mg
Rennie Tablets
Resolve Granules
Respaton
Rheumavit Tablets
Rhuaka Herbal Syrup
Rhuaka Tablets
Rhubarb & Soda Mixture Ammoniated BP
Ribena
Rhubarb Compound Mixture BPC
Rhubarb Mixture Compound Paediatric BPC
Riddovydrin Liquid
Rinurel Linctus
Rinurel Tablets
Rite-Diet Diabetic Fruit Cake
Rite-Diet Gluten-free Baking Powder
Rite-Diet Gluten-free Crunchy Bars
Rite-Diet Gluten-free Muesli Cookies
Rite-Diet Gluten-Free Biscuits (chocolate
    chip cookies; half-coated choco
    late biscuit; custard cream biscuit;
    Lincoln biscuit; shortcake biscuit;
    sultana biscuit; soya bran)
Rite-Diet Gluten-Free Canned Rich Fruit
    Cake
Robaxisal Forte Tablets
Roberts Aspirin & Caffeine Tablets
Robinsons Baby Rice
Robitussin AC Liquid
Robitussin Cough Soother
Robitussin Cough Soother
    Junior Formula
Robitussin Plus Liquid
Robitussin Liquid
Robitussin Syrup
RoC Compact Cleanser
RoC Eye Make-up Remover Lotion
RoC Foundation Cream
RoC Vitamin Cream
Rock Salmon Cough Mixture
Rohypnol Tablets 1 mg
Roscorbic Effervescent Tablets
Roscorbic Tablets 25 mg
Roscorbic Tablets 50 mg
Roscorbic Tablets 200 mg
Roscorbic Tablets 500 mg
Rose Hip C-100 Capsules
Rose Hip C-200 Capsules
Rose Hip Tablets (English Grains)
Rose Hip Tablets (Potters)
Rose Hip Tablets (Roberts)
Rosmax Syrup
Roter Tablets
Rovigon
Rubelix Syrup
Rubraton B Elixir

Ruby Tonic Tablets (Jacksons)
Rum Cough Elixir
Ruthmol
Rutin Plus Tablets (Gerard)

Safapryn Tablets
Safapryn-Co Tablets
Safflower Seed Oil
Sainsbury's Cold Powders with
    Blackcurrant
Sainsbury's Hot Lemon Powders
Sainsbury's Indigestion Tablets
Sainsbury's Junior Soluble Aspirin
    Tablets
Sainsbury's Paracetamol Tablets 500 mg
Sainsbury's Soluble Aspirin Tablets
Sainsbury's Aspirin Tablets 300 mg
Salzone Syrup
Salzone Tablets 500 mg
Sanatogen Junior Vitamins Tablets
Sanatogen Multivitamins Plus Iron
    (Formula One) Tablets
Sanatogen Multivitamins Tablets
Sanatogen Nerve Tonic Powder
Sanatogen Selected Multivitamins Plus
    Iron (Formula Two) Tablets
Sanatogen Tonic
Sancos Compound Linctus
Sancos Syrup
Savant Tablets
Savlon Baby Care Baby Bath
Savlon Baby Care Cream
Savlon Baby Care Lotion
Savlon Baby Care Oil
Savlon Baby Care Powder
Savlon Baby Care Shampoo
Savlon Baby Care Soap
Saxin
SBL Junior Cough Linctus
SBL Soothing Bronchial Linctus
Scholl Foot Refreshment Spray
Scott's Cod Liver Oil Capsules
Scott's Emulsion
Scotts Husky Biscuits
Seaweed Vitamin A Ester BP & Vitamin
    D BP Capsules (Regent
    Laboratories)
Sebbix Shampoo
Seclodin Capsules
Sedazin Tablets 1 mg
Sedazin Tablets 2.5 mg
Selora Sodium-free Salt Substitute
Senlax Tablets
Senna Laxative Tablets (Boots)
Senna Tablets (Potters)
Senokot Tablets
Senotabs Tablets

Serenid D Tablets 10 mg
Serenid D Tablets 15 mg
Serenid Forte Capsules 30 mg
Sertin Tablets
Setamol Soluble Tablets
Setlers Extra Strength Tablets
Setlers Liquid
Setlers Tablets
Seven Seas Cod Liver Oil
Seven Seas Formula 70 Multivitamin-
    Multimineral Capsules
Seven Seas Malt and Cod Liver Oil
Seven Seas Orange Syrup & Cod Liver
    Oil
Seven Seas Pure Cod Liver Oil Capsules
Seven Seas Start Right Cod Liver Oil for
    Babies
Sidros Tablets
Silk-Lax Tablets
Siloxyl Suspension
Siloxyl Tablets
Simeco Suspension
Simeco Tablets
Simple Hair Conditioner
Simple Shampoo
Simple Soap
Sine-Off Tablets
Sinitol Capsules
Sinutab Tablets
Skin Glow Capsules
SMA Gold Cap Powder and Ready-to-
    Feed
SMA Powder and Concentrated Liquid
Snufflebabe Vapour Rub
Soaklens Solution
Softtab Soft Lens Care Tablets
Solis Capsules 2 mg
Solis Capsules 5 mg
Solis Capsules 10 mg
Solmin Tablets
Solpadeine Capsules
Solpadeine Forte Tablets
Solpadeine Tablets Effervescent
Solprin Tablets
Soluble Aspirin Tablets for Children
    (Boots)
Soluble Phensic Tablets
Solusol Solution
Somnite Suspension 2.5 mg/5 ml
Somnite Tablets 5 mg
Soquette Soaking Solution
Sovol Liquid
Sovol Tablets
Soya Powder & Nicotinamide Tablets
Special Stomach Powder (Halls)
SPHP Tablets
Squill Linctus Opiate BP (Gee's Linctus)
Squill Linctus Opiate, Paediatric, BP

Squire's Soonax Tablets
SR2310 Expectorant
Staffords Mild Aperient Tablets
Staffords Strong Aperient Tablets
Steri-Clens Solution
Steri-Solve Soft Lens Solution
Sterling Health Salts Effervescent
Sterling Indigestion Tablets
Sterling Paracetamol Tablets
Sterogyl Alcoholic Solution
Stomach Aids Tablets
Stomach Mixture (Herbal Laboratories)
Stomach Mixture H138 (Southon
    Laboratories)
Stomach Powder (Diopharm)
Stomach Tablets (Ulter)
Street's Cough Mixture
Strengthening Mixture (Hall's)
Stress B Supplement Tablets
Strychnine & Iron Mixture BPC 1963
Strychnine Mixture BPC 1963
Sudafed Co Tablets
Sudafed Expectorant
Sudafed Linctus
Sunerven Tablets
Super Plenamins Tablets
Super Yeast + C Tablets
Superdrug Health Salts
Surbex-T Tablets
Surem Capsules 5 mg
Surem Capsules 10 mg
Surlax Laxative Tablets
Sweetex
Sylopal Suspension
Sylphen Tablets
Syn-Ergel
Syndol Tablets
Syrtussar Cough Syrup

T-Zone Decongestant Tablets
Tabasan Tablets
Tablets No B006
Tablets No B011
Tablets No B015
Tablets No B024
Tablets No B025
Tablets No B029
Tablets No B034
Tablets No B035
Tablets No B036
Tablets No B037
Tablets No B038
Tablets No B040
Tablets No B041
Tablets No B045
Tablets No B048
Tablets No B070

Tablets No 268A (Potters)
Tablets to Formula A10
Tablets to Formula A11
Tablets to Formula A18
Tablets to Formula A19
Tablets to Formula A20
Tablets to Formula A22
Tablets to Formula A23
Tablets to Formula A31
Tablets to Formula A32
Tablets to Formula A33
Tablets to Formula A45
Tablets to Formula A51
Tablets to Formula A63
Tablets to Formula A67
Tablets to Formula A68
Tablets to Formula A69
Tablets to Formula A70
Tablets to Formula A71
Tablets to Formula A105
Tablets to Formula A111
Tablets to Formula A114
Tablets to Formula A120
Tablets to Formula A147
Tablets to Formula A157
Tablets to Formula A158
Tablets to Formula A161
Tablets to Formula A162
Tablets to Formula A164
Tablets to Formula A165
Tablets to Formula A166
Tablets to Formula A167
Tablets to Formula A169
Tablets to Formula A175
Tablets to Formula A183
Tablets to Formula A184
Tablets to Formula A190
Tablets to Formula A195
Tablets to Formula A202
Tablets to Formula A203
Tablets to Formula A213
Tablets to Formula A221
Tablets to Formula A244
Tablets to Formula A245
Tablets to Formula A246
Tablets to Formula A247
Tablets to Formula A248
Tablets to Formula A249
Tablets to Formula A250
Tablets to Formula A264
Tablets to Formula A266
Tablets to Formula A270
Tablets to Formula A271
Tablets to Formula A272
Tablets to Formula A273
Tablets to Formula A274
Tablets to Formula A275
Tablets to Formula A276

Tablets to Formula A277
Tablets to Formula A298
Tablets to Formula A301
Tablets to Formula A316
Tablets to Formula BA6
Tablets to Formula B10
Tablets to Formula B15
Tablets to Formula B18
Tablets to Formula B19
Tablets to Formula B20
Tablets to Formula B21
Tablets to Formula B22
Tablets to Formula B25
Tablets to Formula B26
Tablets to Formula B29
Tablets to Formula B41
Tablets to Formula B48
Tablets to Formula B51
Tablets to Formula B56
Tablets to Formula B58
Tablets to Formula B64
Tablets to Formula B65
Tablets to Formula B66
Tablets to Formula B67
Tablets to Formula B68
Tablets to Formula B70
Tablets to Formula B71
Tablets to Formula B72
Tablets to Formula B73
Tablets to Formula B74
Tablets to Formula B75
Tablets to Formula B76
Tablets to Formula B77
Tablets to Formula B78
Tablets to Formula B79
Tablets to Formula B80
Tablets to Formula B81
Tablets to Formula B82
Tablets to Formula B83
Tablets to Formula B85
Tablets to Formula B86
Tablets to Formula B87
Tablets to Formula B90
Tablets to Formula B91
Tablets to Formula B93
Tablets to Formula B94
Tablets to Formula B96
Tablets to Formula B98
Tablets to Formula B100
Tablets to Formula B102
Tablets to Formula B104
Tablets to Formula B117
Tablets to Formula B118
Tablets to Formula B120
Tablets to Formula B122
Tablets to Formula B124
Tablets to Formula B128
Tablets to Formula B141

Tablets to Formula B143
Tablets to Formula B145
Tablets to Formula B148
Tablets to Formula B156
Tablets to Formula B157
Tablets to Formula B158
Tablets to Formula B160
Tablets to Formula B163
Tablets to Formula B169
Tablets to Formula B178
Tablets to Formula B180
Tablets to Formula B181
Tablets to Formula B182
Tablets to Formula B190
Tablets to Formula B193
Tablets to Formula B207
Tablets to Formula B209
Tablets to Formula B210
Tablets to Formula B211
Tablets to Formula B212
Tablets to Formula B213
Tablets to Formula B214
Tablets to Formula B215
Tablets to Formula B216
Tablets to Formula B217
Tablets to Formula B218
Tablets to Formula B222
Tablets to Formula B223
Tablets to Formula B224
Tablets to Formula B225
Tablets to Formula B227
Tablets to Formula B228
Tablets to Formula B231
Tablets to Formula B234
Tablets to Formula B235
Tablets to Formula B236
Tablets to Formula B243
Tablets to Formula B248
Tablets to Formula B250
Tablets to Formula B251
Tablets to Formula B252
Tabmint Anti-Smoking Chewing Gum Tablets
Tancolin Childrens Cough Linctus
Tedral Expectorant
Tensium Tablets 2 mg
Tensium Tablets 5 mg
Tensium Tablets 10 mg
Tercoda Elixir
Tercolix Elixir
Terpalin Elixir
Terperoin Elixir
Terpoin Antitussive
Terrabron
Three Noughts Cough Syrup
Tidmans Bath Sea Salt
Timotei Herbal Shampoo
Titan Hard Cleanser
Tixylix Cough Linctus

Tolu Solution BP
Tolu Syrup BP
Tolu Compound Linctus Paediatric BP
Tonatexa Mixture
Tonexis HP
Tonic Tablets (Thomas Guest)
Tonic Wines
Tonivitan A & D Syrup
Tonivitan B Syrup
Tonivitan Capsules
Top C Tablets
Toptabs
Total All Purpose Solution
Totavit D R Capsules
Totolin Paediatric Cough Syrup
Tramil Capsules
Trancoprin Tablets
Transclean Cleaning Solution
Transdrop
Transoak Solution
Transol Solution
Tranxene Capsules 7.5 mg
Tranxene Capsules 15 mg
Tranxene Tablets 15 mg
Trimtamyl Gluten-Free Bread Mix
Trifyba
Triocos Linctus
Triogesic Elixir
Triogesic Tablets
Triominic Syrup
Triominic Tablets
Triopaed Linctus
Triotussic Suspension
Triovit Tablets
Triple Action Cold Relief Tablets
Tropium Capsules 5 mg
Tropium Capsules 10 mg
Tropium Tablets 5 mg
Tropium Tablets 10 mg
Tropium Tablets 25 mg
Trufree Crispbran
Tudor Rose Bay Rhum
Tums Tablets
Tusana Linctus
Tussifans Syrup
Tussimed Liquid
Two-A-Day Iron Jelloids Tablets
Tysons Catarrh Syrup

Udenum Gastric Vitamin Powder
Ultracach Analgesic Capsules
Ultradal Antacid Stomach Tablets
Ultralief Tablets
Uncoated Tablets to Formula A323
Uncoated Tablets to Formula A325
Unichem Baby Oil
Uniflu Tablets

Unigesic Capsules
Unigest Tablets
Unisomnia Tablets 5 mg
United Skin Care Programme (Uni
  Derm; Uni-Salve; Uni-Wash)

Valium Capsules 2 mg
Valium Capsules 5 mg
Valium Syrup 2 mg/5 ml
Valium Tablets 2 mg
Valium Tablets 5 mg
Valium Tablets 10 mg
Valonorm Tonic Solution
Valrelease Capsules
Vanamil Tablets
Vapex Inhalent
Vaseline Intensive Care Lotion
Vaseline Intensive Care Lotion Herbal and Aloe
Veganin Tablets
Veno's Adult Formula Cough Mixture
Veno's Cough Mixture
Veno's Honey & Lemon Cough Mixture
Veracolate Tablets
Verdiviton Elixir
Vervain Compound Tablets
Vi-Daylin Syrup
Vicks Coldcare Capsules
Vicks Cremacoat Syrup
Vicks Cremacoat Syrup with Doxylamine
  Cremacoat Syrup with Guaiphene
  sin Vicks Cremacoat Syrup with Paracetamol
  & Dextromethorphan
Vicks Daymed
Vicks Formula 44 Cough Mixture
Vicks Inhaler
Vicks Medinite
Vicks Pectorex Solution
Vicks Sinex Nasal Spray
Vicks Vapo-Lem Powder Sachets
Vicks Vapour Rub
Videnal Tablets
Vigour Aids Tablets
Vigranon B Complex Tablets
Vigranon B Syrup
Vikelp Coated Tablets
Vikonon Tablets
Villescon Liquid
Villescon Tablets
Vikonon Tablets
Virvina Elixir
Visclair Tablets
Vita Diem Multi Vitamin Drops
Vita-Six Capsules
Vitalin Tablets

Vitamin & Iron Tonic (Epitone) Solution
Vitamin A & D Capsules BPC 1968
  (Regent Laboratories)
Vitamin A Ester & Vitamin D2 Capsules
  (Regent Laboratories)
Vitamin A Ester Capsules
  (Regent Laboratories)
Vitamin A Ester Conc, Alpha Tocopherol
  Acetate Nat Capsules
  (Regent Laboratories)
Vitamin A 4500 Units & Vitamin D2
  Capsules (Regent Laboraties)
Vitamin A 6000 Units & Vitamin D2
  Capsules (Regent Laboratories)
Vitamin A, C & D Tablets) Approved
  Prescription Services)
Vitamin A, D & C Tablets
  (Regent Laboratories)
Vitamin B Complex Tablets (English Grains)
Vitamin B Complex with Brewer's Yeast
  Tablets (English Grains)
Vitamin B1 Dried Yeast Powder (Distillers)
Vitamin B1 Yeast Tablets (Distillers)
Vitamin B12 Tablets 0.01 mg
Vitamin B12 Tablets 0.025 mg
Vitamin B12 Tablets 0.05 mg
Vitamin B12 Tablets 0.10 mg
Vitamin B12 Tablets 0.25 mg
Vitamin B12 Tablets 0.5 mg
Vitamin B12 Tablets 1 mg
Vitamin C Tablets Effervescent 1 gramme
Vitamin Capsules (Regent Laboratories)
Vitamin Malt Extract with Orange Juice
  (Distillers)
Vitamin Mineral Capsules
  (Regent Laboratories)
Vitamin Tablets No B077
Vitamin Tablets No B081
Vitamin Tablets No B084
Vitaminised Iron & Yeast Tablets
  (Kirby Warrick Pharmaceuticals)
Vitanorm Malt Extract
Vitanorm Malt Extract Syrup
Vitasafe's CF Kaps Tablets
Vitasafe's WCF Kaps Tablets
Vitathone Chilblain Tablets
Vitatrop Tablets
Vitavel Powder for Syrup
Vitavel Solution
Vitepron Tablets
Vitorange Tablets
Vitrite Multi-Vitamin Syrup
Vykmin Fortified Capsules

W L Tablets
Wallachol Syrup
Wallachol Tablets
Wate-on Emulsion
Wate-on Emulsion Super
Wate-on Tablets
Wate-on Tablets Super
Wate-on Tonic
Waterhouses All Fours
Wines
Woodwards Nursery Cream
Wrights Glucose with Vitamin D Powder
Wrights Vaporizing Fluid

Xanax Tablets 0.25 mg
Xanax Tablets 0.5 mg
Xanax Tablets 1.0 mg

Yeast & B12 Tablets (English Grains)
Yeast Plus Tablets (Thomas Guest)
Yeast-Vite Tablets
Yellow Phenolphthalein Tablets
     (any strength)

Zactirin Tablets
Zefringe Sachets
Zubes Expectorant Cough Syrup
Zubes Original Cough Mixture
Zyriton Expectorant Linctus

PART XVIIIB

DRUGS TO BE PRESCRIBED IN CERTAIN CIRCUMSTANCES
UNDER THE NHS PHARMACEUTICAL SERVICES

Drugs in Column 1 of this part may be prescribed for persons mentioned in Column 2, only for the treatment of the purpose specified in Column 3. The Doctor must endorse the prescription with the reference "S3B".

Drug (1)	Patient (2)	Purpose (3)
Acetylcysteine Granules	Any Patient	Abdominal complications associated with cystic fibrosis
Carbocisteine	A patient under the age of 18 who has undergone a tracheostomy	Any condition which, through damage or disease, affects the air ways and has required a tracheostomy
Clobazam	Any Patient	Epilepsy
Pregnavite Forte F Tablets	A woman who has previously given birth to a child (whether or not born alive) with a defect of the neural tube or aborted a foetus with such a defect	Reduction of the risk of spina bifida or anencephaly in a child which may be born to the patient

PART XVIII C

GUIDANCE ON THE THERAPEUTIC GROUPS OF DRUGS THAT ARE RESTRICTED
UNDER THE NHS PHARMACEUTICAL SERVICES

The restrictions on prescribing and dispensing at public expense which came into effect on 1 April 1985 are limited to the following therapeutic groups.

Indigestion remedies

Laxatives

Analgesics used for mild or moderate pain

Cough and Cold remedies including

    Cough suppressants
    Expectorants, demulcents and compound preparations
    Mucolytics
    Inhalations
    Systemic and Topical Nasal Decongestants

Bitters and Tonics
Vitamins
Benzodiazepine Tranquillisers and Sedatives

0320M/1

INDEX

	Page		Page
Bags (contd)		Betaloc Tablets	29
Plastics (Stoma) Drainable	156	Betaloc – SA	29
Plastics (Stoma) Disposable	156	Beverages	307
Rubber (Stoma)	156	Bi–Aglut Products	308
Balneum Bath Additive	29	Biloptin Capsules	274
Bandages	60	Bioclusive Dressing	75
Basic Price	7	Bisacodyl	
meaning for approved appliances	3,57	Suppositories	36
meaning for chemical reagents	3	Tablets	36
Bath Eye	85	Bisgaard Leg Bandage (see	
Becotide Rotahaler	93	Elastic Web with Foot	
Beeswax	36	Loop Bandages)	
Belladonna		Bismuth Ammonium Citrate	
Mixture, Paediatric	36	Solution	36
and Alkali Mixture	36	Bismuth and Morphine Mixture	36
and Ipecacuanha Mixture,		Bismuth Salicylate	36
Paediatric	36	Bismuth Subcarbonate	36
Plaster	96	Bismuth Subgallate Suppositories	36
Tincture	36	Bismuth Subnitrate	36
Below–Knee Stockings Elastic	80/83	and Iodoform paste	36
Dispensing Fee, Appliance		Bisoprolol Fumarate Tablets	36
Contractors	23	BJ6 Eye Drops	36
Prescription Charge	340	Black Currant Syrup	36
Professional Fee, Pharmacy		"Black List"	353/371
Contractors	11	Bladder/Irrigating Syringe	105
Belts		Blenderm Surgical Tape	101
Incontinence	109	Blood Glucose Strips	276/277
Stoma	157	Appendix	278/278a
Suprapubic	100	Blue Line Bandages	61
Suspender	81/83	BM–Test	276
Umbilical (Infants)	107	Boil Dressings	73
Bendrofluazide Tablets	36	Boots Covering Cream	308
Benoral Suspension	29	Borderline Substances	
Benorylate		List A	307
Mixture	36	List B	322
Oral Suspension	36	List C	339
Tablets	36	(see also under separate names)	
Bentonite	36	Borderline Substance Foods	
Benzalkonium		(entitlement to Zero Discount)	5
Chloride Solution	36	Boric Acid	36
Lozenges	36	Eye Lotion	36
Benzocaine		Lint	94
Lozenges	351	Ointment	36
Benzoic Acid		Breast Reliever	63
Ointment, Compound	36	Breast Shields	63
Solution	36	Bricanyl Syrup	29
Benzoin		Tablets	29
Tincture	36	Broken Bulk – provisions	
Tincture, Compound	36	for payment	9
Benzydamine Mouth–wash	351	Brompton Cough Lozenges	44
Oral spray	351	Brovon Midget Inhaler	59
Benzyl Benzoate	36	Brufen Tablets	29
Application	36	Brushes	
Benzylpenicillin Injection	351	Iodine	63
Betadine Products	308	Throat	63

INDEX

INDEX

0321M/21

INDEX

0321M/25

*Part X Appendix page number

*Part X Appendix page number

INDEX

INDEX

*Part X Appendix Page number

NOTES

NOTES

NOTES

NOTES

NOTES

NOTES

NOTES

NOTES

NOTES

NOTES

NOTES

NOTES

Printed in the United Kingdom for HMSO
Dd 0292340   C400   9/90